Case Studies in Hematology

Case Studies in Hematology

Editor: Aries Green

AMERICAN
MEDICAL PUBLISHERS
www.americanmedicalpublishers.com

AMERICAN
MEDICAL PUBLISHERS
www.americanmedicalpublishers.com

Cataloging-in-Publication Data

Case studies in hematology / edited by Aries Green.
p. cm.
Includes bibliographical references and index.
ISBN 979-8-88740-602-2
1. Hematology. 2. Hematology--Case studies. 3. Blood--Diseases.
4. Blood--Diseases--Treatment. I. Green, Aries.
RC633 .C55 2023
616.15--dc23

American Medical Publishers,
41 Flatbush Avenue,
1st Floor, New York,
NY 11217, USA

ISBN 979-8-88740-602-2 (Hardback)

Contents

Preface

The branch of medicine which is involved in the study, diagnosis, and treatment of disorders related to blood and blood-forming tissues is known as hematology. It encompasses a diverse range of conditions, which include both benign and malignant blood disorders. The diagnosis and management of these disorders involves a combination of clinical assessment, laboratory testing, and specialized procedures. Some of the diagnostic tools which are used to evaluate the composition, function, and structure of blood cells are complete blood counts (CBC), blood smears, bone marrow biopsies and genetic testing. These tests are used to identify abnormalities, determine the type and severity of the disorder, and guide appropriate treatment decisions. The disorders which are studied within this field can be broadly classified into three categories, namely, anemia, bleeding disorders, and blood cancers. This book provides comprehensive insights into the field of hematology. Those in search of information to further their knowledge will be greatly assisted by it.

This book is a comprehensive compilation of works of different researchers from varied parts of the world. It includes valuable experiences of the researchers with the sole objective of providing the readers (learners) with a proper knowledge of the concerned field. This book will be beneficial in evoking inspiration and enhancing the knowledge of the interested readers.

In the end, I would like to extend my heartiest thanks to the authors who worked with great determination on their chapters. I also appreciate the publisher's support in the course of the book. I would also like to deeply acknowledge my family who stood by me as a source of inspiration during the project.

Editor

1

A Rare Cause of Acquired Factor X Deficiency in an 87-Year-Old Female

Ayrton Bangolo,[1] Trupti Waykole,[1] Bilal Niazi,[1] Chandini Sajja,[1] Mahabuba Akhter,[1] Bhavna Gupta,[2] and Sameh Elias[1]

[1]*Department of Internal Medicine, Hackensack Meridian Health Palisades Medical Center, 7600 River Road, North Bergen, NJ 07047, USA*
[2]*Department of Hematology and Oncology, Hackensack Meridian Health Palisades Medical Center, 7600 River Road, North Bergen, NJ 07047, USA*

Correspondence should be addressed to Ayrton Bangolo; ayrtonbangolo@yahoo.com

Academic Editor: Kostas Konstantopoulos

Factor X deficiency is a rare coagulopathy that can be inherited or acquired. Acquired factor X deficiency has been associated with plasma cell dyscrasias, amyloids, and use of vitamin K antagonists. Of plasma cell dyscrasias, most cases in the literature have been associated with multiple myeloma with or without concomitant AL amyloidosis. Here, we present a rare case of acquired isolated factor X deficiency in an elderly patient with immunoglobulin A (Ig A) monoclonal gammopathy of undetermined significance (MGUS). Herein, we highlight a rare cause of acquired factor X deficiency, and we hope to contribute to the growing literature of plasma cell dyscrasias associated with factor X deficiency.

1. Introduction

Factor X is one of the vitamin K-dependent serine proteases. It plays a crucial role in the coagulation cascade, as the first enzyme in the common pathway of thrombus formation [1]. In the presence of factor Va, calcium, and phospholipid membrane, factor X forms the prothrombinase complex that accelerates thrombin formation [2]. Acquired cases of factor X deficiency can be seen in patients with plasma cell dyscrasias as well as amyloidosis [3]. Patients with factor X values less than 10 percent can have a high risk of spontaneous major bleeding, and those with more than 40 percent are usually asymptomatic [4]. The most common bleeding symptom reported at all levels of severity of the deficiency is epistaxis [2]. The inherited form affects one person in every one million [5, 6]. Here, we present an asymptomatic 87-year-old female with monoclonal gammopathy of undetermined significance (MGUS) who was incidentally found to have isolated factor X deficiency during a preoperative evaluation. With this case report, we hope to contribute to the growing literature of plasma cell dyscrasias associated with factor X deficiency.

2. Case Presentation

This case is about an 87-year-old female with a past medical history of thyroid cancer, primary hyperparathyroidism, and monoclonal gammopathy of undetermined significance (MGUS). The patient was referred to the hematology office by the primary care physician for evaluation of prolonged prothrombin time (PT) and partial thromboplastin time (PTT) during surgical preoperative evaluation. Notably, the patient was diagnosed with papillary thyroid cancer two months prior to presentation and was scheduled to undergo a thyroidectomy the month following our office encounter. She was diagnosed with immunoglobulin A (IgA) MGUS 3 years prior to presentation during evaluation of hypercalcemia (workup for multiple myeloma was done at the time, but the patient was found to have primary hyperparathyroidism). An

Table 1: Coagulation factors, prothrombin time, and partial thromboplastin time activities before and upon mixing studies.

	Laboratory values	Laboratory values upon mixing
Prothrombin time	15.6 seconds (9.1–12)	10.2 seconds
Partial thromboplastin time	36 seconds (24–33)	28 seconds
International normalized ratio	1.5 (0.9–1.2)	
von Willebrand factor antigen	153% (50–200)	
von Willebrand factor activity	119% (50–200)	
Factor II activity	85% (50–154)	
Factor VII activity	110% (51–186)	
Factor VIII activity	115% (56–140)	
Factor IX activity	83% (60–177)	
Factor X activity	15% (76–183)	83%
Factor XI activity	83% (60–150)	
Factor XII activity	102% (50–150)	
Factor XIII activity	124%	

immunofixation 6 months prior revealed a lower level of IgA with kappa light chain, consistent with stable MGUS. She denies any hematuria, epistaxis, postmenopausal vaginal bleeding, or easy bruising. The patient had prior surgeries without preoperative prolongation of PT and PTT or excessive intraoperative bleeding.

On physical examination, she was found to be hemodynamically stable without any signs of bleeding. Laboratory workup revealed a prolonged PT, PTT, and an isolated decrease in the activity of factor X which corrected upon mixing studies as seen in Table 1. A diagnosis of factor X deficiency was made, and no therapy was indicated given the patient was asymptomatic at the time of diagnosis.

The patient received 25 international units per kilogram (IU/Kg) of factor X concentrate on the day of thyroidectomy and the next 2 days following the surgery without any major bleeding complications.

3. Discussion

Acquired factor X deficiency is a rare coagulopathy that can be seen in patients with plasma cell dyscrasias as well as amyloidosis [3, 7]. Coagulopathy, with clinically relevant bleeding events, is not an unusual phenomenon for patients with systemic amyloidosis secondary to multiple myeloma (MM) [7]. However, clinically relevant bleeding in patients with symptomatic MM, without associated amyloidosis, has been recently reported in the literature [7]. Monoclonal gammopathy of undetermined significance (MGUS) cells are characterized by the same primary genetic mutations as in myeloma and represent a precursor condition with an average 1%/year risk of progression into myeloma or other lymphoproliferative disorders [8]. Some cases of essential monoclonal gammopathy can cause acquired coagulopathy as the immunoglobulin can interact with coagulation factors [9]. To our knowledge, this will be the first case report of acquired factor X deficiency associated with MGUS without concomitant MM or AL amyloidosis.

Factor X deficiency is associated with bleeding in individuals who have a factor X activity of less than 10 percent. This includes excessive bleeding after invasive procedures and intracranial, umbilical cord, joint, and muscle bleeding [10]. The risk of bleeding correlates relatively well with factor X activity levels in plasma [11]. Our patient's factor X activity level was 15% and thus she did not have any bleeding symptoms. But, she was scheduled to receive prophylactic treatment before and after surgery.

Plasma-derived factor X concentrates are used for treating bleeding. Dosing is 25 international units/kg, repeated daily until bleeding stops [12]. In institutions where a factor X concentrate is not available, bleeding can be treated with a 3-factor or 4-factor prothrombin complex concentrate or fresh frozen plasma [12]. Single-factor replacement therapy is preferred over multifactor therapy as reported in the series of study by Peyvandi et al. [13]. The aim of treatment should be maintaining a factor X level that is at least 10% to 20% normal for minor bleeding. For more serious hemorrhage, a factor X level that is greater than 40% of normal should be the goal [2]. Our patient had a factor X activity of 15%, and she did not report any bleeding symptoms; thus, she did not need any therapy at the time of our encounter. However, she received prophylactic therapy with factor X concentrate before and after the thyroidectomy, given the invasive nature of the procedure, with good outcome.

4. Conclusion

Acquired factor X deficiency is a rare coagulopathy that has been associated with amyloidosis, secondary to multiple myeloma (MM). Only recently, cases of acquired factor X deficiency in MM patients, without concomitant amyloidosis, have been reported. Circulating immunoglobulins in plasma cell dyscrasias interact with coagulation factors and lead to the deficiency. Monoclonal gammopathy of undetermined significance (MGUS) has been associated with acquired coagulopathies by the same mechanism. However, to our knowledge, no case of factor X deficiency in the setting of MGUS has been previously reported in the literature. With this case report, we portray a rare, acquired cause of factor X deficiency and we aim to contribute to the growing literature of plasma cell dyscrasias-associated coagulopathies.

Consent

Written informed consent was obtained from the patient for publication of this case report and any accompanying images.

Disclosure

Sameh Elias and Bhavna Gupta are the study's guarantors.

Authors' Contributions

Ayrton Bangolo searched the literature, wrote, and revised the manuscript. Trupti Waykole, Bilal Niazi, Chandini Sajja, and Mahabuba Akther revised and edited the manuscript. Sameh Elias and Bhavna Gupta revised and approved the final version. All authors certify that they contributed sufficiently to the intellectual content and data analysis. Each author has reviewed the final version of the manuscript and approved it for publication.

References

[1] J. Uprichard and D. J. Perry, "Factor X deficiency," *Blood Reviews*, vol. 16, no. 2, pp. 97–110, 2002.

[2] F. Peyvandi and M. Menegatti, "Inherited deficiencies of coagulation factors II, V, V+VIII, VII, X, XI, and XIII.," in *Williams Hematology, 10e*, K. Kaushansky, J. T. Prchal, L. J. Burns, M. A. Lichtman, M. Levi, and D. C. Linch, Eds., McGraw-Hill Education, New York, NY, USA, 2021.

[3] S. B. Reynolds, D. P. Maghavani, and H. Hashmi, "Acquired factor X deficiency in a patient with multiple myeloma: a rare case highlighting the significance of comprehensive evaluation and the need for antimyeloma therapy for bleeding diathesis," *BMJ Case Reports*, vol. 12, no. 9, 2019.

[4] E. M. Van Cott and M. Laposata, "Bleeding and thrombotic disorders," in *Laposata's Laboratory Medicine: Diagnosis of Disease in the Clinical Laboratory*, M. Laposata, Ed., McGraw-Hill Education, New York, NY, USA, 2019.

[5] F. Peyvandi and M. Menegatti, "Treatment of rare factor deficiencies in 2016," *Hematology*, vol. 2016, no. 1, pp. 663–669, 2016.

[6] M. Menegatti and F. Peyvandi, "Factor X deficiency," *Seminars in Thrombosis and Hemostasis*, vol. 35, no. 4, pp. 407–415, 2009.

[7] W. Liu, M. Xuan, F. Xue, and R. Yang, "Acquired coagulation factor X deficiency: three cases report and literature review," *Zhonghua Xue Ye Xue Za Zhi*, vol. 35, no. 7, pp. 633–636, 2014.

[8] G. Bianchi, E. K. O'Donnell, and K. Anderson, "Plasma cell neoplasms: general considerations," in *Williams Hematology, 10e*, K. Kaushansky, J. T. Prchal, L. J. Burns, M. A. Lichtman, M. Levi, and D. C. Linch, Eds., McGraw-Hill Education, New York, NY, USA, 2021.

[9] M. A. Lichtman, "Essential monoclonal gammopathy," in *Williams Hematology, 10e*, K. Kaushansky, J. T. Prchal, L. J. Burns, M. A. Lichtman, M. Levi, and D. C. Linch, Eds., McGraw-Hill Education, New York, NY, USA, 2021.

[10] C. Romagnolo, S. Burati, S. Ciaffoni et al., "Severe factor X deficiency in pregnancy: case report and review of the literature," *Haemophilia*, vol. 10, no. 5, pp. 665–668, 2004.

[11] F. Peyvandi, R. Palla, M. Menegatti et al., "Coagulation factor activity and clinical bleeding severity in rare bleeding disorders: results from the European Network of Rare Bleeding Disorders," *Journal of Thrombosis and Haemostasis*, vol. 10, no. 4, pp. 615–621, 2012.

[12] M. Hunault and K. A. Bauer, "Recombinant factor VIIa for the treatment of congenital factor VII deficiency," *Seminars in Thrombosis and Hemostasis*, vol. 26, no. 4, pp. 401–405, 2000.

[13] F. Peyvandi, G. Auerswald, S. K. Austin, R. Liesner, and K. Kavakli, "Álvarez Román MT, diagnosis, therapeutic advances, and key recommendations for the management of factor X deficiency," *Blood Reviews*, vol. 50, Article ID 100833, 2021.

2

Intermediate between Idiopathic Hypereosinophilia and Chronic Eosinophilic Leukemia: A Report of Two Hypereosinophilic Cases with Possible Novel Molecular Mutations

Jui Choudhuri,[1] Mohammad Eskandari,[2] Yang Shi,[1] and Yanhua Wang[1]

[1]*Department of Pathology, Montefiore Medical Center/Albert Einstein College of Medicine, 111 East 210th Street, Bronx 10467, NY, USA*
[2]*Department of Pathology, Altru Health System, 1200 S. Columbia Rd., Grand Forks 58201, ND, USA*

Correspondence should be addressed to Yanhua Wang; ywang@montefiore.org

Academic Editor: Sudhir Tauro

To distinguish a reactive eosinophilia from its malignant counterpart is challenging. Establishing clonality of the eosinophils is crucial and considered the determining factor for establishing a diagnosis. Cases of hypereosinophilia without clear reactive etiologies, no evidence of end-organ damage, normal cytogenetics, and no molecular mutations are termed as "Idiopathic Hypereosinophilia (IHE)." For cases which lie between the spectrum of chronic eosinophilic leukemia (CEL) and IHE, identification of underlying molecular abnormalities might be helpful in better understanding the disease process and prognosis. Here, we report two cases of hypereosinophilia in which five possible novel molecular mutations were identified by targeted next-generation sequencing (NGS) analysis. They were FBXW7, KM2A, TCF3, ERBB4, and MET. With multiple genetic mutations, these cases could be classified as chronic eosinophilic leukemia. Both these young patients responded well to steroid therapy. While targeted NGS is a useful tool in identifying new molecular mutation associated with hypereosinophilia, our cases raise the question of further investigating this entity and if there is a possibility of an intermediate category lying between the spectrum of CEL and IHE. Defining hypereosinophilia with clonal molecular abnormality as a malignant process may need to be revisited. Even though attempts are being made to identify mutations in IHE, it might be more significant clinically to differentiate them based on response to steroid therapy and prognosis.

1. Introduction

Idiopathic hypereosinophilic syndrome (HES) is defined as eosinophilia ($>1.5\times10^9$/L) that persists for at least 6 months with no identifiable causes and is associated with end-organ damage and dysfunction in multiple organs [1–3]. Chronic eosinophilic leukemia (CEL) is a myeloproliferative neoplasm with autonomous and clonal proliferation of eosinophil precursors resulting in increased numbers of eosinophils in the peripheral blood (PB), bone marrow (BM), and/or peripheral tissues [4]. Myeloid and lymphoid neoplasms with eosinophilia, in contrast, are associated with gene rearrangements of PDGFRA, PDGFRB, FGFR1, or PCM1-JAK2 [4]. These neoplasms have different clinical and hematological findings, influenced by the partner genes involved [5]. HES and CEL are diagnoses of exclusion and rendered after ruling out reactive processes and hypereosinophilia associated with myeloid and lymphoid neoplasms such as acute myeloid leukemia (AML), myelodysplastic syndrome (MDS), and systemic mastocytosis (SM) [4, 6].

Distinguishing HES and CEL is sometimes challenging. CEL differs from HES by showing clonality and/or increased blasts by the 2016 World Health Organization (WHO) criteria [4]. The clonality in these cases is mainly evaluated by conventional karyotyping and/or identifying specific mutations for myeloid neoplasms. In cases of hypereosinophilia without clear reactive etiologies, no evidence of end-organ damage, normal cytogenetics, and no molecular mutations, the term "idiopathic hypereosinophilia (IHE)" is warranted [4]. Recent studies on IHE patients have identified mutation in 28–53% of patients in various studies [7, 8]. The range of gene mutation and most frequently mutated genes has varied in studies.

Here, we reported two cases of persistent hypereosinophilia in which possible novel gene mutations were identified and these have not been reported previously in literature; however, the response to treatment made the diagnoses challenging.

2. Case Presentation

The first patient, a 17-year-old female, with no significant past medical history, presented with 1.5 months of facial angioedema, shortness of breath, chest pain, pleural effusion, acne-type rash, and visual loss. There was no history of recent medication prior to onset of symptoms, and a complete blood count was significant for eosinophilia. C1 esterase quantitative was normal. She had received antibiotics and antihistaminic at another facility. Imaging demonstrated diffuse lymphadenopathy and bilateral pleural effusions. Tuberculosis, autoimmune etiology including hereditary angioedema, rheumatologic etiology including sarcoidosis or systemic lupus erythematosus (SLE), and an oncologic process including lymphoma were excluded. 81% eosinophils were identified in the pleural fluid. Bone marrow biopsy was normocellular with trilineage hematopoiesis and approximately 30% eosinophils with some trilobed and multilobated forms. There was no increase in blasts, and some small hypolobated megakaryocytes were present (Figure 1). She was treated subsequently with steroid (prednisone, 60 mg/day and weaned gradually over seven months) alone, and the eosinophil counts dropped rapidly. Her overall eosinophil count remained slightly above the normal range afterwards. She still had some vision and sinus symptoms, but other symptoms resolved. Her absolute eosinophil count declined from 12.9 k/ul (normal 0.1–0.3 k/ul) to 0.4 k/ul over the course of the treatment and continued to remain within the normal range at one-year follow-up.

The second patient was a 33-year-old female with past medical history of multiple sclerosis, who presented with abdominal pain for three weeks and was diagnosed and treated for colitis. She was noted to have ~60% eosinophils on complete blood count. Infection and nonhematological malignancy were ruled out. A pleural effusion was noted incidentally on an abdominal X-ray. A thoracentesis was performed, and the pleural fluid analysis was notable for 86% eosinophils. A bone marrow biopsy revealed a relatively normocellular marrow (overall 60% cellularity) with trilineage hematopoiesis and marked increase in eosinophils (25% on aspirate); rare eosinophils showed abnormal lobation (trilobed forms) (Figure 2). The patient was placed on intravenous methylprednisolone 70 mg per day. Her eosinophil count decreased, from 7.4 k/ul to 0.1 k/ul, and she was discharged from the hospital 4 days later (Figure 3). She did have a recurrence two years later with an eosinophil count of 3.3 k/ul but responded promptly to steroid treatment and has been asymptomatic since then with normal eosinophil count.

Both patients showed normal karyotype and were negative for PDGFRA/B or FGFR1 rearrangements by cytogenetics/fluorescence in situ hybridization methods. Next-generation sequencing (NGS) for both showed different mutations (allele burden >5%) with no overlapping genes. The first patient showed four mutations: FBXW7 (c.566_567delAAinsGT; p.K189S), KMT2A (c.3634 + 4G > A), TCF3 (c.1357G > A; p.A453T), and TCF3 (c.635C > T; p.A212V), and the second patient showed three mutations: ASXL1 (c.2866C > T; p.L956F), ERBB4 (c.644A > C; p.E215A), and MET (c.467C > T; p.S156L). While ASXL1 and FBXW7 have been reported previously [7, 8], the other mutations identified, KM2A and TCF3 in the first patient and ERBB4 and MET in the second patient, have not been reported previously in patients with eosinophilia to the best of our knowledge; however, they are categorized as tier 1 according to the Catalogue of Somatic Mutations in Cancer (COSMIC) [9] (Table 1).

3. Discussion

Eosinophilia can coincide with different nonhematologic and hematologic disorders and carries potential for end-organ damage. The normal count of eosinophils in the peripheral blood is 3–5% which corresponds to an absolute eosinophil count (AEC) of 350–500/mm^3 [10]. In the clinical setting, eosinophilia can be divided into mild (500 < AEC < 1500), moderate (1500 < AEC < 5000), and severe (AEC > 5000) [10, 11]. Diagnosis of primary eosinophilia relies on multiple steps, including exclusion of secondary etiologies of eosinophilia, as well as morphologic review of the peripheral blood and bone marrow, cytogenetics, FISH, flow cytometry, and clonal T-cell gene rearrangement studies to detect histopathologic or clonal evidence of an acute or chronic myeloid or lymphoproliferative disorder.

The 2008 World Health Organization defined a semimolecular classification scheme of disease subtypes including myeloid and lymphoid neoplasms with eosinophilia and abnormalities of PDGFRA, PDGFRB, or FGFR1, chronic eosinophilic leukemia-not otherwise specified (CEL-NOS), lymphocyte-variant hypereosinophilia, and idiopathic hypereosinophilic syndrome (HES), which was categorized as a diagnosis of exclusion [12]. The 2016 WHO classification revision added a provisional entity of PCM1-JAK2 rearrangement neoplasms [4, 13]. Mattis et al. in their recent work have described the algorithm for diagnosis of IHE/HES and CEL and have emphasized that IHE and HES are two distinct entities separated by organ damage and the terms should not be used interchangeably [3].

While various studies have tried identifying mutations for IHE, few common mutations have been identified. Wang et al. in their work on HES found 28% of patients carrying somatic mutations and with the most frequent being ASXL1 [7]. Their study showed that mutations frequently affect genes involving DNA methylation and chromatin modification. HES patients with verified mutations showed several clinical, laboratory, and bone marrow histomorphologic features resembling those of CEL-NOS. Their findings suggested that molecular and genetic status was critical for leukemogenesis, most likely to be correlated with morphologic abnormalities; integrating

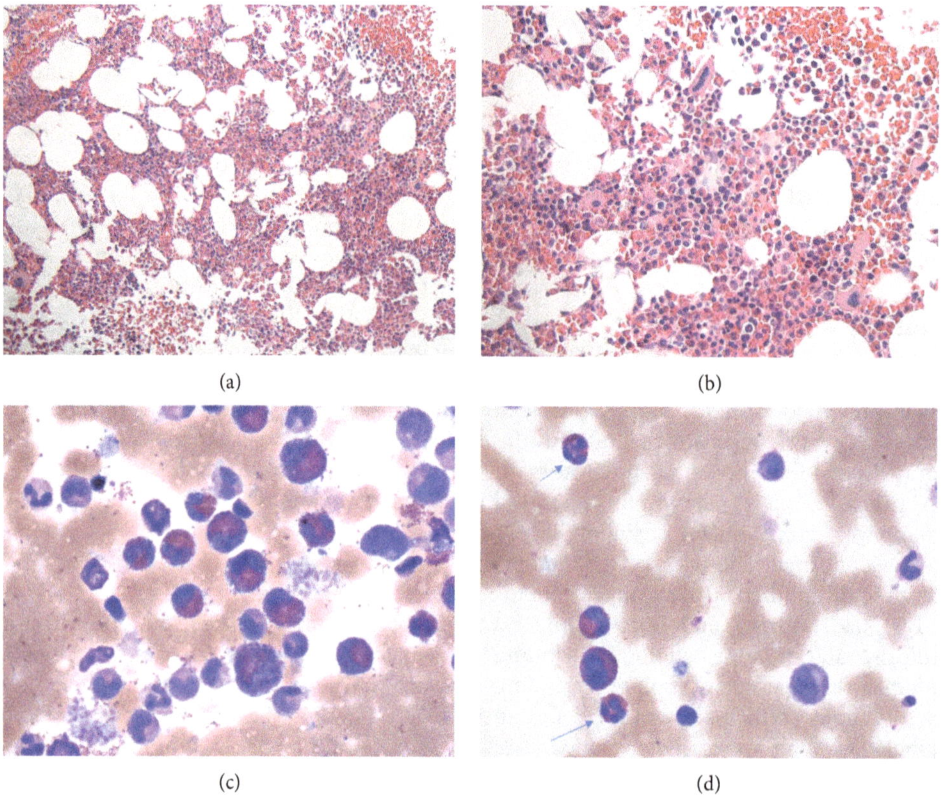

FIGURE 1: Bone marrow biopsy in a 17-year-old female with no significant past medical history. (a) H&E (400X magnification) section of the bone marrow biopsy, with trilineage hematopoiesis and a significant increase in eosinophils. (b) H&E (400X magnification) section of the bone marrow biopsy. (c), (d) Aspirate at high power (1000X magnification) showing an increase in mature eosinophils with occasional trilobed nuclei (arrow) and no increase in blasts.

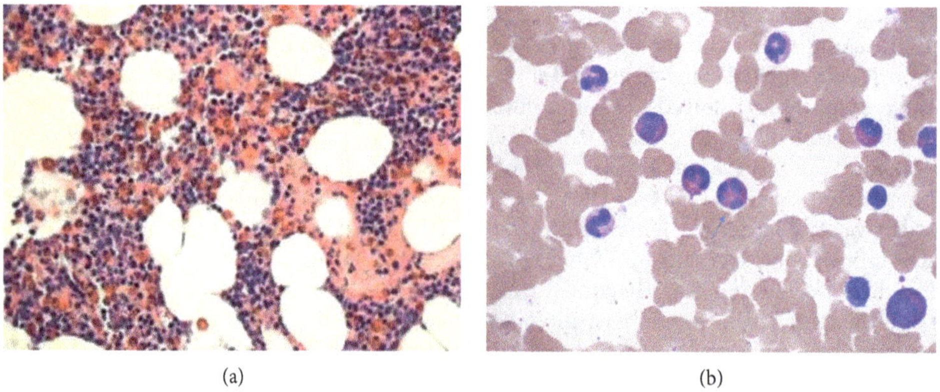

FIGURE 2: Bone marrow biopsy in a 33-year-old female with a past medical history of multiple sclerosis. (a) H&E (400X magnification) section of the bone marrow biopsy, with trilineage hematopoiesis and a significant interstitial increase in eosinophils. (b) Aspirate at high power (1000X magnification) showing mature eosinophils with rare trilobed nuclei (arrow) and no increase in blasts.

morphological assessment into the interpretation of genetic data might aid to distinguish a true neoplasm from nonneoplastic hypereosinophilia [7, 14]. Another study by Lee et al. identified 53% patients with IHE/HES to have somatic mutations and the most frequent was NOTCH1, having hidden T-cell malignancy potential. They saw more dysplastic eosinophils in patients with mutations and concluded that somatic mutations are likely to be associated with clonal proliferation of eosinophils, possibly including myeloproliferative neoplasm [8] (Table 2).

Andersen et al. performed whole exome sequencing and genome-wide methylation analysis on purified eosinophils from patients with idiopathic HES. They found somatic missense mutations in cancer-related genes in three patients. The genes included spliceosome PUF60 and the cadherin gene CDH17 [15]. In our patient population, we identified two of 16 patients diagnosed with IHE having possible somatic mutations (unpublished data). A germline mutation is considered to have an allele frequency of 50 to 100% [16].

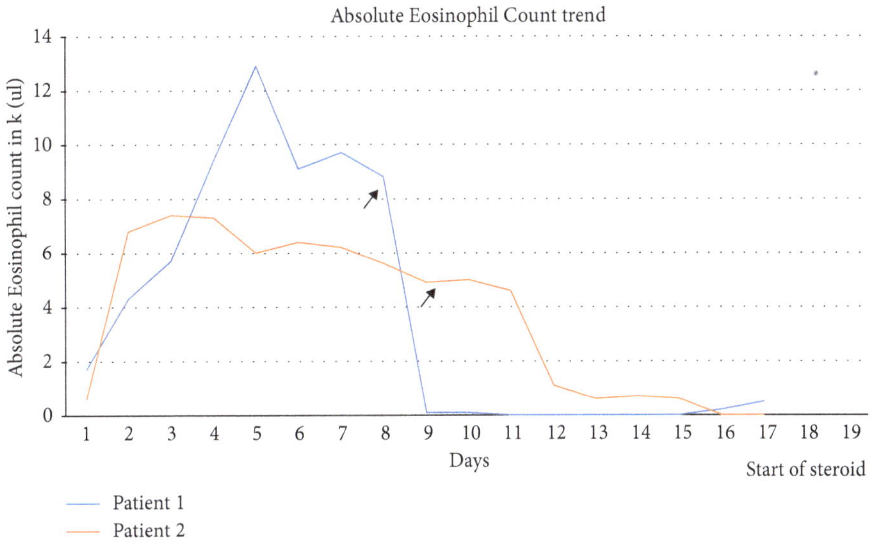

Figure 3: Trend of absolute eosinophil counts (k/ul) of both patients over time following treatment with steroid. Blue line: patient 1; orange line: patient 2. The arrows indicated steroid usage.

Table 1: Demographic and mutation analysis result in two cases of idiopathic hypereosinophilia.

Age (years)/ gender	Mutations	Nucleotide change	Allele frequency (%)	Tier	Karyotype/FISH analysis
17/F	FBXW7	c.566_567delAAinsGT; p.K189S	45	1	46, XX
	KMT2A	c.3634 + 4G > A	48	1	No rearrangement of PDGFRA (4q12) and PDGFRB (5q31)
	TCF3	c.1357G > A; p.A453T	51	1	FGRFR1 (8p11)
	TCF3	c.635C > T; p.A212V	51		MDS/MPN FISH panel: negative*
33/F	ASXL1	c.2866C > T; p.L956F	47	1	46, XX
	MET	c.467C > T; p.S156L	49	1	FGRFR1 (8p11)
	ERBB4	c.644A > C; p.E215A	53	1	No rearrangement of PDGFRA (4q12) and PDGFRB (5q31)

* FISH panel for MDS/MPN includes the following probes: EGR1, D7Z1, D7S486 (7q31), D8Z2 (8 CEN), KMT2A (MLL), TP53, D17Z1 (17CEN), D20S1157 (20PTEL18), D20S108 (20q12), PDGFRA, PDGFRB, CSF1R, FGFR1, CEP 9, ABL1, BCR, D13S319 (13q14.3), and LAMP1 (13q34) (Vysis FISH Probes, Abbott Molecular).

A somatic mutation is usually present with a lower allele frequency because it is not present in all cells [17]. Four mutations were identified in the first patient's sample, and three mutations were identified in the second patient's sample. Most likely, it is because the samples contained a very high percentage of neoplastic eosinophils, and these eosinophils showed heterozygous mutations. Therefore, the VAF is approximately 50%. It is less likely that the patients had three or four germline mutations at the same time. However, germline mutations cannot be completely ruled out due to lack of oral epithelial cell controls. The next-generation sequencing panel with a larger array of mutations revealed novel mutations which have not been identified previously. These genes include KMT2A, TCF3, ERBB4, and MET. Three of these mutations were missense, including ERBB4 (c.644A > C; p.E215A), MET (c.467C > T; p.S156L), and TCF3 (c.1357G > A; p.A453T and c.635C > T; p.A212V). The KMT2A gene has a splice-region alteration (c.3634 + 4G > A).

KMT2A is also known as myeloid/lymphoid or mixed-lineage leukemia (MLL), a gene which encodes a transcriptional coactivator playing an essential role in hematopoiesis. Mutation of this gene has been seen in acute lymphoblastic leukemia and acute myeloid leukemia [18]. A variant of KMT2A (MLL) was also reported in Wiedemann–Steiner Syndrome (WSS), an abnormality in facial and skeletal growth, as well as intellectual development delay [19]. KMT2A can translocate to many different partners; some translocations might be associated with eosinophilia; however, the exact mechanism has not been elucidated [20].

TCF3 encodes a member of helix-loop-helix transcription factors. It is required for B- and T-lymphocyte development. Deletion or mutation of this gene may play an important role in lymphoid malignancies. It has been reported involving in several chromosomal translocations in different leukemias or lymphomas, such as with PBX1 in *t*(1; 19) reported in pre-B acute lymphoblastic leukemia, with TFPT in *t*(19; 19) seen in pediatric leukemia and with

Table 2: Mutations identified in the literature.

Author	Frequency of mutation	Genes involved
Wang et al.	28%	ASXL1, TET2, EZH2, SETBP1, CBL, NOTCH1 DNMT3A, NRAS, JAK2 exon 13, and GATA2
Lee et at.	53%	NOTCH1, TP53, TET2, EZH2, FLT3, IKZF1, ITPKB, SAMHD1, SF3A1, STAG2, ZMYM3, CDKN2A, ATRX, DIS3, BRD4, CARD6, GATA2, NFKBIE, SMC1A, ASXL1, ATM, BIRC3, CBL, CCND1, CEBPA, FAM46 C, FAT4, FBXW7, GATA1, MAPK1, MPL, NF1, PRKD3, PRPF40 B, RUNX1, SCRIB, SF1, SF3B1, SH2B3, SMC3, WT1, PTEN, MED12, BCOR, CSF1R, CSF3R, DNMT3A, EGR2, HIST1H1E, JAK2, LRP1B, POLG, PRKD3, PRPF40 B, RB1, SETBP1, SMARCA2, SMC3, TGM7, U2AF2, and ZRSR2
Choudhuri et al.	—	FBXW7, KMT2A, TCF3, ASXL1, ERBB4, and MET

ZNF384 in *t*(12; 19) in acute leukemia [21–23]. However, its association with eosinophilia has not been reported yet.

ERBB4 is a member of the tyrosine kinase family and the epidermal growth factor receptor subfamily. It maintains a critical role in regulating cell proliferation and differentiation, as well as cell migration and organogenesis. Mutations in this gene have been associated with different malignancies, including sarcoma, cancer, and lymphoma [24–27]. Different expression patterns of EGF, EGFR, and ERBB4 in the nasal polyp can be associated with an increase of eosinophilic infiltrate, indicating a cytokine role related to ERBB4 [28]. However, its role in pathologic eosinophilia is not fully understood. More cases with this mutation might be needed to characterize its mechanism.

MET is another member of the receptor tyrosine kinase family. It plays a role in cellular survival, embryogenesis, and cellular migration and invasion. Mutations of the gene with amplification and overexpression have been found to be associated with several human malignancies, such as papillary renal cell carcinoma, hepatocellular carcinoma, and various head and neck cancers [29–31]. However, the relationship of MET mutation with eosinophilia has not been reported yet.

According to the 2008 WHO classification, our two cases are classified as IHE. However, the 2016 WHO revision stated clearly that idiopathic hypereosinophilia is defined as eosinophilia with no evidence of eosinophil clonality [4, 32]. If multiple mutations are considered evidence of eosinophilic clonality, then our cases are classified as CEL, not otherwise specified, according to the 2016 WHO revision. Both our patients were young, with bone marrow involvement but responded well to steroids and did not require chemotherapy. They did not have any organ damage. This leads to a dilemma in classifying them as CEL which is a rare, aggressive disease with a high risk of acute transformation [33]. Patients with hypereosinophilia that mostly involves the bone marrow might present with anemia and thrombocytopenia, while patients with hypereosinophilia that mostly involves extramedullary organs might present with symptoms related to cytokine release, such as sinusitis, gastroenteritis, neuritis, pleural effusions, abdominal pain, and shortness of breath. The two scenarios might have different disease mechanisms and presentations. Treatment options include high-dose steroids followed by other agents such as hydroxycarbamide, interferon-alpha, and imatinib, for corticosteroid-resistant or corticosteroid-sparing cases. Patients with bone marrow disease might benefit from chemotherapy and bone marrow transplant.

In the previous literature, idiopathic hypereosinophilia has been reported as a rare chronic condition which can sometimes be fatal in the older age group and prognosis depends on organs involved [1, 34]. Our cases bring up the question if these should be classified based on mutations or good response to steroid, also raising the possibility of an intermediate category with clonality and yet excellent prognosis and responsiveness to steroid. These cases highlight that, for IHE patients, even though attempts are being made to identify mutations, the relevance of mutations is still not well understood, and it might be imperative to investigate them further or classify clinically for patients and clinicians. Further studies will help clarify both the overlapping and unique features of these two entities and to understand if there are entities lying within this spectrum which can be classified separately. This information will be extremely relevant for clinicians, pathologists, and patients.

4. Conclusions

In summary, we present two cases of IHE with possible novel mutations identified on NGS and that have not been previously reported. Some of these mutations have undetermined clinical significance at this point. However, the excellent response to steroid for both patients make it important to study this disease entity and investigate it based on both either molecular mutations or clinical profile.

References

[1] A. Osowo, J. Fetten, and S. Navaneethan, "Idiopathic hypereosinophilic syndrome: a rare but fatal condition presenting with common symptoms," *Southern Medical Journal*, vol. 99, no. 2, pp. 188-189, 2006.

[2] S. A. Wang, "The diagnostic work-up of hypereosinophilia," *Pathobiology*, vol. 86, no. 1, pp. 39–52, 2019.

[3] D. M. Mattis, S. A. Wang, and C. M. Lu, "Contemporary classification and diagnostic evaluation of hypereosinophilia," *American Journal of Clinical Pathology*, vol. 154, no. 3, pp. 305–318, 2020.

[4] WHO, *WHO Classification of Tumours of Haematopoietic and Lymphoid Tissues. Revised Fourth Edition*, WHO, Geneva, Switzerland, 4 edition, 2017.

[5] N. Savage, T. I. George, and J. Gotlib, "Myeloid neoplasms associated with eosinophilia and rearrangement ofPDGFRA, PDGFRB, andFGFR1: a review," *The International Journal of Literary Humanities*, vol. 35, no. 5, pp. 491–500, 2013.

[6] J. Gotlib, "World Health Organization-defined eosinophilic disorders: 2015 update on diagnosis, risk stratification, and management," *American Journal of Hematology*, vol. 90, no. 11, pp. 1077–1089, 2015.

[7] S. A. Wang, W. Tam, A. G. Tsai et al., "Targeted next-generation sequencing identifies a subset of idiopathic hypereosinophilic syndrome with features similar to chronic eosinophilic leukemia, not otherwise specified," *Modern Pathology*, vol. 29, no. 8, pp. 854–864, 2016.

[8] J.-S. Lee, H. Seo, K. Im et al., "Idiopathic hypereosinophilia is clonal disorder? Clonality identified by targeted sequencing," *PLoS One*, vol. 12, no. 10, Article ID e0185602, 2017.

[9] Data from: COSMIC Catalogue of Somatic Mutations in Cancer.94.

[10] M. Brigden and C. Graydon, "Eosinophilia detected by automated blood cell counting in ambulatory North American outpatients. Incidence and clinical significance," *Archives of Pathology and Laboratory Medicine*, vol. 121, no. 9, pp. 963–967, 1997.

[11] A. Tefferi, M. M. Patnaik, and A. Pardanani, "Eosinophilia: secondary, clonal and idiopathic," *British Journal of Haematology*, vol. 133, no. 5, pp. 468–492, 2006.

[12] S. H. Swerdlow, E. Campo, N. L. Harris et al., *WHO Classification of Tumours of Haematopoietic and Lymphoid Tissues*p. 439, Fourth edition, WHO, Geneva, Switzerland, 2008.

[13] A. Reiter and J. Gotlib, "Myeloid neoplasms with eosinophilia," *Blood*, vol. 129, no. 6, pp. 704–714, 2017.

[14] S. A. Wang, R. P. Hasserjian, W. Tam et al., "Bone marrow morphology is a strong discriminator between chronic eosinophilic leukemia, not otherwise specified and reactive idiopathic hypereosinophilic syndrome," *Haematologica*, vol. 102, no. 8, pp. 1352–1360, 2017.

[15] C. L. Andersen, H. M. Nielsen, L. S. Kristensen et al., "Whole-exome sequencing and genome-wide methylation analyses identify novel disease associated mutations and methylation patterns in idiopathic hypereosinophilic syndrome," *Oncotarget*, vol. 6, no. 38, pp. 40588–40597, 2015.

[16] M. M. He, Q. Li, M. Yan et al., "Variant Interpretation for Cancer (VIC): a computational tool for assessing clinical impacts of somatic variants," *Genome Medicine*, vol. 11, no. 1, p. 53, 2019.

[17] C. Baer, W. Walter, S. Hutter et al., ""Somatic" and "pathogenic"—is the classification strategy applicable in times of large-scale sequencing?" *Haematologica*, vol. 104, no. 8, pp. 1515–1520, 2019.

[18] M. J. Thirman, H. J. Gill, R. C. Burnett et al., "Rearrangement of the MLL gene in acute lymphoblastic and acute myeloid leukemias with 11q23 chromosomal translocations," *New England Journal of Medicine*, vol. 329, no. 13, pp. 909–914, 1993.

[19] S. P. Strom, R. Lozano, H. Lee et al., "De Novo variants in the KMT2A (MLL) gene causing atypical Wiedemann-Steiner syndrome in two unrelated individuals identified by clinical exome sequencing," *BMC Medical Genetics*, vol. 15, no. 1, p. 49, 2014.

[20] M. A. Sanders, F. G. Kavelaars, A. Zeilemaker et al., "RNA sequencing reveals a unique fusion of the lysine (K)-specific methyltransferase 2A and smooth muscle myosin heavy chain 11 in myelodysplastic syndrome and acute myeloid leukemia," *Haematologica*, vol. 100, no. 1, pp. e1–e3l, 2015.

[21] N. Yuan, L. Song, W. Lin et al., "Autophagy collaborates with ubiquitination to downregulate oncoprotein E2A/Pbx1 in B-cell acute lymphoblastic leukemia," *Blood Cancer Journal*, vol. 5, no. 1, p. e274, 2015.

[22] A. S. Gabriel, F. M. Lafta, E. C. Schwalbe et al., "Epigenetic landscape correlates with genetic subtype but does not predict outcome in childhood acute lymphoblastic leukemia," *Epigenetics*, vol. 10, no. 8, pp. 717–726, 2015.

[23] J. Piao, S. Takai, T. Kamiya et al., "Poly (ADP-ribose) polymerase inhibitors selectively induce cytotoxicity in TCF3-HLF-positive leukemic cells," *Cancer Letters*, vol. 386, pp. 131–140, 2017.

[24] C. J. A. Ramachandra, A. Mehta, C. H. Lua, A. Chitre, K. P. M. M. Ja, and W. Shim, "ErbB receptor tyrosine kinase: a molecular switch between cardiac and neuroectoderm specification in human pluripotent stem cells," *Stem Cells*, vol. 34, no. 10, pp. 2461–2470, 2016.

[25] J. Edenfield, C. Schammel, J. Collins, D. Schammel, and W. J. Edenfield, "Metaplastic breast cancer: molecular typing and identification of potential targeted therapies at a single institution," *Clinical Breast Cancer*, vol. 17, no. 1, pp. e1–e10, 2017.

[26] A. Mendoza-Naranjo, A. El-Naggar, D. H. Wai et al., "ERBB 4 confers metastatic capacity in ewing sarcoma," *EMBO Molecular Medicine*, vol. 5, no. 7, pp. 1087–1102, 2013.

[27] I. Scarfò, E. Pellegrino, E. Mereu et al., "Identification of a new subclass of ALK-negative ALCL expressing aberrant levels of ERBB4 transcripts," *Blood*, vol. 127, no. 2, pp. 221–232, 2016.

[28] C. Duan, C. W. Li, L. Zhao et al., "Differential expression patterns of EGF, EGFR, and ERBB4 in nasal polyp epithelium," *PLoS One*, vol. 11, no. 6, Article ID e0156949, 2016.

[29] W. Sterlacci, M. Fiegl, M. Gugger, L. Bubendorf, S. Savic, and A. Tzankov, "MET overexpression and gene amplification: prevalence, clinico-pathological characteristics and prognostic significance in a large cohort of patients with surgically resected NSCLC," *Virchows Archiv*, vol. 471, no. 1, pp. 49–55, 2017.

[30] W. Y. Kim, S.-H. Shim, H. Y. Jung, M. Dong, S.-N. Kim, and S. J. Lee, "The gene copy number of c-MET has a significant impact on progression-free survival in Korean patients with ovarian carcinoma," *Human Pathology*, vol. 64, pp. 98–105, 2017.

[31] S. K. Tey, E. Y. T. Tse, X. Mao et al., "nuclear met promotes hepatocellular carcinoma tumorigenesis and metastasis by upregulation of TAK1 and activation of NF-κB pathway," *Cancer Letters*, vol. 411, pp. 150–161, 2017.

[32] S. H. Swerdlow, E. Campo, S. A. Pileri et al., "The 2016 revision of the World Health Organization classification of lymphoid neoplasms," *Blood*, vol. 127, no. 20, pp. 2375–2390, 2016.

[33] G. Helbig, A. Soja, A. Bartkowska-Chrobok, and S. Kyrcz-Krzemień, "Chronic eosinophilic leukemia-not otherwise specified has a poor prognosis with unresponsiveness to conventional treatment and high risk of acute transformation," *American Journal of Hematology*, vol. 87, no. 6, pp. 643–645, 2012.

[34] F. Khalid and F. Holguin, "Idiopathic hypereosinophilic syndrome in an elderly female: a case report," *American Journal of Case Reports*, vol. 20, pp. 381–384, 2019.

3

Juvenile Myelomonocytic Leukemia in a Child: A Case Report of Palliative Chemotherapy and Literature Review Applied to Limited Resources Centers

Natharina Yolanda,[1] Stefanus Gunawan,[1] Max F. J. Mantik,[1] and Anjo J. P. Veerman[2]

[1]*Department of Child Health, Faculty of Medicine, Sam Ratulangi University, Manado, Indonesia*
[2]*Amsterdam University Medical Center, VU University, Amsterdam, Netherlands*

Correspondence should be addressed to Natharina Yolanda; natharinayolanda@hotmail.com

Academic Editor: Chihaya Imai

Juvenile myelomonocytic leukemia (JMML) is a rare hematopoietic malignancy in children, with an incidence of 1.2 per million children per year. At this moment, we present a case report and a brief literature review of JMML in a child, primarily focused on its applicability in low-middle income countries. A 3.5-year-old male was referred to our tertiary center due to pallor, enlarging abdomen and neck mass, recurrent fever, and chronic diarrhea. Initial laboratory workup showed hemoglobin of 6.4 g/dl, white blood cell of $315.62 \times 10^3/\mu L$, and platelet of $17 \times 10^3/\mu L$. Blood smears showed 10% suspected blasts, 17% myelocytes, and 17% metamyelocytes with thrombocytopenic crisis. The HbF level was 5.8%. BCR-ABL gene tested negative. The patient was diagnosed with juvenile myelomonocytic leukemia. Considering that HSCT could not be done in our center and lack other financial possibilities to seek treatment abroad, the family agreed to do the palliative treatment. The patient was treated with oral 6-mercaptopurine and subcutaneous cytarabine. Four weeks after receiving 6-mercaptopurine, the white blood cell count decreased to $10.6 \times 10^3/\mu L$ and the spleen size was half of the original size. The patient continued chemotherapy until week 15, chemotherapy was stopped, but 16 weeks after the diagnosis of JMML, he developed severe thrombocytopenia, endophthalmitis, and sepsis and passed away. As a conclusion, in JMML cases in developing countries without HSCT, palliative chemotherapy is acceptable, and palliative care is an important aspect.

1. Introduction

Juvenile myelomonocytic leukemia (JMML) is a rare hematopoietic malignancy in children with features characteristic of myelodysplastic and myeloproliferative disorders [1]. In 2008, the World Health Organization (WHO) classified JMML as myelodysplastic syndrome (MDS) or myeloproliferative neoplasms (MPN) [2]. This rare disease has an incidence rate of 1.2 per million children per year or 1% of all childhood leukemias [3]. JMML is associated with two inherited diseases: neurofibromatosis type 1 (NF-1) and Casitas B-lineage (CBL)-syndrome [1]. There are five subtypes of JMML: PTPN11-mutated JMML, NRAS-mutated JMML, KRAS-mutated JMML, NF-1-mutated JMML, and CBL-mutated JMML [4]. Cytogenetic analysis of JMML patients showed monosomy 7 in 24–33% of patients, other chromosomal abnormalities in 10–27%, and normal karyotype in 40–60% [5].

JMML affects young children, with a median age at diagnosis of 20–24 months and a significant male predominance (2.5 : 1) [5, 6]. The symptoms of JMML are fever and general malaise, plus symptoms due to infiltration of organs by malignant cells, infection, pallor, lymphadenopathy, marked hepatosplenomegaly, cutaneous lesions, and hemorrhagic manifestations. Hematologic abnormalities are caused by hyperactivation of signal transduction in the RAS pathway [7]. Leukocytosis with monocytosis, myeloid/erythroid precursors, anemia, and thrombocytopenia are common findings in peripheral blood. The median blast cell percentage in peripheral blood is less than 2% and the blast count does not exceed 20%. Bone marrow abnormalities are nonspecific and less informative than peripheral blood smears [5]. JMML patients respond poorly to chemotherapy, and the probability of survival of most patients without allogeneic hematopoietic stem cell transplantation (HSCT) is low. Even after HSCT, the 5-year event survival rate is only 44–53% [8]. At this moment, we present a case report and a brief literature review of JMML in a child, primarily focused on its applicability in low-middle income countries.

2. Case Report

A 3.5-year-old male was referred to our tertiary center, Estella Clinic for Children with Cancer and Blood Diseases, Manado, Indonesia, due to pallor and enlarging abdomen and neck mass noticed over the last year. The mother also mentioned recurrent fever and diarrhea for the previous two years. The patient's weight was 9.4 kg and his height was 76 cm (weight for age $<P_3$, height for age $<P_3$, and weight for height P_{15-50}). Physical examination showed anemia, breathing difficulty, enlarged unilateral neck, lymph node with a diameter of 3 cm, enlarged liver 7 cm below the costal margin, spleen length 10 cm, and peripheral edema. He was diagnosed with tuberculosis and treated with triple tuberculostatic therapy; probably, this was a false diagnosis and JMML being the cause of his symptoms.

The initial routine blood test showed a hemoglobin content of 6.4 g/dl, white blood cell counts of $315.62 \times 10^3/\mu L$, neutrophils of $180.5 \times 10^3/\mu L$, lymphocytes of $23.4 \times 10^3/\mu L$, monocytes of $77.93 \times 10^3/\mu L$, and platelets of $17 \times 10^3/\mu L$. Blood smears showed normocytic anemia and leukocytosis with various stages of cell maturation, i.e., 10% suspected blast, 17% myelocyte, and 17% metamyelocytes, with a thrombocytopenic crisis. The HbF level was 5.8%. BCR-ABL gene tested negative. Chest X-ray and echocardiography were within normal limits. An abdominal ultrasound showed enlargement of the liver, spleen, peripancreatic, and paraaortic lymph nodes.

Our patient was diagnosed with juvenile myelomonocytic leukemia, accompanied by cachexia. Considering that HSCT was not able to be done in our center, the lack of financial possibilities to seek treatment abroad, and the complex condition of the patient, the family agreed to do palliative treatment to keep him in a reasonably good clinical condition for as long as possible. He had received hydroxyurea shortly before the diagnosis of JMML was made. The patient was treated with oral 6-mercaptopurine (6-MP) and subcutaneous cytarabine. The treatment plan consisted of 4 cycles of a 4-weeks regimen of 3 weeks 6MP daily and 1 dose of cytarabine weekly, with one week of no chemotherapy. Doses were to be increased if well tolerated, but to be decreased, if counts dropped too low. 6-MP was given daily, started with a dose of 10 mg/m^2/day, and increased 20% every cycle, if tolerated, until a maximum of 20 mg/m^2/day. Subcutaneous cytarabine 10 mg/m^2 was given every week, except for the very first week. The chemotherapy was well tolerated, and the patient's general condition was improving; his weight increased to 10.2 kg. He survived a bout of COVID infection with a mild cough and a positive COVID antigen test. There was no fever, bleeding signs, or breathing difficulty. Four weeks after receiving 6-MP, the white blood cell count decreased to $10.6 \times 10^3/\mu L$, and the spleen size was half of the original size (categorized as a complete clinical response). The 6-MP dose was increased by 20% in the second cycle and was also well tolerated. The patient continued the chemotherapy at home until week 16, and chemotherapy was stopped, but 16 weeks after the diagnosis of JMLL, he developed severe thrombocytopenia, endophthalmitis, and sepsis and passed away. The protocol of palliative chemotherapy for JMML at our center and the patient's laboratory findings during treatment are shown in Table 1.

3. Discussion

The presenting clinical picture of this patient with pallor, persistent fever, cervical lymphadenopathy, hepatosplenomegaly, and hyperleukocytosis directed to hematological malignancy. The peripheral blood smear showed less than 20% blasts. The myeloblast predominance in the blood smear suggested a diagnosis of the myeloid lineage. This patient was initially diagnosed with chronic myeloid leukemia and shortly treated with hydroxyurea, until further workups showed a negative BCR-ABL gene and increased HbF. The diagnosis of JMML is based on diagnosis criteria per the 2016 revision of the World Health Organization Classification (Table 2) [9, 10].

This patient fulfilled all items in category 1 (peripheral blood monocyte count $>1000/\mu L$, blasts in peripheral blood $<20\%$, splenomegaly, absence of BRC-ABL gene) and two items in category 3 (circulating myeloid precursors and increased HbF with age). This patient also had the epidemiologic characteristics of JMML, i.e., male sex and age less than six years old. The pathogenesis of JMML involves hyperactivation of signal transduction along the RAS pathway, with a resultant selective hypersensitivity of JMML cells to GM-CSF. Unfortunately, we could not perform laboratory tests to find aberrations in the RAS pathway.

Marked splenomegaly and hepatomegaly are usually found and may cause abdominal discomfort and breathing difficulty. Lymphadenopathy is observed in about half of the patients, and leukemic infiltrates may give rise to enlarged tonsils. Peribronchial and interstitial pulmonary infiltrates may be evident on the chest X-ray and manifest as cough and respiratory distress. Central nervous system involvement is uncommon in JMML. Cutaneous involvement is frequent and most often appears as eczematous eruptions or indurated raised lesions with a main pale area [11].

Allogenic hematopoietic stem cell transplantation (HSCT) is the only curative regimen for most patients with JMML. HSCT can achieve long-treatment-free survival in about 50% of patients, but it still has a high relapse rate of 30–40% [12]. In the absence of treatment, the progression of JMML is highly variable, including blast crisis, acute leukemia, or even spontaneous partial or complete remission [13].

AML protocols for intensive chemotherapy can induce temporary remission in JMML, but this approach is also very

Table 1: Protocol of palliative chemotherapy for juvenile myelomonocytic leukemia at our center and patient's laboratory findings during treatment.

	Week																
	1	2	3	4	5	6	7	8	9	10	11	12	13	14	15	16	17
6-MP					*				*				*				
ARA-C		↓	↓	↓		↓	↓	↓		↓	↓	↓		↓	↓	↓	
	6-MP (6-mercaptopurine): $10\,mg/m^2/day$; ARA-C (cytarabine): $10\,mg/m^2/week$ for 3 weeks.																
	* If 6-MP is well tolerated, and WBC still high, the doses may be increased by 20% every next phase, until a maximum of 200%																
Hb (gr/dL)	8.3	6.5	6.1	7.8	10.4	10	10.8										9.6
Ht (%)	21.2	18.3	17.2	24.5	32.4	29.5	30	Patient at home, no lab data									28
WBC (/μL)	236,700	99,700	11,900	7,800	10,600	26,700	47,100										30,500
Platelet (/μL)	22,000	69,000	57,000	11,000	45,000	34,000	30,900										11,000
Chemotherapy	6-MP	6-MP ARA-C	6-MP ARA-C	6-MP ARA-C		6-MP ARA-C increase 20%	6-MP ARA-C	6-MP ARA-C		6-MP ARA-C	6-MP ARA-C	6-MP ARA-C		6-MP ARA-C	6-MP ARA-C	6-MP ARA-C	Patient died

6-MP, 6-mercaptopurine; ARA-C, cytarabine.

TABLE 2: Diagnosis criteria for juvenile myelomonocytic leukemia (JMML) per the 2016 revision to the World Health Organization classification [10].

Category 1 (all are required)	Clinical and hematologic features	Absence of the BCR-ABL1 fusion gene $>1 \times 10$/L circulating monocytes $<20\%$ blasts in the peripheral blood and bone marrow Splenomegaly
Category 2 (one is sufficient)	Genetic studies	Somatic mutation in KRAS, NRAS, or PTPN11 (germline mutations need to be excluded) Clinical diagnosis of NF-1 or NF-1 gene mutation Germline CBL mutation and loss of heterozygosity of CBL
Category 3 (patients without genetic features must have the following in addition to category 1)	Other features	Monosomy 7 or other chromosomal abnormality or at least 2 of the criteria given as follows: circulating myeloid or erythroid precursors, increased hemoglobin F for age, hyperphosphorylation of STAT-5, GM-CSF hypersensitivity

NF-1, neurofibromin-1; CBL, casitas B-lineage lymphoma; PTPN11, protein tyrosine phosphatase nonreceptor type; KRAS, Kirsten rat sarcoma; NRAS, neuroblastoma rat sarcoma.

toxic. The European Working Group of MDS (EWOG-MDS) trial reported no significant difference in event survival rate and mortality of AML-type chemotherapy compared to less intensive treatment [12]. For many decades, cytoreductive therapy with 6-MP at 50 mg/m^2 or low dose, i.e., cytarabine in a 40 mg/m^2 dose for five days has been used to control the JMML symptoms before HSCT [13]. In aggressive cases, high-dose fludarabine 30 mg/m^2 and cytarabine 2 g/m^2 daily for five consecutive days have been adopted by some centers [14]. JMML sometimes was sensitive to 6-MP, and cytosine arabinoside (Ara-C) was added because of its efficacy in AML. However, neither intensive nor low-dose chemotherapy has been demonstrated to improve the outcome of patients with JMML [15]. Various combinations of busulfan (BU), melphalan (MRL), cyclophosphamide (CY), and fludarabine (FLU) have been tested as conditioning regimens [15]. Sakashita et al. found that BU/L-PAM/CY and BU/L-PAM/FLU combinations were associated with a higher overall survival rate than total body irradiation or BU alone [7]. Due to the unavailability of HSCT in our center, we opted for chemotherapy to control the disease. We used mercaptopurine and cytarabine due to their exhaustive studies and availability in our center.

Jin Kang et al. in Korea proposed a novel regimen for newly diagnosed JMML lacking access to transplantation. They offered a standard regimen in 3-week intervals consisting of a combination of chemotherapy (Ara-C, etoposide, and vincristine) and differentiation therapy (isotretinoin). If the disease relapsed or progressed, they continued to salvage the regimen of chemotherapy (Ara-C, etoposide) and differentiation therapy (low-dose Ara-C) in 3-4 weeks intervals. This regimen was safe and effective, but the study was only done on 5 JMML patients [16]. Another regimen was tested by Feng et al. in China, consisting of decitabine, cytarabine, and fludarabine. They reported that this regimen is safe, effective, and feasible with a response rate of 97%. Although, the complete remission rate was low and primarily partial [17]. Given that DNA hypermethylation of specific genes is contributing to the aggressiveness of JMML, azacytidine (AZA), a DNA hypomethylating agent, has been tested as a potential treatment for JMML. Cseh et al. in their retrospective study treated 9 JMML patients with low-dose azacytidine before HSCT and highlighted two complete remissions and two partial remissions. However, there were several adverse events (severe neutropenia, skin rash, and gastrointestinal problems) [18].

The Food and Drug Administration (FDA) currently approved azacitidine for JMML therapy in March 2022. Azacitidine has been shown to induce complete clinical remission in some JMML patients. A study by Niemeyer et al. stated that azacitidine monotherapy is a suitable option for children with newly diagnosed JMML [19]. Fabri et al. in Slovakia tested a novel approach using azacytidine 75 mg/m^2, i.e., on days 1–7 of a 28-day cycle as a bridging therapy before HSCT and reported a good response and favorable toxicity [20]. Some studies report sustained remission after azacitidine therapy [21] and the disappearance of the monosomy 7 clones in JMML without HSCT [22]. Azacitidine is currently the standard of care for most patients with JMML prior to HSCT.

Age, platelet count, and percentage of HbF at diagnosis are the main prognostic factors in JMML. Age >2 years at diagnosis, platelet count $<33 \times 10^6$/mm^3, and HbF >10% are related to short survival [5]. This patient had a bad prognosis due to his age at diagnosis, being older than two years old, initial low platelet count, and cachexia. In most patients, JMML can be a rapidly progressive and fatal disorder if left untreated. Most untreated patients die from respiratory failure due to pulmonary infiltration with leukemic cells, and progression to acute leukemia is observed in less than 20% of patients [5].

In a terminal illness with limited available therapy, palliative care is appropriate. Palliative care is a patient-centered approach that aims to improve the quality of life of patients and their families through the prevention and relief of suffering using early identification and treatment of pain and other physical, psychosocial, and spiritual problems [23]. Palliative care may or may not include cytostatic drugs to improve clinical conditions and extend life. However, this approach has the risk of severe side effects too. The provision of palliative care for children differs from that for adults for several reasons: (1) evaluation of pain severity and quality of life is complex and (2) communication with children about disease, treatment, and death is influenced by their developmental stages [24]. The application of palliative care in cancer patients can decrease the number of unnecessary procedures, length of hospital stay, and need for intensive care, facilitate pain management, and improve communication between parents and the healthcare teams [25].

Our patient's history suggested he had been suffering from JMML for about one year before he reached the Estella Clinic for Children with Cancer and Blood Diseases. He came from a small town about 400 km or 10 hours car drive away from Manado. After making the diagnosis of JMML, when he was in cachectic condition, he was treated with a simple palliative chemotherapy course: 6 MP orally daily plus cytarabine subcutaneously weekly. He improved significantly, both clinically and in laboratory values. After two months, he came home with his family and had a good quality of life until, in the end, low WBC counts and low platelets led to his death four months after the start of palliative chemotherapy. His home health care was provided by his parents and a local health care provider. At the end of his life, with use of antibiotics and analgetics, he passed away with minimal pain and breathing difficulty. In retrospect, the increases of 20% of 6-MP and cytarabine was maybe not indicated, since his WBC had come down already. Also, a check of his hematological data should have been performed at least before starting the third course of cytostatic drugs in order to prevent neutropenia and sepsis.

Unfortunately, access to pediatric palliative care in low- or middle-income countries is limited and primarily focused on adult patients. Lack of knowledge about the principles of palliative care and misperceptions about palliative care are significant barriers that limit the development of palliative services in low- and middle-income countries [25]. Therefore, providing education and training to clinicians in the pediatric oncology department is one of the initial steps necessary to develop palliative care for pediatric cancer patients. In countries with limited pediatric oncologists, it is important to train primary care pediatricians and family physicians in pediatric palliative care [26].

Consent

A written informed consent to participate in this study was provided by the participant's legal guardian/next of kin.

Authors' Contributions

NY was involved in patient care, drafting the initial manuscript, and project administration, as well as revising the manuscript. SG and MM were involved in the patient's treatment decision as well as reviewing the initial manuscript. AV was involved in the patient care and review and modification of the initial manuscript. All authors have approved the final manuscript submission and have agreed to be accountable for all aspects of the study.

Acknowledgments

The authors thank the patient's family for providing consent and granting permission to draft and publish this case report. The authors acknowledge the medical staff of Estella Clinic for Children with Cancer and Blood Diseases, Manado, Indonesia, who were associated with this patient in the preparation of this manuscript.

References

[1] A. Yoshimi, S. Kojima, and N. Hirano, "Juvenile myelomonocytic leukemia: epidemiology, etiopathogenesis, diagnosis, and management considerations," *Pediatric Drugs*, vol. 12, no. 1, pp. 11–21, 2010.

[2] A. Tefferi and J. W. Vardiman, "Classification and diagnosis of myeloproliferative neoplasms: the 2008 World Health Organization criteria and point-of-care diagnostic algorithms," *Leukemia*, vol. 22, no. 1, pp. 14–22, 2008.

[3] R. J. Chan, T. Cooper, C. P. Kratz, B. Weiss, and M. L. Loh, "Juvenile myelomonocytic leukemia: a report from the 2nd international JMML symposium," *Leukemia Research*, vol. 33, no. 3, pp. 355–362, 2009.

[4] A. Wintering, C. C. Dvorak, E. Stieglitz, and M. L. Loh, "Juvenile myelomonocytic leukemia in the molecular era: a clinician's guide to diagnosis, risk stratification, and treatment," *Blood Advances*, vol. 5, no. 22, pp. 4783–4793, 2021.

[5] C. M. Niemeyer, M. Arico, G. Basso et al., "Chronic myelomonocytic leukemia in childhood: a retrospective analysis of 110 cases European working group on myelodysplastic syndromes in childhood (EWOG-MDS)," *Blood*, vol. 89, no. 10, pp. 3534–3543, 1997.

[6] N. Yoshida, S. Hirabayashi, S. Watanabe et al., "Prognosis of 75 patients with juvenile myelomonocytic leukemia: prospective study by MDS committee in the Japanese society of pediatric hematology," *The Japanese Journal of Clinical Hematology*, vol. 52, no. 12, pp. 1853–1858, 2011.

[7] K. Sakashita, K. Matsuda, and K. Koike, "Diagnosis and treatment of juvenile myelomonocytic leukemia," *Pediatrics International*, vol. 58, no. 8, pp. 681–690, 2016.

[8] M. Yabe, Y. Ohtsuka, K. Watanabe et al., "Transplantation for juvenile myelomonocytic leukemia: a retrospective study of 30 children treated with a regimen of busulfan, fludarabine, and melphalan," *International Journal of Hematology*, vol. 101, no. 2, pp. 184–190, 2015.

[9] C. C. Dvorak and M. L. Loh, "Juvenile myelomonocytic leukemia: molecular pathogenesis informs current approaches to therapy and hematopoietic cell transplantation," *Frontiers in Pediatrics*, vol. 25, 2014.

[10] D. A. Arber, A. Orazi, R. Hasserjian et al., "The 2016 revision to the World Health Organization classification of myeloid neoplasms and acute leukemia," *Blood*, vol. 127, no. 20, pp. 2391–2405, 2016.

[11] F. Locatelli, M. Algeri, P. Merli, and L. Strocchio, "Novel approaches to diagnosis and treatment of juvenile myelomonocytic leukemia," *Expert Review of Hematology*, vol. 11, no. 2, pp. 129–143, 2018.

[12] F. Locatelli, P. Nolke, M. Zecca et al., "Hematopoietic stem cell transplantation (HSCT) in children with juvenile myelomonocytic leukemia (JMML): results of the EWOG-MDS/EBMT trial," *Blood*, vol. 105, no. 1, pp. 410–419, 2005.

[13] E. Bergstraesser, H. Hasle, T. Rogge et al., "Non-hematopoietic stem cell transplantation treatment of juvenile myelomonocytic leukemia: a retrospective analysis and definition of response criteria," *Pediatric Blood and Cancer*, vol. 49, no. 5, pp. 629–633, 2007.

[14] C. M. Niemeyer and C. Kratz, "Juvenile myelomonocytic leukemia," *Current Oncology Reports*, vol. 5, no. 6, pp. 510–515, 2003.

[15] A. K. Gupta, J. P. Meena, A. Chopra, P. Tanwar, and R. Seth, "Juvenile myelomonocytic leukemia-a comprehensive review and recent advances in management," *American Journal of Blood Research*, vol. 11, pp. 1–21, 2021.

[16] H. J. Kang, H. Y. Shin, H. S. Choi, and H. S. Ahn, "Novel regimen for the treatment of juvenile myelomonocytic leukemia (JMML)," *Leukemia Research*, vol. 28, no. 2, pp. 167–170, 2004.

[17] X. Feng, Z. Peng, Y. He et al., "Improvement of survival in JMML by induction regimen of decitabine + cytarabine + fludarabine before hematopoietic stem cell transplantation: study of 33 cases in single center," *Blood*, vol. 134, no. Supplement_1, p. 4267, 2019.

[18] A. Cseh, C. M. Niemeyer, A. Yoshimi et al., "Bridging to transplant with azacitidine in juvenile myelomonocytic leukemia: a retrospective analysis of the EWOG-MDS study group," *Blood*, vol. 125, no. 14, pp. 2311–2313, 2015.

[19] C. M. Niemeyer, C. Flotho, D. B. Lipka et al., "Response to upfront azacitidine in juvenile myelomonocytic leukemia in the AZA-JMML-001 trial," *Blood Advances*, vol. 5, no. 14, 2021.

[20] O. Fabri, J. Horakova, I. Bodova et al., "Diagnosis and treatment of juvenile myelomonocytic leukemia in slovak republic: novel approache," *Neoplasma*, vol. 66, no. 5, pp. 818–824, 2019.

[21] S. K. Hashmi, J. N. Punia, A. N. Marcogliese et al., "Sustained remission with azacitidine monotherapy and an aberrant

precursor B-lymphoblast population in juvenile myelomonocytic leukemia," *Pediatric Blood and Cancer*, vol. 66, no. 10, Article ID e27905, 2019.

[22] I. Furlan, C. Batz, C. Flotho et al., "Intriguing response to azacitidine in a patient with juvenile myelomonocytic leukemia and monosomy 7," *Blood*, vol. 113, no. 12, pp. 2867-2868, 2009.

[23] World Health Organization, *Definitions of Palliative Care*, World Health Organization, Geneva, Switzerland, 2002.

[24] Committee on Hospital Care and Institute for Patient- and Family-Centered Care, "Patient- and family-centered care and the pediatrician's role," *Pediatrics*, vol. 129, no. 2, pp. 394–404, 2012.

[25] C. Feudtner, S. Friebert, J. Jewell et al., "Pediatric palliative care and hospice care commitments, guidelines, and recommendations," *Pediatrics*, vol. 132, no. 5, pp. 966–972, 2013.

[26] M. Doherty and C. Thabet, "Development and implementation of a pediatric palliative care program in a developing country," *Frontiers in Public Health*, vol. 6, p. 106, 2018.

4

Pure Red Cell Aplasia with Del(20q) Sensitive for Immunosuppressive Treatment

Anh Khoi Vo,[1] Hilde Kollsete Gjelberg,[2] Randi Hovland,[3,4] Marte Karen Lindstad Brattås,[5] Øystein Bruserud,[1,6] and Håkon Reikvam[1,6]

[1]*Section Hematology, Department of Medicine, Haukeland University Hospital, Bergen, Norway*
[2]*Department of Pathology, Haukeland University Hospital, Bergen, Norway*
[3]*Department of Medical Genetics, Haukeland University Hospital, Bergen, Norway*
[4]*Department of Biological Sciences, University of Bergen, Bergen, Norway*
[5]*Department of Medicine, Haraldsplass Deaconess Hospital, Bergen, Norway*
[6]*Department of Clinical Science, University of Bergen, Bergen, Norway*

Correspondence should be addressed to Håkon Reikvam; hakon.reikvam@med.uib.no

Academic Editor: Yusuke Shiozawa

Pure red cell aplasia (PRCA) is a rare syndrome that only affects the erythroid lineage. It is defined by a normocytic, normochromic anemia with a marked reticulocytopenia and severe reduction or absence of erythroid precursors in the bone marrow. Treatment of primary, idiopathic PRCA is immunosuppressive therapy. Although it is rare, isolated cytogenetic abnormalities can be seen in PRCA, and abnormal karyotype is associated with poor response to immunosuppressive therapy and poor prognosis. We describe a 77-year-old male with primary, idiopathic PRCA and a deletion of chromosome 20q, del(20q), in the bone marrow cells. He was successfully treated with immunosuppressive therapy and became transfusion-independent. The same cytogenetic abnormality has also been described in a few other reports; taken together, these observations suggest that del(20q) may represent a recurrent cytogenetic abnormality in PRCA. Our case report clearly illustrates that even patients with primary PRCA and an abnormal karyotype can respond to immunosuppression and become transfusion-independent.

1. Introduction

Pure red cell aplasia (PRCA) is a rare syndrome that solely affects erythroid lineage. It is defined by a normocytic, normochromic anemia with a marked reticulocytopenia and severe reduction or absence of erythroid precursors from the bone marrow [1, 2]. The disease is classified into congenital (also known as Diamond-Blackfan anemia) and acquired PRCA. The acquired form is usually an acute and self-limiting disease that mainly occurs in children, whereas the chronic variant is most common in adults. Although acquired PRCA in adults may present as a primary, idiopathic disease, it can also be secondary to other underlying conditions.

The primary form of PRCA is considered to be an autoimmune disease with immune-mediated inhibition of the differentiation and maturation of erythroid precursors [1–3]. On the contrary, secondary PRCA can be associated with various disorders including lymphoproliferative disorders (e.g., leukemia, Hodgkin's and non-Hodgkin's lymphoma, and thymoma), solid tumors, viral infections (e.g., parvovirus B19 infections), other autoimmune disorders, and certain pharmacologic agents [1, 2]. Although usually not considered to be a preleukemic condition [2], it may be a prodrome to myelodysplastic syndrome (MDS) [4, 5]. Several case reports have described a number of recurring cytogenetic aberrations, e.g., isolated i(17q) and del(5q); most of these cases are patients with MDS with PRCA(5). Isolated del(20q) has also been reported in cases of both PRCA with MDS and primary, idiopathic PRCA [4, 6]. Taken together, these previous reports indicate a potential association between PRCA and certain cytogenetic abnormalities. Here, we describe a case of PRCA with an isolated del(20q) with no evidence for any concomitant hematologic disorders.

2. Case Presentation

A 77-year-old man was undergoing follow-up at his primary hospital due to chronic kidney disease stage 4. In addition, he had abnormal levels of liver and pancreas serum markers of unknown etiology. His medical history included hypertension, hypercholesterolemia, Barrett's esophagus, and stenting of the left carotid artery due to a transient ischemic attack. During routine follow-up, blood tests revealed a progressive normocytic, normochromic anemia. The patient did not respond to the initial treatment with iron supplements and erythropoietin injections. There was a gradual progression until the blood tests showed hemoglobin (Hb) 6.0 g/dL (normal range: 13.4–17.0), mean corpuscular volume (MCV) 101 fL (82–98), reticulocytes $<0.010 \times 10^{12}$/L (0.03–0.1), thrombocytes 445×10^9/L (145–348), and total leukocytes 6.8×10^9/L (3.5–11.0). The peripheral blood differential count showed neutrophils, 4.8×10^9/L (1.7–8.2), lymphocytes, 0.9×10^9/L (0.7–5.3), monocytes, 0.7×10^9/L (0.04–1.30), eosinophils, 0.4×10^9/L (0.0–0.7), and basophils, $<0.1 \times 10^9$/L (0.0–0.3). Thus, the patient had a normocytic, normochromic anemia with low reticulocyte counts but no evidence for a general bone marrow failure.

A bone marrow biopsy showed total absence of erythropoiesis with normal megakaryocytes and normal granulocytopoiesis with large amounts of iron in the bone marrow (Figure 1). This was also confirmed by cytomorphology of the bone marrow aspirate, demonstrating total absence of erythropoiesis, without signs of dysplasia in the granulocytopoiesis or megakaryocytopoiesis (Figure 2). No definitive signs of dysplasia were detected. Thus, absence of erythropoiesis was the only abnormality demonstrated by the bone marrow examination, and the patient was treated with regular erythrocyte transfusions.

Further investigations included serological tests for B19 parvovirus, Epstein–Barr virus (EBV), cytomegalovirus (CMV), hepatitis A, hepatitis B, hepatitis C, and human immunodeficiency virus (HIV), but there was no evidence for any of these infections being the cause of the hematological disease. A computed tomography (CT) scan of the chest showed no signs of thymoma, and flowcytometric analyses of the bone marrow did not detect any evidence for monoclonal B-cell or T-cell populations. Karyotyping of bone marrow cells revealed a deletion at the long arm of chromosome 20 and the karyotype 46,XY,del(20) (q11)[6]/46,XY[14] (Figure 3).

The findings justified the diagnosis of PRCA with the chromosomal abnormality del(20q). Previous studies suggest treatment with cyclosporine A to be superior to corticosteroids and cyclophosphamide with regard to response rate and relapse-free survival [1, 7]. This was not the preferred choice of treatment in the present case due to the patient's chronic kidney disease and the risk of nephrotoxicity. Oral prednisolone was therefore initiated with a dosage of 1 mg/kg/day in addition to regular erythrocyte transfusions (Figure 4). The patient responded to the steroid treatment; increasing peripheral blood reticulocyte counts were observed after two weeks, and after three weeks of treatment, the patient was transfusion-independent with stable hemoglobin levels corresponding to 10-11 g/dL. Initially, no major side effects of the steroid treatment were reported.

Tapering of corticosteroids was initiated after six weeks and was initially without any complications (Figure 4). Hemoglobin levels remained stable, although the reticulocyte counts decreased at a later point. After discontinuation of corticosteroids (Figure 4), the patient suffered a relapse and treatment was reinitiated but with a lower prednisolone starting a dose of 30 mg/day. He responded to this treatment, and the dose was slowly tapered over months until he could continue with a maintenance dose of prednisolone 7.5 mg daily. During this period, he had a stable hemoglobin level above 10 g/dL. However, the patient had a second relapse and was hospitalized for erythrocyte transfusions. A new bone marrow aspiration demonstrated normal granulocytopoiesis, normal megakaryocytes, and total absence of erythropoiesis, coinciding with the initial findings. Mutational analysis of the bone marrow with the Truesight Myeloid Sequencing Panel (Illumina®) did not reveal mutations and strengthened the suspicion of a nonclonal myeloid disorder. Hence, PRCA remained the most likely diagnosis. The patient had then used oral prednisolone for 16 months, and as the response to steroid treatment was assumed to decline and given the potential serious side effects of long term steroid treatment, we changed the immunosuppressive treatment to cyclosporine A with tapering of steroid treatment. He ultimately received cyclosporine A at a dose of 200 mg/day with careful monitoring of his kidney and liver functions. His reticulocyte count and hemoglobin level was rapidly increasing (Figure 4).

3. Discussion

In this case report, we present a PRCA patient with a deletion of chromosome 20q in the bone marrow cells, and no evidence was found for concomitant hematologic disorders or other disorders commonly associated with PRCA (e.g., viral infections and solid tumors) [1, 2]. The diagnosis was based on peripheral blood and bone marrow examination, immunohistochemistry, and G-banding analysis of bone marrow cells.

Although the associations with other conditions and differences in the responsiveness to various therapeutic strategies suggest a diverse pathophysiology of PRCA [1, 7, 8], the role of cytogenetic abnormalities in the pathogenesis of PRCA remains unknown. A small number of studies have reported PRCA patients with isolated cytogenetic abnormalities; most of these patients had PRCA together with other hematologic disorders. Inui et al. reported a case of isolated isochromosome i(17)q in MDS with PRCA; two similar cases had been reported earlier, and these findings suggest that i(17)q is a recurrent cytogenetic abnormality in MDS with PRCA. Another possible recurring abnormality described in MDS with PRCA is del(5q). Park

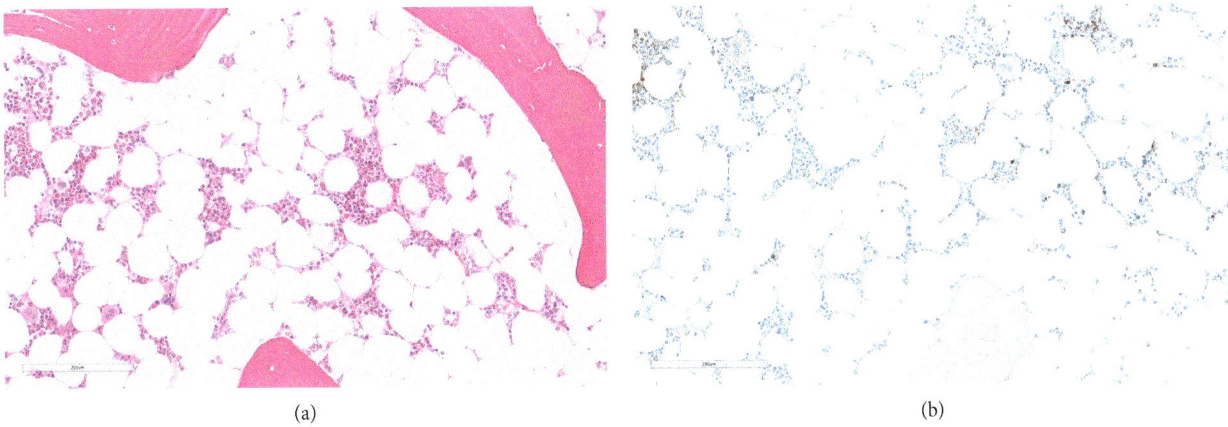

FIGURE 1: Histopathological features of the bone marrow in PRCA. (a) The bone marrow core biopsy section shows a slightly hypocellular marrow with intact granulocytic and megakaryocytic cells but the absence of erythroid colonies (hematoxylin and eosin, scale bar: 200 μm). (b) Immunoperoxidase staining for hemoglobin A highlights only scattered positive cells (dark brown) with no colony formation (scale bar: 200 μm). Most of the brownish appearing cells represent iron-laden macrophages.

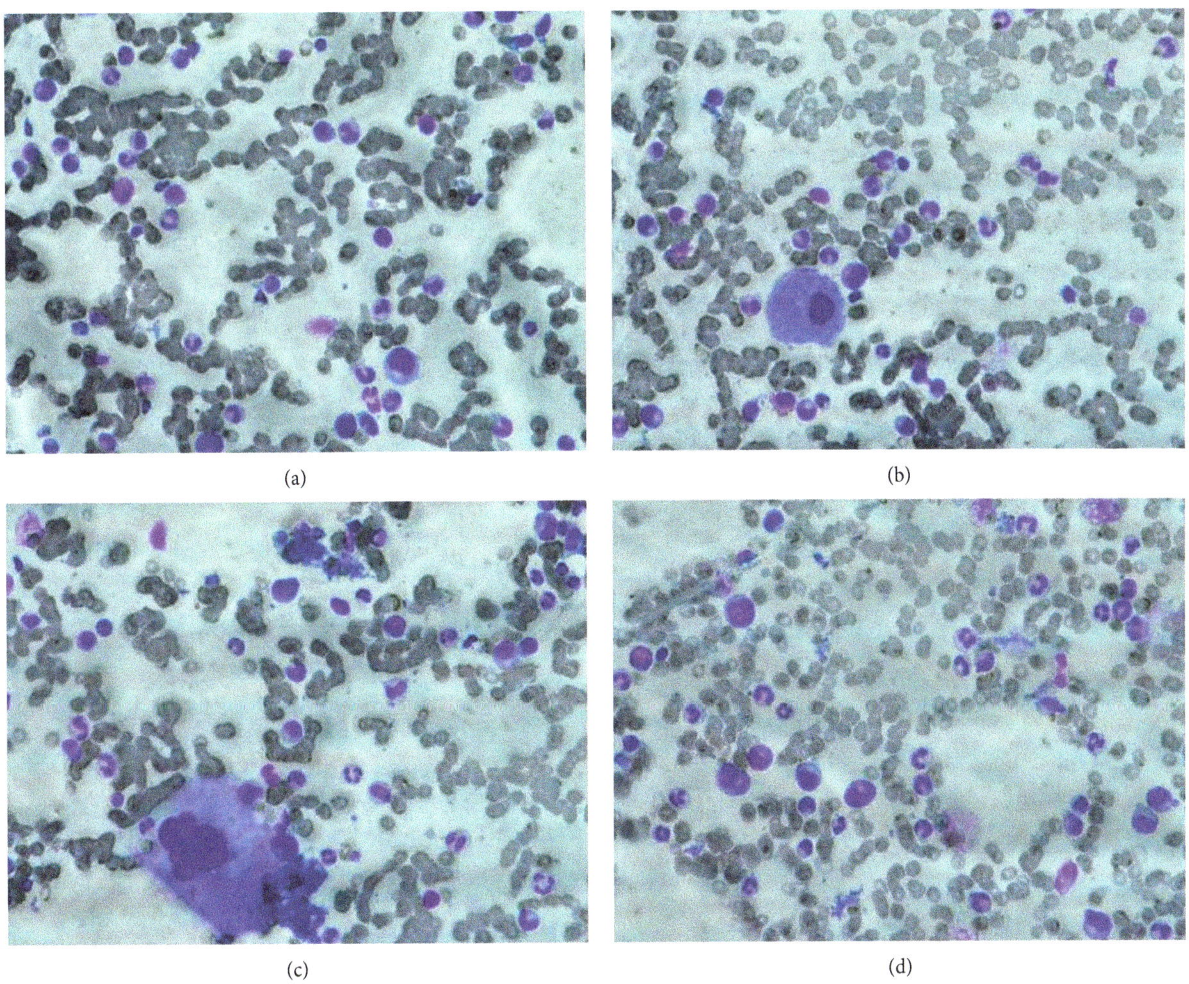

FIGURE 2: Cytomorphology of the bone marrow aspirate. Bone marrow aspirate at the time of diagnosis was stained with May-Grunwald-Giemsa (MGG). The smear confirmed the total absence of erythropoiesis, without signs of dysplasia in granulocytopoiesis or megakaryocytopoiesis. Four different areas are demonstrated in the figure.

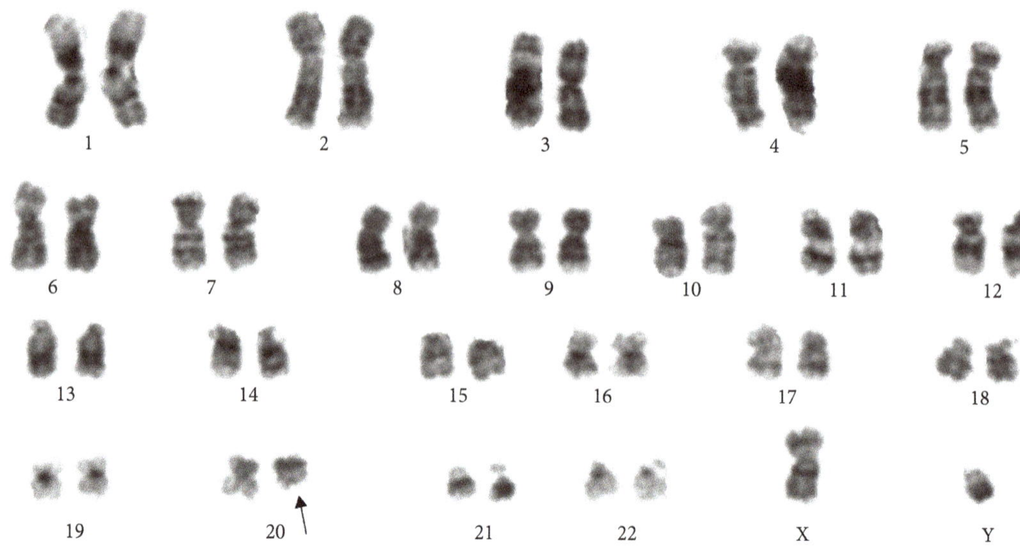

FIGURE 3: Karyotyping of bone marrow cells using G-banding. G-banding analysis after unstimulated culture of bone marrow showed the karyotype 46,XY del(20)(q11.2).

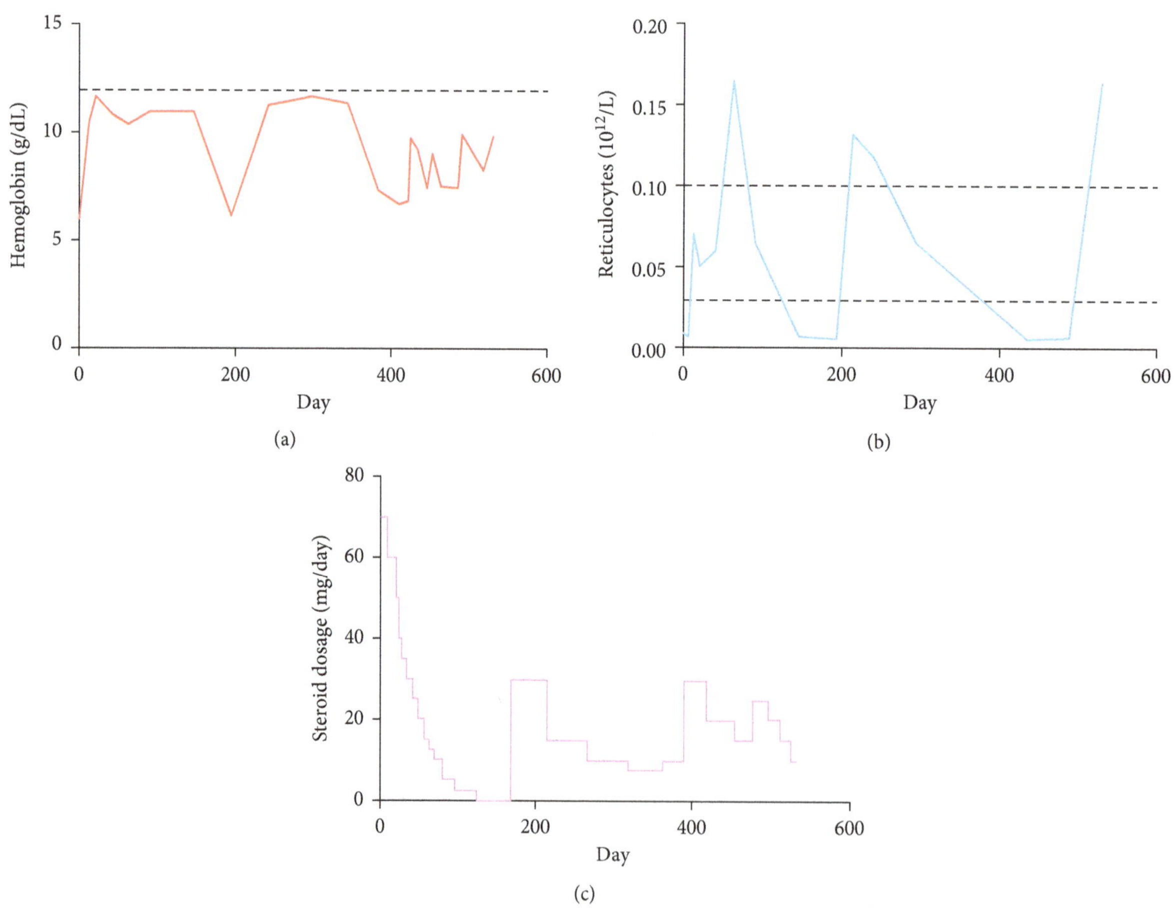

FIGURE 4: The response to immunosuppressive treatment. The figure shows the levels of hemoglobin (a) and reticulocytes (b) in peripheral blood after initiation of corticosteroid therapy. The corticosteroid treatment was gradually tapered (c). Days on the X-axis indicate days after initial diagnosis. The stippled horizontal lines indicate the normal range for hemoglobin and reticulocytes.

et al. reported del(5q) in four of six patients with MDS with PRCA [9]. This abnormality is commonly seen in the context of MDS alone [5, 10, 11]. These MDS patients frequently show erythroid hypoplasia, i.e., a marked decrease and maturation arrest of erythroid precursors; such hypoplasia is uncommon in MDS and has been proposed to represent a distinct entity referred to as MDS with PRCA [4, 9, 12]. The present patient had no cytopenias in other lines, and he had no mutations in the most common genes associated with MDS. The diagnosis of MDS or development of frank MDS hence seems unlikely, strengthening the diagnosis of PRCA.

Our patient had an isolated deletion of chromosome 20q which has only been reported in a few cases of PRCA. Kurtin et al. reported two such PRCA cases with no other hematologic disorders, and they postulated an association between this karyotypic abnormality and PRCA [6]. Wang et al. [4] reported two PRCA patients with this abnormality together with MDS. Lacy et al. [11] also reported a PRCA patient with del(20q), but it is not clear whether this patient had any additional hematologic disorders.

The del(20q) abnormality is associated with dyserythropoiesis and dysmegakaryocytopoiesis and is thought to represent an early aberration in hematologic malignancies due to the loss of the *L3MBTL1* polycomb tumor suppressor protein; this has been shown to cause replicative stress and genomic instability *in vitro* [6, 10, 13]. Knockdown of *L3MBTL1* represses human-induced pluripotent stem cells (iPSCs) for hematopoietic differentiation and enhances commitment toward the erythroid lineage [14]. Del(20q) is more common in various myeloid disorders [6, 13, 15] and in the rare Shwachman–Diamond syndrome [16], whereas it is uncommon in aplastic anemia (AA) [17]. However, its role in the development of these disorders are yet to be further clarified. In a study with patients who acquired isolated del(20q) after cytotoxic therapy, approximately two-thirds did not develop therapy-related myeloid neoplasms. The subset of patients who developed therapy-related myeloid neoplasms often presented with del(20q) in a higher percentage of metaphases, terminal deletion rather than interstitial, and a longer persisting deletion [18]. The abnormality has been more extensively studied in MDS where it is associated with a favorable prognosis when no other cytogenetic abnormalities are present [19]. Besides *L3MBTL1*, it is not known which of the lost genes are involved in the development of MDS and other myeloid disorders [20]. At the time of diagnosis and after several relapses, our patient did not have any evidence for MDS or any other myeloid disorders, though it should be emphasized that some reports have suggested that PRCA might be a pre-MDS disorder [1, 4, 12, 21, 22].

PRCA is a very diverse and rare disease with no standardized therapeutic strategy. The treatment is mainly based on experience and case reports [8]. The first-choice treatment for primary, idiopathic PRCA is immunosuppressive therapy. Corticosteroids are usually preferred [1, 7, 23], and the reported response rates are 27–62%, but the relapse rate is substantial [1, 7, 11, 23]. Cyclosporine A has also been reported to be effective with a response rate of 65–87% [7], but the experience with this drug is more limited, and there are uncertainties regarding relapse rate. Maintenance therapy is required to prevent relapse for most patients. In spite of this, cyclosporine A is currently considered to be the first line of treatment granted among the patients who does not present with contraindications [7, 8, 24]. It has also been reported to be effective in patients with refractory PRCA [3]. In the present case, corticosteroid therapy was chosen due to chronic kidney disease of unknown etiology. Corticosteroid therapy also has a high rate of second remission in relapsed patients [25] and was successful in our patient even though it was reinitiated at a lower dose. However, immunosuppressive therapy generally seems to be less effective in relapsed PRCA compared with treatment naïve PRCA [26], and patients may develop refractory PRCA [3].

Monoclonal antibodies such as alemtuzumab and rituximab are other alternatives commonly used for patients with refractory PRCA. Varying results have been reported for these drugs [24, 27, 28], possibly due to the pathophysiological heterogeneity of PRCA with the majority of the idiopathic cases being T-cell-mediated, while cases responsive to rituximab may represent B-cell-mediated etiology [8].

PRCA with abnormal karyotype seems to be associated with poor response to immunosuppressive therapy and consequently poor prognosis. Lacy et al. [11] reported three patients with abnormalities involving chromosome 5 and one with del(20q), none of which responded to immunosuppressive treatment. Similar observations have been made by others [29, 30]. This lack of responsiveness possibly reflects the heterogeneity of PRCA patients with regard to the pathogenesis. In contrast to previous reports, our patient responded to two modalities of immunosuppression even after several relapses. However, there are few studies on idiopathic PRCA with isolated cytogenetic abnormalities, and our present case emphasizes the need for further studies to further elucidate the role of del(20q) in PRCA. Our case report clearly shows that response to immunosuppression is possible also for PRCA patients with cytogenetic abnormalities.

4. Conlusion

To conclude, PRCA is a rare disease, and cytogenetic abnormalities are detected for a subset of these patients. The role of such abnormalities in the pathogenesis of PRCA remains elusive. However, even patients with cytogenetic abnormalities may respond to immunosuppressive treatment and become transfusion-independent. For this reason, detection of an abnormal karyotype should not exclude immunosuppression as the first-line treatment.

Consent

The provided information is deidentified, and no health protected information is shared on this publication. Written consent was provided by the patient.

Acknowledgments

The study was supported by Helse Vest.

References

[1] R. T. Means, "Pure red cell aplasia," *Blood*, vol. 128, no. 21, pp. 2504–2509, 2016.

[2] P. Fisch, R. Handgretinger, and H. E. Schaefer, "Pure red cell aplasia," *British Journal of Haematology*, vol. 111, no. 4, pp. 1010–1022, 2000.

[3] R. T. Means Jr., E. N. Dessypris, and S. B. Krantz, "Treatment of refractory pure red cell aplasia with cyclosporine A: disappearance of IgG inhibitor associated with clinical response," *British Journal of Haematology*, vol. 78, no. 1, pp. 114–119, 1991.

[4] S. A. Wang, G. Yue, L. Hutchinson et al., "Myelodysplastic syndrome with pure red cell aplasia shows characteristic clinicopathological features and clonal T-cell expansion," *British Journal of Haematology*, vol. 138, no. 2, pp. 271–275, 2007.

[5] Y. Inui, K. Yamamoto, A. Okamura et al., "Isolated isochromosome 17q in myelodysplastic syndromes with pure red cell aplasia and basophilia," *Internal Medicine*, vol. 51, no. 12, pp. 1579–1584, 2012.

[6] P. J. Kurtin, G. W. Dewald, D. J. Shields, and C. A. Hanson, "Hematologic disorders associated with deletions of chromosome 20q: a clinicopathologic study of 107 patients," *American Journal of Clinical Pathology*, vol. 106, no. 5, pp. 680–688, 1996.

[7] K. Sawada, N. Fujishima, and M. Hirokawa, "Acquired pure red cell aplasia: updated review of treatment," *British Journal of Haematology*, vol. 142, no. 4, pp. 505–514, 2008.

[8] S. K. Balasubramanian, M. Sadaps, S. Thota et al., "Rational management approach to pure red cell aplasia," *Haematologica*, vol. 103, no. 2, pp. 221–230, 2018.

[9] S. Park, A. Merlat, M. Guesnu et al., "Pure red cell aplasia associated with myelodysplastic syndromes," *Leukemia*, vol. 14, no. 9, pp. 1709-1710, 2000.

[10] M. F. Zahid, U. A. Malik, M. Sohail, I. N. Hassan, S. Ali, and M. H. S. Shaukat, "Cytogenetic abnormalities in myelodysplastic syndromes: an overview," *International Journal of Hematology-Oncology and Stem Cell Research*, vol. 11, no. 3, pp. 231–239, 2017.

[11] M. Q. Lacy, P. J. Kurtin, and A. Tefferi, "Pure red cell aplasia: association with large granular lymphocyte leukemia and the prognostic value of cytogenetic abnormalities," *Blood*, vol. 87, no. 7, pp. 3000–3006, 1996.

[12] J. García-Suárez, T. Pascual, M. A. Muñoz, B. Herrero, and A. Pardo, "Myelodysplastic syndrome with erythroid hypoplasia/aplasia: a case report and review of the literature," *American Journal of Hematology*, vol. 58, no. 4, pp. 319–325, 1998.

[13] R. P. Hasserjian and P. Dal Cin, "Deletion of chromosome 20q: friend or foe?" *Leukemia Research*, vol. 35, no. 7, pp. 844-845, 2011.

[14] F. Perna, L. P. Vu, M. Themeli et al., "The polycomb group protein L3MBTL1 represses a SMAD5-mediated hematopoietic transcriptional program in human pluripotent stem cells," *Stem Cell Reports*, vol. 4, no. 4, pp. 658–669, 2015.

[15] J. Grinfeld, J. Nangalia, E. J. Baxter et al., "Classification and personalized prognosis in myeloproliferative neoplasms," *New England Journal of Medicine*, vol. 379, no. 15, pp. 1416–1430, 2018.

[16] R. Valli, A. Minelli, M. Galbiati et al., "Shwachman-diamond syndrome with clonal interstitial deletion of the long arm of chromosome 20 in bone marrow: haematological features, prognosis and genomic instability," *British Journal of Haematology*, vol. 184, no. 6, pp. 974–981, 2019.

[17] J. P. Maciejewski, A. Risitano, E. M. Sloand, O. Nunez, and N. S. Young, "Distinct clinical outcomes for cytogenetic abnormalities evolving from aplastic anemia," *Blood*, vol. 99, no. 9, pp. 3129–3135, 2002.

[18] C. C. Yin, J. Peng, Y. Li et al., "Clinical significance of newly emerged isolated del(20q) in patients following cytotoxic therapies," *Modern Pathology*, vol. 28, no. 8, pp. 1014–1022, 2015.

[19] J. Schanz, H. Tüchler, F. Solé et al., "New comprehensive cytogenetic scoring system for primary myelodysplastic syndromes (MDS) and oligoblastic acute myeloid leukemia after MDS derived from an international database merge," *Journal of Clinical Oncology*, vol. 30, no. 8, pp. 820–829, 2012.

[20] J. Huh, R. V. Tiu, L. P. Gondek et al., "Characterization of chromosome arm 20q abnormalities in myeloid malignancies using genome-wide single nucleotide polymorphism array analysis," *Genes, Chromosomes and Cancer*, vol. 49, no. 9, pp. 390–399, 2010.

[21] P. J. Williamson, D. G. Oscier, A. J. Bell, and T. J. Hamblin, "Red cell aplasia in myelodysplastic syndrome," *Journal of Clinical Pathology*, vol. 44, no. 5, pp. 431-432, 1991.

[22] H. D. Kim, K. W. Kim, S. Y. Park et al., "Myelodysplastic syndrome with erythroid aplasia following pure red cell aplasia," *The Korean Journal of Internal Medicine*, vol. 19, no. 3, pp. 193–195, 2004.

[23] R. J. Charles, K. M. Sabo, P. G. Kidd, and J. L. Abkowitz, "The pathophysiology of pure red cell aplasia: implications for therapy," *Blood*, vol. 87, no. 11, pp. 4831–4838, 1996.

[24] Z. Long, F. Yu, Y. Du et al., "Successful treatment of refractory/relapsed acquired pure red cell aplasia with sirolimus," *Annals of Hematology*, vol. 97, no. 11, pp. 2047–2054, 2018.

[25] D. A. Clark, E. N. Dessypris, and S. B. Krantz, "Studies on pure red cell aplasia. XI. Results of immunosuppressive treatment of 37 patients," *Blood*, vol. 63, no. 2, pp. 277–286, 1984.

[26] M. Hirokawa, K. Sawada, N. Fujishima et al., "Long-term outcome of patients with acquired chronic pure red cell aplasia (PRCA) following immunosuppressive therapy: a final report of the nationwide cohort study in 2004/2006 by the Japan PRCA collaborative study group," *British Journal of Haematology*, vol. 169, no. 6, pp. 879–886, 2015.

[27] H. W. Auner, A. Wolfler, C. Beham-Schmid, D. Strunk, W. Linkesch, and H. Sill, "Restoration of erythropoiesis by rituximab in an adult patient with primary acquired pure red cell aplasia refractory to conventional treatment," *British Journal of Haematology*, vol. 116, no. 3, pp. 727-728, 2002.

[28] M. Dungarwalla, J. C. W. Marsh, J. A. Tooze et al., "Lack of clinical efficacy of rituximab in the treatment of autoimmune neutropenia and pure red cell aplasia: implications for their pathophysiology," *Annals of Hematology*, vol. 86, no. 3, pp. 191-197, 2007.

[29] P. H. Fitzgerald and J. W. Hamer, "Primary acquired red cell hypoplasia associated with a clonal chromosomal abnormality and disturbed erythroid proliferation," *Blood*, vol. 38, no. 3, pp. 325–335, 1971.

[30] E. N. Dessypris, A. Fogo, M. Russell, E. Engel, and S. B. Krantz, "Studies on pure red cell aplasia. X. Association with acute leukemia and significance of bone marrow karyotype abnormalities," *Blood*, vol. 56, no. 3, pp. 421–426, 1980.

5

Successful Treatment of Pediatric Refractory/Relapsed AML with KIR-Ligand-Mismatched Cord Blood Transplant after FLAG-IDA Reinduction Therapy with or without the GO Regimen

Daisuke Toyama, Ryosuke Matsuno, Yumiko Sugishita, Ryota Kaneko, Naoko Okamoto, Masaya Koganesawa, Sachio Fujita, Kosuke Akiyama, Keiichi Isoyama, and Shohei Yamamoto

Department of Pediatrics, Showa University Fujigaoka Hospital, Yokohama, Japan

Correspondence should be addressed to Shohei Yamamoto; shohei-y@med.showa-u.ac.jp

Academic Editor: Chihaya Imai

Prognosis in pediatric patients with refractory/relapsed acute myeloid leukemia (AML) is grim, and there is no standard treatment for such patients. Combined treatment with intensive chemotherapy and gemtuzumab ozogamicin (GO), a monoclonal anti-CD33 antibody conjugated with calicheamicin, is useful as reinduction therapy in refractory/relapsed AML. Here, we describe three cases of pediatric refractory/relapsed AML that were successfully managed with FLAG-IDA (fludarabine, cytarabine, granulocyte colony-stimulating factor, and idarubicin), with or without GO, as reinduction therapy before a KIR-ligand-mismatched cord blood transplant. This strategy relies on the fact that killer cell immunoglobulin-like receptors (KIR) on cord blood natural killer (NK) cells recognize human leukocyte antigen (HLA) class I alleles, and that donor KIR-ligand incompatibility may be associated with lower incidence of relapse and improved survival in AML, as cells that lack these inhibitory HLA ligands can activate NK cells. All three patients are currently alive and have been disease-free for 24–65 months, although one patient developed severe sinusoidal obstructive syndrome (SOS). Thus, our strategy can result in excellent outcomes in pediatric patients with refractory/relapsed AML.

1. Introduction

Outcomes in children with refractory/relapsed acute myeloid leukemia (AML) are extremely poor [1]. Fludarabine, cytarabine, granulocyte colony-stimulating factor (G-CSF), and idarubicin (FLAG-IDA) is a commonly used reinduction regimen in AML patients [2], and FLAG-IDA combined with gemtuzumab ozogamicin (GO) is a feasible reinduction regimen for relapsed AML [3, 4]. Killer cell immunoglobulin-like receptor (KIR)-ligand incompatibility is thought to be associated with reduced incidence of relapse and better leukemia-free survival [5, 6] because clinically beneficial graft versus leukemia effects might be mediated by donor-recipient inhibitory KIR-mismatched natural killer (NK) cells [7]. Here, we describe the cases of three patients with pediatric refractory/relapsed AML who were treated using the FLAG-IDAregimen, with or without GO, as a reinduction therapy before KIR-ligand-mismatched cord blood transplant (KIR-CBT).

2. Case Presentations

Between April 2011 and December 2015, one male and two female pediatric patients with relapsed or refractory AML were treated with one course of FLAG-IDA, with or without GO, after which they underwent KIR-CBT. Patient characteristics are listed in Table 1. All three patients displayed one or more poor prognostic factors, as identified by previous studies [1, 8]. One patient (case 1) suffered from refractory (induction failure) AML, while the other two (cases 2 and 3) had relapsed AML. Among the 2 cases of relapsed AML, case 2 underwent HSCT after the first

Table 1: Characteristics of the three patients with pediatric refractory/relapsed acute myeloid leukemia.

	Case 1	Case 2	Case 3
Age of induction failure or relapse/gender	2 years/female	18 years/female	13 years/male
Diagnosis (FAB classification)	M2	M0	M2
CD33 expression level (%)	90	18	84
Karyotype	46, XX	46, XX. Del (5)	46, XY
FLT3-ITD	None	None	None
Disease status	Induction failure	1st relapse	1st relapse
Poor prognostic factor(s)			
Induction failure	Yes	No	No
Age >10 years at relapse	No	Yes	Yes
Early relapse (1 year from diagnosis)	—	No	Yes (11 months)
HSCT at 1st CR	No	Yes	No
Adverse cytogenetics	No	Yes	No

FAB, French-British-American classification; HSCT, hematopoietic stem-cell transplantation; 1 CR, first complete remission; 2 CR, second complete remission, FLAG, fludarabine, cytarabine, granulocyte colony-stimulating factor; IDA, idarubicin; GO, gemtuzumab ozogamicin.

Table 2: Characteristics of KIR-CBT in the three patients.

	Case 1	Case 2	Case 3
Disease status at HSCT	1 CR	2 CR	2 CR
Interval between GO and HSCT (days)	36	—	56
Conditioning	TBI + CY	LPAM + Flu + TBI2Gy	TBI + CY
Donor source	UR-CB	UR-CB	UR-CB
HLA match (DNA typing)	5/8 (B, C, DR)	5/8 (B, C)	5/8 (B, C, DR)
HLA-C			
Patient	C08 : 01/12 : 03 (C1/C1)	C03 : 04/14 : 02 (C1/C1)	C03 : 03/07 : 02 (C1/C1)
Donor	C08 : 01/04 : 01 (C1/C2)	C01 : 02/04 : 01 (C1/C2)	C04 : 01/07 : 02 (C1/C2)
KIR-HLA			
GVH direction mismatch	KIR2DL1 (inhibitory KIR)	KIR2DL1 (inhibitory KIR)	KIR2DL1 (inhibitory KIR)
NCC ($\times 10^7$/kg)	6.1	3.2	2
Engraftment (Neutro $> 0.5 \times 10^9$/L)	Day 36	Day 32	Day 30
SOS prophylaxis	Ursodeoxycholic acid + LMWH	Ursodeoxycholic acid + LMWH + rTM	Ursodeoxycholic acid + LMWH + rTM
SOS	Very severe	—	—
GVHD			
GVHD prophylaxis	Tacrolimus + MTX	Tacrolimus + MTX	Tacrolimus + MTX
aGVHD	Grade I (skin: stage 2)	—	Grade III (skin: stage 3, gut: stage 3)
cGVHD	Limited (skin)	—	—
Treatment of aGVHD	PSL	—	PSL
Infection	—	CMV viremia	—
Prognosis	Alive (65 months)	Alive (34 months)	Alive (24 months)

KIR-CBT, KIR-ligand-mismatched cord blood transplant; HSCT, hematopoietic stem-cell transplantation; GO, gemtuzumab ozogamicin; HLA, human leukocyte antigen; GVH, graft-versus-host; NCC, nucleated cord blood cells; SOS, sinusoidal obstruction syndrome; GVHD, graft-versus-host disease; aGVHD, acute GVHD, cGVHD, chronic GVHD; CR, complete remission; TBI, total body irradiation; CY, cyclophosphamide; LPAM, melphalan; Flu, fludarabine; UR, unrelated; CB, cord blood; rTM, recombinant human soluble thrombomodulin: LMWH, low-molecular-weight heparin; tacrolimus; MTX, methotrexate; PSL, prednisolone; CMV, cytogenesis virus.

complete remission (1 CR) because she had a high-risk karyotype (5q-), while case 3 suffered an early relapse. Cases 1 and 3 were administered FLAG-IDA with GO as reinduction therapy prior to KIR-CBT, while case 2 was given only FLAG-IDA as only 18% of her leukemic cells expressed CD33. The FLAG-IDA protocol comprised 30 mg/m^2 fludarabine and 2 g/m^2 cytarabine on days 2–6, 10 mg/m^2 idarubicin on day 6, and 300 μg/m^2 G-CSF on days 1–6. GO was administered at a dose of 3 mg/m^2 on day 7 of treatment, and its use was approved by the institutional review board of the Showa University Fujigaoka Hospital, Japan. All cases achieved CR after reinduction therapy (Table 1) and promptly underwent KIR-CBT (Table 2). KIR-ligand mismatching was defined based on KIR-ligand incompatibility, as initially described by Leung [9]. All three patient-donor pairs were KIR-ligand-incompatible in the graft-versus-host (GVH) direction and were all donor-mismatched for KIR2DL1 with HLA-C missing from the recipient. Cases 1 and 3 received full-intensity conditioning cyclophosphamide (120 mg/kg) and total body irradiation (TBI: 12 Gy), while case 2 received melphalan (140 mg/m^2), fludarabine (125 mg/m^2), and TBI (2 Gy), as this was her 2nd HSCT. Anti-thymocyte globulin (ATG) was not used in any of the patients, and tacrolimus (0.02 mg/kg/day) and short-term methotrexate were used for prophylaxis against graft-versus-host disease (GVHD). Ursodeoxycholic acid (UDCA) and low-molecular-weight heparin (LMWH) were administered for prophylaxis against sinusoidal obstruction syndrome (SOS) in case 1, while cases 2 and 3 received prophylactic recombinant human soluble thrombomodulin (rTM; 380 U/kg per day for 7 days from days 7 to 13), in addition to UDCA and LMWH [10]. All three cases underwent KIR-CBT within 2 months of reinduction therapy. In case 1, extremely severe SOS developed on day 8 which was treated with rTM; however, this was ineffective, and continuous hemodiafiltration was initiated to maintain hydration and remove any inflammatory cytokines. This resulted in a gradual improvement in her SOS by day 20. Additionally, Grade I acute GVHD (stage 2 skin rash) and limited chronic GVHD (affecting the skin alone) developed in this patient, which were successfully treated with prednisolone (PSL). Tacrolimus was suspended at 9 months after KIR-CBT. In cases 2 and 3, prophylactic rTM was successful and they did not develop SOS. In case 2, no acute or chronic GVHD occurred, and the administration of tacrolimus was stopped at 5 months after KIR-CBT. In case 3, grade III acute GVHD (stage 3 skin rash and stage 3 diarrhea) developed, and it responded well to PSL treatment. Chronic GVHD did not occur in this patient, and the administration of tacrolimus was stopped at 5 months after KIR-CBT. All three patients are currently alive without any evidence of relapse at 24–65 months after KIR-CBT.

3. Discussion

Prognosis in pediatric patients with refractory/relapsed AML is poor at best and known prognostic factors for poor survival include early relapse, undergoing HSCT during 1 CR, age of >10 years at relapse, and adverse cytogenetics [1]. Since April 2011, our strategy for treating patients with refractory or relapsed AML having poor prognostic factors has been one course of FLAG-IDA, with or without GO, followed by KIR-CBT. This strategy has two major implications for the treatment of pediatric patients with refractory/relapsed AML, especially those with poor prognostic factors. First, the FLAG-IDA regimen, with or without GO, might be a feasible reinduction therapy. This is because, among pediatric patients with relapsed AML, those who do not achieve 2 CR exhibit significantly lower 5-year OS rate than the patients who achieve 2 CR [1, 8]. A European study group has reported that FLAG, with or without an anthracycline, can induce 2 CR in 78% of the cases, which is an excellent rate of induction [1]. GO, a monoclonal anti-CD33 antibody conjugated with calicheamicin, has been shown to be effective in relapsed AML [11], and FLAG-IDA, combined with low-dose GO (3 mg/m^2), is a feasible induction therapy option in younger patients with primary AML [3, 4]. All three of our patients also achieved CR after being treated with FLAG-IDA, with or without GO. Second, we used KIR-CBT (a type of HSCT) in pediatric refractory/relapsed AML patients with poor prognostic factors because of the following rationale. NK cells express inhibitory KIR on their surface, and NK cell alloreactivity after allogeneic transplantation is determined by the specificity of the KIR on the donor NK cells for the recipient's MHC (major histocompatibility complex) class I antigens [12]. Ruggeri et al. were the first to report good clinical results, i.e., no relapse, rejection, or acute GVHD in AML patients who underwent HLA-mismatched transplantation involving KIR-ligand incompatibility in the GVH direction [5]. In a study wherein approximately 80% of the patients were administered ATG, Willemze et al. have reported that KIR-ligand incompatibility had a beneficial effect on outcomes after CBT [13]. In contrast, in a study in which only 30% of the patients were administered ATG, Brunstein et al. have reported that KIR-ligand incompatibility had no effect on outcomes after CBT [14]. It is possible that in vivo T-cell depletion, secondary to ATG administration, contributed to the posttransplant expansion of functional NK cells which then favored alloreactivity in the presence of KIR-ligand mismatching. Although none of our patients were given ATG, there were no relapses, and acute GVHD remained under control. This may be because many Japanese express HLA-C1 and few episodes of acute GVHD have been recorded after KIR-ligand-mismatched HSCT in Japan [15]. Rubnitz et al. have reported no relapses in pediatric AML patients who underwent KIR-ligand-mismatched HSCT after achieving CR [16]. As these results suggest that NK cell alloreactivity affects the extent of minimal residual disease, KIR-CBT should be performed as soon as possible after CR has been achieved. Although all three of our patients successfully achieved CR, evidence for the efficacy of including GO during induction therapy and KIR-CBT in pediatric AML remains inconclusive. Recent advances in AML treatment have identified several promising modalities, such as anti-methylating agents, immune checkpoint inhibitors (ICIs), and chimeric antigen receptor-T cells (CAR-T). Daver et al. have reported that Azacitidine, in combination with ICIs, may be safe and effective in patients with relapsed AML [17], while Li et al. have stated that CD33 CAR-T is effective against AML cells and that it prolongs survival in a mouse xenograft model [18]. Those new drugs can alter the treatment landscape of pediatric refractory/relapsed AML and provide new treatment opportunities in the future.

In conclusion, the FLAG-IDA reinduction therapy described here, with or without GO, when used before KIR-CBT, appears to be a feasible treatment strategy in pediatric patients with refractory/relapsed AML. However, definitive conclusions about the efficacy of this approach cannot be made because of the very small number of patients included in this study. Therefore, additional prospective studies are required to evaluate the same.

Authors' Contributions

D. T. wrote the paper, and S. Y., R. M., Y. S., R. K., N. O., M. K., S. F., K. A., K.I, and S. Y treated the patients.

References

[1] A. Sander, M. Zimmermann, M. Dworzak et al., "Consequent and intensified relapse therapy improved survival in pediatric AML: results of relapse treatment in 379 patients of three consecutive AML-BFM trials," *Leukemia*, vol. 24, no. 8, pp. 1422–1428, 2010.

[2] Fleischhack, Hasan, Graf, Mann, and Bode, "IDA-FLAG (idarubicin, fludarabine, cytarabine, G-CSF), an effective remission-induction therapy for poor-prognosis AML of childhood prior to allogeneic or autologous bone marrow transplantation: experiences of a phase II trial," *British Journal of Haematology*, vol. 102, no. 3, pp. 647–655, 1998.

[3] W. J. Kell, A. K. Burnett, R. Chopra et al., "A feasibility study of simultaneous administration of gemtuzumab ozogamicin with intensive chemotherapy in induction and consolidation in younger patients with acute myeloid leukemia," *Blood*, vol. 102, no. 13, pp. 4277–4283, 2003.

[4] N. Yoshida, H. Sakaguchi, K. Matsumoto, and K. Kato, "Successful treatment with low-dose gemtuzumab ozogamicin in combination chemotherapy followed by stem cell transplantation for children with refractory acute myeloid leukaemia," *British Journal of Haematology*, vol. 158, no. 5, pp. 666–668, 2012.

[5] L. Ruggeri, M. Capanni, E. Urbani et al., "Effectiveness of donor natural killer cell alloreactivity in mismatched hematopoietic transplants," *Science*, vol. 295, no. 5562, pp. 2097–2100, 2002.

[6] L. Moretta, F. Locatelli, D. Pende, E. Marcenaro, M. C. Mingari, and A. Moretta, "Killer Ig-like receptor-mediated control of natural killer cell alloreactivity in haploidentical hematopoietic stem cell transplantation," *Blood*, vol. 117, no. 3, pp. 764–771, 2011.

[7] K. C. Hsu, C. A. Keever-Taylor, A. Wilton et al., "Improved outcome in HLA-identical sibling hematopoietic stem-cell transplantation for acute myelogenous leukemia predicted by KIR and HLA genotypes," *Blood*, vol. 105, no. 12, pp. 4878–4884, 2005.

[8] H. Nakayama, K. Tabuchi, A. Tawa et al., "Outcome of children with relapsed acute myeloid leukemia following initial therapy under the AML99 protocol," *International Journal of Hematology*, vol. 100, no. 2, pp. 171–179, 2014.

[9] W. Leung, "Use of NK cell activity in cure by transplant," *British Journal of Haematology*, vol. 155, no. 1, pp. 14–29, 2011.

[10] S. Yamamoto, R. Matsuno, Y. Sugishita et al., "Sinusoidal obstructive syndrome prophylaxis with recombinant human soluble thrombomodulin is feasible in gemtuzumab ozogamicin-treated patients undergoing allogeneic hematopoietic cell transplantation," *Bone Marrow Transplantation*, vol. 52, no. 7, pp. 1068–1070, 2017.

[11] E. L. Sievers, R. A. Larson, E. A. Stadtmauer et al., "Efficacy and safety of gemtuzumab ozogamicin in patients with CD33-positive acute myeloid leukemia in first relapse," *Journal of Clinical Oncology*, vol. 19, no. 13, pp. 3244–3254, 2001.

[12] J. S. Miller, "How killers kill," *Blood*, vol. 112, no. 2, p. 213, 2008.

[13] R. Willemze, C. A. Rodrigues, M. Labopin et al., "KIR-ligand incompatibility in the graft-versus-host direction improves outcomes after umbilical cord blood transplantation for acute leukemia," *Leukemia*, vol. 23, no. 3, pp. 492–500, 2009.

[14] C. G. Brunstein, J. E. Wagner, D. J. Weisdorf et al., "Negative effect of KIR Alloreactivity in recipients of umbilical cord blood transplant depends on transplantation conditioning intensity," *Blood*, vol. 113, no. 22, pp. 5628–5634, 2009.

[15] K. C. Hsu, T. Gooley, M. Malkki et al., "KIR ligands and prediction of relapse after unrelated donor hematopoietic cell transplantation for hematologic malignancy," *Biology of Blood and Marrow Transplantation*, vol. 12, no. 8, pp. 828–836, 2006.

[16] J. E. Rubnitz, H. Inaba, R. C. Ribeiro et al., "NKAML: a pilot study to determine the safety and feasibility of haploidentical natural killer cell transplantation in childhood acute myeloid leukemia," *Journal of Clinical Oncology*, vol. 28, no. 6, pp. 955–959, 2010.

[17] N. Daver, G. Garcia-Manero, S. Basu et al., "Efficacy, safety, and biomarkers of response to azacitidine and nivolumab in relapsed/refractory acute myeloid leukemia: a non-randomized, open-label, phase II study," *Cancer Discovery*, vol. 9, no. 3, pp. 370–383, 2019.

[18] S. Li, Z. Tao, Y. Xu et al., "CD33-Specific chimeric antigen receptor T cells with different Co-stimulators showed potent anti-leukemia efficacy and different phenotype," *Human Gene Therapy*, vol. 29, no. 5, pp. 626–639, 2018.

6

Association of Immune Thrombocytopenia and T-Lymphoblastic Lymphoma in a Pediatric Patient

Ryan A. Denu,[1,2] Daniel R. Matson,[3] Matthew J. Davis,[2,4] Natalie J. Tedford,[4] Christine E. Brichta,[4] Carol A. Diamond,[2,4] and Margo L. Hoover-Regan[2,4]

[1]*Medical Scientist Training Program, School of Medicine and Public Health, University of Wisconsin-Madison, Madison, WI, USA*
[2]*Carbone Cancer Center, University of Wisconsin, Madison, WI, USA*
[3]*Department of Pathology and Laboratory Medicine, School of Medicine and Public Health, University of Wisconsin-Madison, Madison, WI, USA*
[4]*Department of Pediatrics, School of Medicine and Public Health, University of Wisconsin-Madison, Madison, WI, USA*

Correspondence should be addressed to Margo L. Hoover-Regan; mhooverregan@wisc.edu

Academic Editor: Håkon Reikvam

Immune thrombocytopenia (ITP) is characterized by isolated thrombocytopenia of unclear etiology. We present a unique case of an 8-year-old girl with chronic ITP who was subsequently diagnosed with T-lymphoblastic lymphoma at age 11. The clinical course was complicated by the occurrence of nonepileptiform events with bizarre behavior changes following the administration of nelarabine and intrathecal and high-dose systemic methotrexate. This case highlights an unusual co-occurrence of hematologic malignancy and chronic ITP in an otherwise healthy child. We speculate that underlying genetic or immunologic lesions may predispose a subset of pediatric ITP patients to the development of hematologic malignancies.

1. Introduction

Immune thrombocytopenia (ITP) is a disorder characterized by isolated thrombocytopenia secondary to an aberrant antiplatelet antibody response. This results in a significantly shortened lifespan of circulating platelets with otherwise normal peripheral blood counts. The disease classically manifests with cutaneous and mucosal purpura; bone marrow examination typically shows increased megakaryocytes and normal numbers of other hematopoietic progenitors [1, 2]. Most cases of ITP are idiopathic and believed to reflect an autoimmune process secondary to perturbations in immune homeostasis (e.g., infections and autoimmune diseases) with resulting loss of peripheral tolerance [3].

Most children with ITP require only regular monitoring and will recover without treatment. However, treatment is indicated in a subset of patients with clinically significant disease, and this may include glucocorticoids, intravenous immunoglobulin, and anti-D immunoglobulin [4]. Treatment refractory cases may respond to rituximab and thrombopoietin receptor agonists (e.g., eltrombopag and romiplostim). Splenectomy is reserved for patients with chronic severe ITP who fail medical therapy [5]. Regardless of treatment regimen, about 10–30% will go on to develop chronic ITP, defined as thrombocytopenia greater than 12 months. [6–8] Risk factors for chronic ITP include older age, less severe thrombocytopenia at diagnosis, insidious onset of symptoms, and lack of a clear preceding/inciting event [7, 9, 10].

In adults, ITP is often associated with a concurrent hematological malignancy, most commonly chronic lymphocytic leukemia [11]. However, a formal relationship between hematologic malignancies and ITP has not been demonstrated in children. Herein, we report a rare case of chronic ITP that preceded the development of T-lymphoblastic lymphoma in a pediatric patient.

2. Case Presentation

An 8-year-old girl presented with bilateral, nonblanching facial petechiae following an episode of emesis. Her medical history was notable only for eczema. She was found to have thrombocytopenia with a platelet count of 96,000/μL (reference 160,000–370,000/μL). Three weeks later, a repeat complete blood count (CBC) demonstrated a borderline normal platelet count of 155,000/μL. She then experienced a second episode of postemesis facial petechiae after which she underwent a 15-month period of observation. During this time, her platelet count remained between 30,000/μL and 40,000/μL. She then presented with petechiae on her trunk and extremities, and her platelet count was noted to be 14,000/μL. She denied any bleeding episodes, including hematuria or hematochezia, but did complain of easy bruising on her extremities. No hepatosplenomegaly was noted on an otherwise normal physical examination; however, her parents felt she seemed more fatigued than her peers. Furthermore, they reported four years of intermittent febrile episodes associated with occasional syncope. Additional workup included an antinuclear antibody and erythrocyte sedimentation rate that were both within normal limits. A presumptive diagnosis of ITP was made. Because she had no active bleeding and her platelet count remained >10,000/μL, she continued a period of observation only (Figure 1(a)).

Three years after her initial episode, she remained thrombocytopenic, and in consultation with her parents, she underwent bone marrow biopsy to rule out a bone marrow failure syndrome. This showed only linear and orderly trilineage hematopoiesis with increased numbers of morphologically normal megakaryocytes (Figures 1(b) and 1(c)).

Two months later, she presented to her pediatrician's office with postprandial retrosternal and epigastric pain. She had been experiencing 1-2 weeks of poor appetite and intermittent vomiting with tender right cervical adenopathy and a four-pound weight loss. A chest X-ray demonstrated a right pleural effusion and bilateral hilar lymphadenopathy, at which point she was transferred to our hospital. On admission, her lactate dehydrogenase was elevated to 1302 U/L (ref 157–283 U/L), and uric acid was 12.7 mg/dL (ref 2.8–6 mg/dL). Platelets were 152,000/μL, white blood cells were 7.5 K/μL, and hemoglobin was 12.6 g/dL. CT of her neck, chest, abdomen, and pelvis demonstrated a right anterior mediastinal mass ($9 \times 6 \times 18$ cm) with extension through the thoracic inlet, encasement of the great vessels, and compression of the superior vena cava (Figure 2(a)). There was also diffuse thoracic and abdominal lymphadenopathy and bilateral renal infiltrates. Core biopsy of an enlarged lymph node showed medium-sized overtly malignant lymphoid cells with blastic chromatin, which were diffusely positive for TdT and CD3 by immunohistochemistry (Figure 2(b)). A diagnosis of T-lymphoblastic lymphoma was rendered. Concurrent flow cytometry of pleural fluid was remarkable for abundant medium- to large-size blasts, consistent with T-lymphoblastic lymphoma, whereas a bone marrow biopsy and lumbar puncture both showed no evidence of involvement by T lymphoblasts. These findings established a diagnosis of stage III T-ALL according to St. Jude staging criteria.

She was treated per Children's Oncology Group (COG) AALL1231, Arm A. She achieved a complete remission at the end of the induction phase of treatment. Nelarabine was added to the consolidation, delayed intensification, and maintenance phases, in light of this drug conferring benefit on a previous COG study for patients with T-cell acute lymphoblastic leukemia and T-lymphoblastic lymphoma, AALL 0434. Rasburicase and allopurinol were used to manage tumor lysis syndrome. Treatment was complicated by encephalopathy, which developed after nelarabine administration and later after intrathecal and high-dose systemic methotrexate administration. This was characterized by intermittent nonepileptiform events (assessed by electroencephalogram) lasting between 10 and 90 minutes. These events were quite bizarre; for example, our patient would speak in British or Creole accents, recite Disney quotes or songs repeatedly, or make animal noises. She was aware of the events and could sense their onset but seemingly had no control of what she said. These events were mitigated with the use of dextromethorphan rescue, which has previously been reported to abrogate methotrexate-induced neurotoxicity in pediatric patients [12].

The patient remains in remission and has continued to receive treatment per AALL1231. She is currently 15 months into treatment and has completed induction, consolidation, two cycles of interim maintenance, delayed intensification, and two cycles of maintenance chemotherapy. Her platelet count has increased since starting chemotherapy and is currently within normal limits (Figure 1).

3. Discussion

We report here an interesting association of chronic ITP with the development of T-lymphoblastic lymphoma in a child. In a literature search, we identified very few reported cases of concurrent ITP and T-cell malignancies in children and even fewer cases in which chronic ITP preceded the development of lymphoma or leukemia [13–16]. In one such case, a 13-month-old otherwise asymptomatic boy was found to be thrombocytopenic on routine blood work and 10 months later developed a large facial and periorbital hematoma after head trauma [15]. His platelets were reduced at 20,000/μL and flow cytometry confirmed T-ALL with 63% circulating blasts. In another case, a 1-year-old boy was diagnosed with ITP, treated with low-dose prednisone, and then developed T-ALL three years later. His platelet counts returned to normal after completing chemotherapy [13].

Our reports and others raise the possibility that chronic ITP may serve as a predisposing factor for the development of hematologic malignancies in children, specifically acute lymphoblastic leukemias and lymphomas. This would not be entirely surprising, as ITP is associated with hematologic malignancies in adults. However, to date, such a relationship has not been formally demonstrated in the pediatric setting. Emerging data provide several possible mechanisms by which this could occur. First, there is growing evidence that ITP results in significant T-cell dysfunction. This includes a

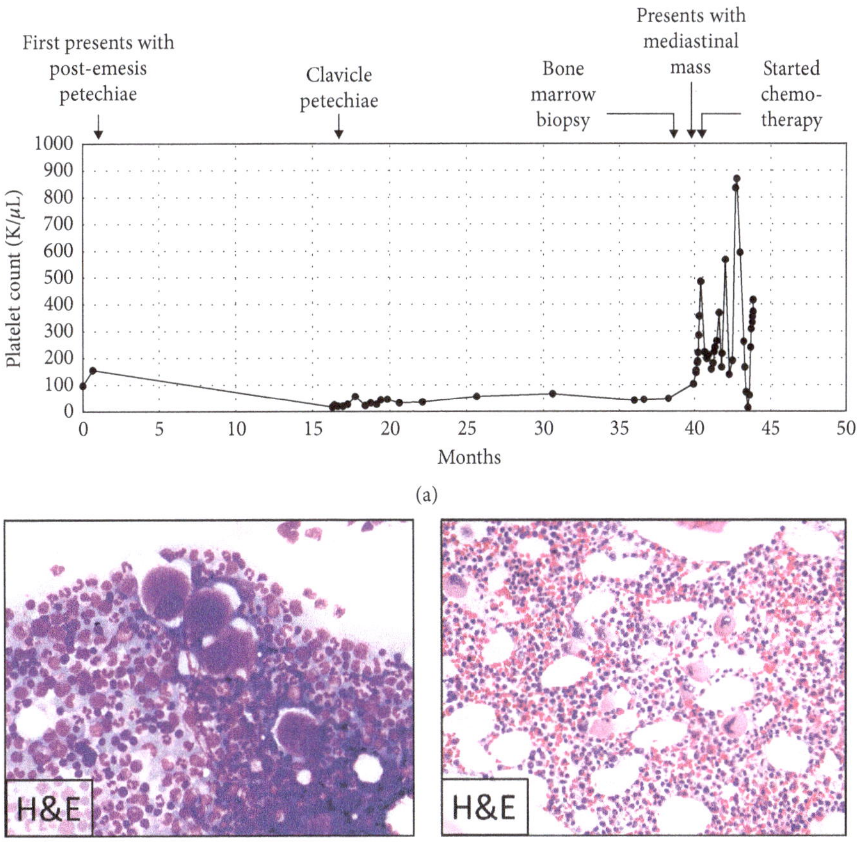

Figure 1: Trend of platelet count over time. (a) The patient's first platelet count was taken 37.1 months prior to the first point on the curve and was within normal limits at 292,000/μL. (B-C) Bone marrow aspirate (b) and biopsy (c) demonstrating increased numbers of morphologically normal megakaryocytes.

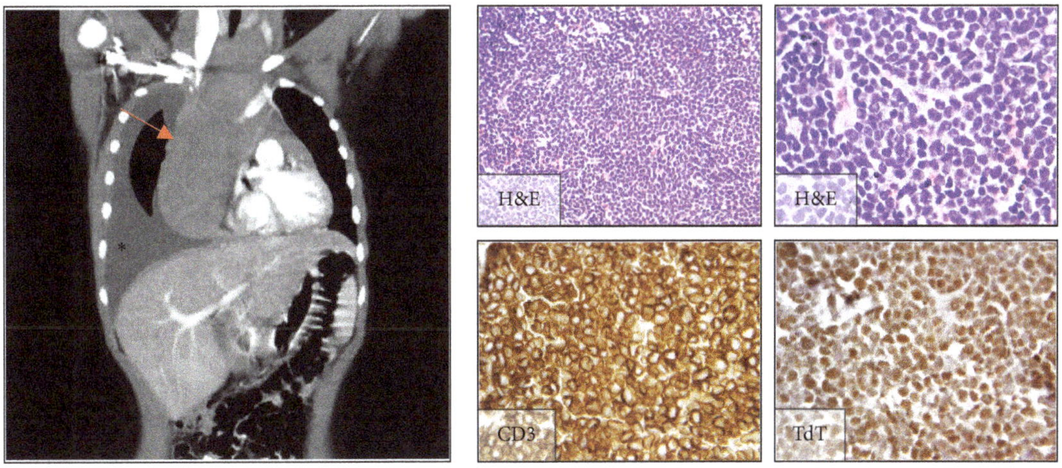

Figure 2: Imaging of mediastinal mass and pathology of lymph node biopsy sample. (a) Coronal view of CT scan of the chest, abdomen, and pelvis demonstrating right anterior mediastinal mass (arrow) measuring $9 \times 6 \times 18$ cm and large right pleural effusion (asterisk). (b) Representative images showing sheets of large overtly malignant cells with blastic chromatin. Immunohistochemistry was strongly positive for CD3 and terminal deoxynucleotidyl transferase (TdT).

reduction in the number and function of T-regulatory cells and a concurrent increase in the number of T-helper cells [17–19]. These changes occur alongside increased levels of interferon γ, tumor necrosis factor α, and interleukin-2 and decreased levels of interleukin-4 [20]. These data suggest that T-cell-related proinflammatory cytokines are central to the pathogenesis of ITP and that children with ITP may have broadly dysregulated T-cell function.

We also consider whether a subset of children with ITP may harbor predisposing genetic factors, which could also put them at risk for the development of hematological malignancies. In such cases, the child's chronic ITP would in fact represent an undiagnosed inherited disorder of thrombocytopenia. There are known mutations that predispose to thrombocytopenia; ANKRD26, RUNX1, and ETV6-related thrombocytopenias are among several recently described entities that are speculated to predispose patients to hematologic malignancies [21]. ANKRD26 mutations are typically in the 5′ untranslated region (UTR) and prevent RUNX1 and FLI1 from binding and silencing ANKRD26, resulting in inappropriate ANKRD26 expression and increased signaling via the myeloproliferative leukemia (MPL) oncogenic pathway [22]. RUNX1 is a transcription factor required for hematopoietic stem cell differentiation, and loss-of-function mutations prevent differentiation into platelets and perpetuate a dedifferentiated state, leading to leukemic transformation [23]. ETV6 is a transcriptional repressor that is required for survival of hematopoietic stem cells and for promoting late phases of megakaryopoiesis [24]. Further work will be needed to assess these potential mechanisms.

Our case raises a question of whether or not children with chronic ITP are predisposed to lymphoblastic lymphomas/leukemias. Additional research into the immunology and genetics of children with chronic ITP should consider a propensity for the development of hematologic malignancies.

Abbreviations

ITP: Immune thrombocytopenia
T-ALL: T-cell acute lymphoblastic leukemia/lymphoma.

Consent

Written informed consent was obtained from the guardian of the patient for publication of this case report.

Acknowledgments

RAD is supported by F30CA203271 and T32GM008692.

References

[1] J. A. D'Orazio, J. Neely, and N. Farhoudi, "ITP in children: pathophysiology and current treatment approaches," *Journal of Pediatric Hematology/Oncology*, vol. 35, no. 1, pp. 1–13, 2013.

[2] L. W. Diggs and J. S. Hewlett, "A study of the bone marrow from thirty-six patients with idiopathic hemorrhagic (thrombopenic) purpura," *Blood*, vol. 3, no. 10, pp. 1090–1104, 1948.

[3] D. B. Cines, J. B. Bussel, H. A. Liebman, and E. T. L. Prak, "The ITP syndrome: pathogenic and clinical diversity," *Blood*, vol. 113, no. 26, pp. 6511-6521, 2009.

[4] C. E. Neunert, "Management of newly diagnosed immune thrombocytopenia: can we change outcomes?," *Blood Advances*, vol. 1, no. 24, pp. 2295–2301, 2017.

[5] S. G. Sandler, "The spleen and splenectomy in immune (idiopathic) thrombocytopenic purpura," *Seminars in Hematology*, vol. 37, no. 1, pp. 10–12, 2000.

[6] F. Demircioğlu, M. Saygi, S. Yilmaz, H. Ören, and G. İrken, "Clinical features, treatment responses, and outcome of children with idiopathic thrombocytopenic purpura," *Pediatric Hematology and Oncology*, vol. 26, no. 7, pp. 526–532, 2009.

[7] K. M. J. Heitink-Pollé, J. Nijsten, C. W. B. Boonacker, M. de Haas, and M. C. A. Bruin, "Clinical and laboratory predictors of chronic immune thrombocytopenia in children: a systematic review and meta-analysis," *Blood*, vol. 124, no. 22, pp. 3295–3307, 2014.

[8] K. M. J. Heitink-Pollé, C. S. P. M. Uiterwaal, L. Porcelijn et al., "Intravenous immunoglobulin vs observation in childhood immune thrombocytopenia: a randomized controlled trial," *Blood*, vol. 132, no. 9, pp. 883–891, 2018.

[9] M. Bruin, M. Bierings, C. Uiterwaal et al., "Platelet count, previous infection and FCGR2B genotype predict development of chronic disease in newly diagnosed idiopathic thrombocytopenia in childhood: results of a prospective study," *British Journal of Haematology*, vol. 127, no. 5, pp. 561-567, 2004.

[10] J. Glanz, E. France, S. Xu, T. Hayes, and S. Hambidge, "A population-based, multisite cohort study of the predictors of chronic idiopathic thrombocytopenic purpura in children," *Pediatrics*, vol. 121, no. 3, pp. e506–e512, 2008.

[11] C. Visco, M. Ruggeri, M. L. Evangelista et al., "Impact of immune thrombocytopenia on the clinical course of chronic lymphocytic leukemia," *Blood*, vol. 111, no. 3, pp. 1110–1116, 2008.

[12] M. Afshar, D. Birnbaum, and C. Golden, "Review of dextromethorphan administration in 18 patients with subacute methotrexate central nervous system toxicity," *Pediatric Neurology*, vol. 50, no. 6, pp. 625–629, 2014.

[13] T. Tonouchi, Y. Toyoda, J. Mimaya, and S. Kojima, "T-cell type acute lymphoblastic leukemia developing during the course of chronic idiopathic thrombocytopenic purpura in a child," *Rinsho Ketsueki*, vol. 26, no. 6, pp. 943–950, 1985.

[14] K. Tokeji, S. Sakaguchi, T. Kurimoto, J. Fujimura, and T. Shimizu, "Immune thrombocytopenia in a child with T cell lymphoblastic lymphoma," *Case Reports in Hematology*, vol. 2016, Article ID 2897325, 2 pages, 2016.

[15] H. Shaukat, J. O'Mara, and M. Neier, "A pediatric case of persistent thrombocytopenia in a patient who developed all," *Journal of Pediatric Hematology/Oncology*, vol. 39, no. 8, pp. e512–e514, 2017.

[16] V. S. Kanwar and E. Bhagat, "Immune thrombocytopenic purpura in two patients with Acute Lymphoblastic Leukemia," *Pediatric Hematology Oncology Journal*, vol. 3, no. 3, p. S32, 2018.

[17] B. Liu, H. Zhao, M. C. Poon et al., "Abnormality of CD4(+) CD25(+) regulatory T cells in idiopathic thrombocytopenic purpura," *European Journal of Haematology*, vol. 78, no. 2, pp. 139–143, 2006.

[18] M. Sakakura, H. Wada, I. Tawara et al., "Reduced Cd4+Cd25+ T cells in patients with idiopathic thrombocytopenic purpura," *Thrombosis Research*, vol. 120, no. 2, pp. 187–193, 2007.

[19] J. Yu, S. Heck, V. Patel et al., "Defective circulating CD25 regulatory T cells in patients with chronic immune thrombocytopenic purpura," *Blood*, vol. 112, no. 4, pp. 1325–1328, 2008.

[20] X. H. Guo, F. Zhao, W. Shi et al., "Detection and clinical significance of Th1/Th2 cytokines in patients with idiopathic thrombocytopenic purpura," *Xi Bao Yu Fen Zi Mian Yi Xue Za Zhi*, vol. 28, no. 11, pp. 1185–1187, 2012.

[21] F. Melazzini, F. Palombo, A. Balduini et al., "Clinical and pathogenic features of ETV6 -related thrombocytopenia with predisposition to acute lymphoblastic leukemia," *Haematologica*, vol. 101, no. 11, pp. 1333–1342, 2016.

[22] D. Bluteau, A. Balduini, N. Balayn et al., "Thrombocytopenia-associated mutations in the ANKRD26 regulatory region induce MAPK hyperactivation," *Journal of Clinical Investigation*, vol. 124, no. 2, pp. 580–591, 2014.

[23] N. Asou, "The role of a Runt domain transcription factor AML1/RUNX1 in leukemogenesis and its clinical implications," *Critical Reviews in Oncology/Hematology*, vol. 45, no. 2, pp. 129–150, 2003.

[24] H. Hock, E. Meade, S. Medeiros et al., "Tel/Etv6 is an essential and selective regulator of adult hematopoietic stem cell survival," *Genes & Development*, vol. 18, no. 19, pp. 2336–2341, 2004.

7

Homozygous CALR Mutation in Primary Myelofibrosis and its Effect on Disease Phenotype: A Case Report and Review of the Literature

Qurratulain Rizvi,[1] Uzma Zaidi,[1] Saba Shahid,[2] Shariq Ahmed,[2] and Tahir Shamsi[1]

[1]*Department of Clinical Haematology, National Institute of Blood Diseases & Bone Marrow Transplantation, P.O. Box-75300, Karachi, Pakistan*
[2]*Department of Genomics, National Institute of Blood Diseases & Bone Marrow Transplantation, P.O. Box-75300, Karachi, Pakistan*

Correspondence should be addressed to Saba Shahid; sabashahid_dbt@yahoo.com

Academic Editor: Eduardo Arellano-Rodrigo

Somatic mutations in *CALR* gene have been reported in 60%–88% of patients with essential thrombocythemia (ET) and primary myelofibrosis (PMF) who are negative for *JAK2* and *MPL* mutations. Most of the *CALR* mutations analyzed to date are heterozygous mutations in exon 9 of the gene. Homozygosity in *CALR* gene is rarely reported, and its association with clinical behavior of disease and impact on outcome of patients is not studied so far. We herein report a case of intermediate-2 risk PMF (according to IPSS) diagnosed with homozygous mutation (c.1139delA p.E380fs*50) in *CALR* gene having severe disease manifestations at presentation.

1. Introduction

Primary myelofibrosis (PMF) is a classical Philadelphia-negative myeloproliferative neoplasm (MPN) characterized by abnormal proliferation of predominantly megakaryocytes and granulocytes. The disease involves remodeling of bone marrow, including progressive myelofibrosis, exaggerated angiogenesis, and extramedullary hematopoiesis manifested by leukoerythroblastic blood smear and hepatosplenomegaly [1]. A number of molecular pathways and mutations play role in the pathogenesis of the disease making it a complex disorder.

Approximately, 50% of patients with PMF carry the *JAK2*-V617F mutation, whereas mutations of *MPL* are found in an additional 5%. Somatic mutations in *CALR* gene were detected in 70% to 84% of *JAK2* nonmutated MPN [2]. An entity defined as triple-negative primary myelofibrosis with absent *JAK2*, *CALR*, and *cMPL* mutation is identified, being associated with reduced overall survival [3]. Most of the *CALR* mutations analyzed to date are heterozygous mutations in exon 9 of the gene. Patients with heterozygous *CALR*-mutant PMF have distinct clinical features, an indolent clinical course, and better survival compared with PMF patients carrying *JAK2* (V617F) or an *MPL* exon 10 mutation [4, 5]. Due to the high prevalence of *CALR* mutation in PMF, WHO has incorporated its presence in the revised diagnostic criteria of prefibrotic and overt myelofibrosis [6]. Homozygosity in *CALR* gene is rarely reported, and its association with clinical behavior of disease and impact on outcome of patients is not studied so far [7]. We herein report a case of PMF diagnosed with homozygous mutation in *CALR* gene having severe disease manifestations at presentation.

2. Case Scenario

A 57-year-old gentleman, known diabetic, presented with complaints of easy fatigability, loss of appetite, low-grade fever, and left hypochondrial discomfort for the past 2 months. Physical examination revealed splenomegaly (8 fingers below the left costal margin). Complete blood count showed Hb of 9.4 g/dl, TLC of 5.8×10^9/L, and Plt count of 337×10^9/L with leukoerythroblastic picture and absent circulating blasts. Bone marrow findings were consistent with primary myelofibrosis, exhibiting hypercellularity with marked increase in reticulin fibrosis (MF grade 2, according to EUMNET consensus, Figure 1) and atypical, hypolobated megakaryocytes forming loose clusters (Figure 2). Blast percentage was less than 5%. Cytogenetic analysis showed normal male karyotype. BCR-ABL translocation via PCR, *JAK2*-V617F, and *MPL* mutation were not detected. Associated *CALR* mutations were not determined via next-generation sequencing due to resource constraints. Serum erythropoietin level was 200 U/L. According to the International Prognostic Scoring System (IPSS), the patient was falling into intermediate-2 risk category. He was initially prescribed ruxolitinib 10 mg twice daily (gradually escalated to 15 mg twice daily) along with erythropoietin 20,000 IU weekly for correction of anemia.

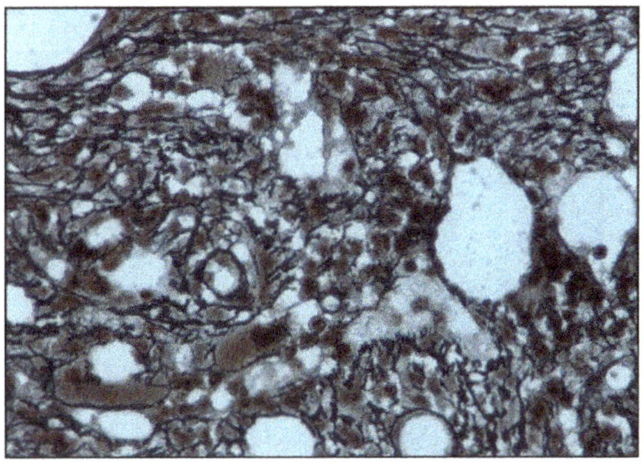

FIGURE 1: Reticulin stain showing MF grade 2 fibrosis.

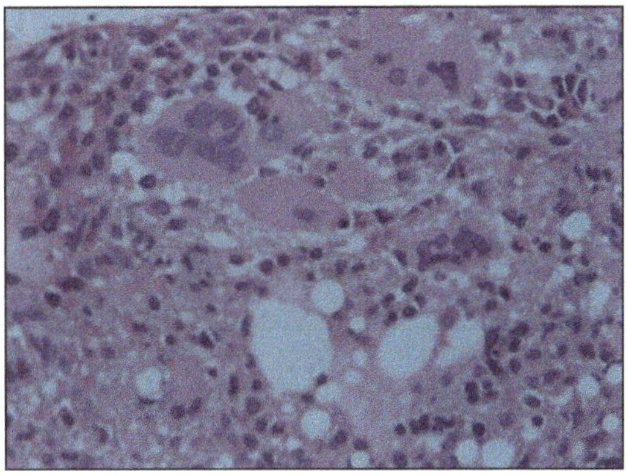

FIGURE 2: Trephine biopsy showing atypical megakaryocytes.

3. Methodology

The research protocol was approved by the Institutional Review Board (ERC/IRB) and conformed to the tenets of the Declaration of Helsinki. Written informed consent was obtained from the patient. The diagnosis was established according to the 2016 WHO criteria, and the clinical and laboratory data were reviewed from medical record.

3.1. Mutation Analysis. The DNA was extracted from the peripheral blood sample of the MPN patient using a QIAamp DNA Mini Kit (Qiagen, Hilden, Germany) according to the manufacturer's instructions. The *JAK2* and *MPL* mutations were analyzed by using the ARMS PCR for *JAK2*-V617F and *MPL* W515L/K mutations as previously described [8]. Sanger sequencing was performed to screen *CALR* gene for exon 9. The genomic region of interest was amplified by PCR. Amplification of *CALR* exon 9 was performed by using previously reported primers *CALR*. –F (5′-ACAACTTCCTCATCACCAACG-3′) and *CALR*–R (5′-GGCCTCAGTCCAGCCCTG -3′) [8]. The total reaction volume of 20 μl contained approximately 50 ng of DNA, 200 nmol/l for forward and reverse primers, deoxynucleotide triphosphates (dNTPs, 200 μmol/l each), 1 unit of Dream Taq DNA Polymerase (Thermo Scientific, Life Technologies Inc, Carlsbad, California 92008). Samples were amplified using the following PCR conditions: 94°C for 10 minutes; 30 cycles of 94°C for 30 seconds; 59°C for 30 seconds; 72°C for 30 seconds with final extension of 72°C for 10 minutes and hold at 4°C. PCR products were analyzed using 2% agarose gel electrophoresis. Sequencing products were purified, and the sequencing reaction was performed using the BigDye terminator cycle sequencing kit, v3.1 (Applied Biosystems®, California, USA) and was analyzed on an automated DNA analyzer (ABI, 3500).

4. Results and Discussion

Sanger sequencing for *CALR* exon 9 mutation identified a homozygous mutation (c.1139delA p.E380fs*50) in this case as shown in Figure 3. The same mutation has been reported in Chinese population in heterozygous state which disturbed the reading frame shift and significantly altered C-terminal domain of *CALR* protein [9]. This is a unique finding, as homozygosity in *CALR* gene has been exclusively associated with type 2 mutation (5 bp insertion; 1). Basically, *CALR* mutations do not alter the primary structure of the *CALR* binding site for glycoproteins but affect the C-terminal domain, which contains a KDEL motif and a Ca^{2+} binding domain [10].

The advent of mutation in *CALR* gene changed the landscape of MPNs. It was first recognized as a somatic mutation in patients with MPNs who had no mutations in either *JAK2* or *MPL* by Klampfl et al. in 2013 [7]. Calreticulin is a protein found in endoplasmic reticulum, cytoplasm, or cell surface, which maintains the calcium hemostasis, regulates the cell proliferation, phagocytosis, and apoptosis, and also ensures proper glycoprotein folding [11]. Patients with heterozygous *CALR*-mutated PMF are usually males, younger as compared to *JAK2*-mutated cases, and they have myeloproliferation more specific to the megakaryocytic lineage, thus presenting with a more pronounced thrombocytosis. They usually have low hemoglobin and white cell counts. There is low incidence of thrombotic complications and longer survival reported in this group of patients. This prognostic impact of *CALR* in PMF is limited to type 1 mutation, with type 2 having similar prognosis as that of *JAK2*-mutated PMF [12].

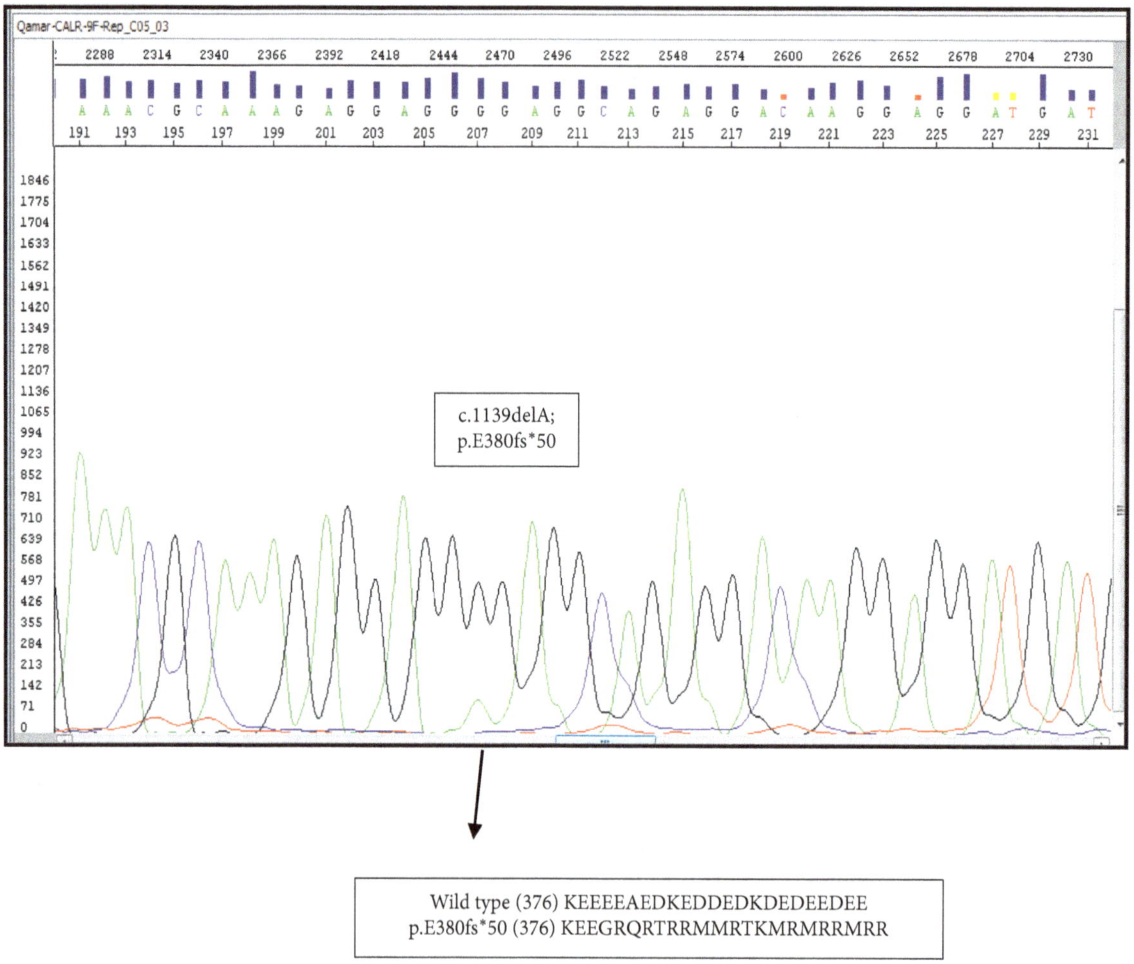

FIGURE 3: Electropherogram of *CALR* exon 9 homozygous mutation (c.1139delA; p.E380fs*50) and the new peptide sequence.

Mutated *CALR* homozygosity seems to be a rare event in MPNs and is reported with type 2 mutations in exon 9. In the study by Klampfl et al., three of 289 *CALR*-mutated patients were homozygous for the mutation, and all had type 2 mutations [7]. Similar frequencies of acquired 19pUPD for both *CALR* insertions and deletions were found by Nangalia et al. [13]. There is not much literature to provide specific evidence concerning homozygous *CALR* mutations and its impact on the phenotypic behavior of the disease as well as on the type of *CALR* mutation.

Homozygous *CALR* mutation in PMF has been associated with acquired myeloperoxidase (MPO) deficiency as reported by Alexandre et al. [14]. An individual case report of homozygous *CALR* type 1 mutation has been described in a patient with an atypical BCR-ABL1-positive MPN [15].

Our index case was diagnosed in the fibrotic phase of PMF. He was found to be in intermediate-2 risk category according to IPSS. His molecular mutation profile was negative for *JAK2*, *MPL*, and BCR-ABL translocation. Interestingly, the mutation in *CALR* gene detected in this patient was homozygous mutation (c.1139delA p.E380fs*50), which seems to be a type 2-like mutation based on the classification according to the absence of (KDEL) motif in the wild type and modification in the alpha helix structure. These mutations produce a new C-terminus which results in loss of endoplasm reticulum (ER) retention signals but maintain the structural integrity of protein. The resultant mutant *CALR* was found in ER without accumulation on the cell surface or Golgi apparatus [13]. This structural modification affects the function and leads to decrease in Ca^{+2} export from the ER and causes downregulation of the calreticulin-NFAT signaling pathway which is directed more towards myeloid lineage commitment [16].

In contrast to the clinical findings associated with heterozygous mutations, i.e., lesser disease severity, thrombocytosis at baseline, and overall good prognosis, our patient with homozygous mutation presented in the advanced phase of disease with constitutional symptoms including weight loss, anorexia, fatigue and low-grade fever, and massive splenomegaly requiring treatment. His platelet count was within normal range at presentation. He was offered *JAK2* inhibitor and erythropoiesis-stimulating agent. After a period of 6 months, the patient was reevaluated using dynamic IPSS (DIPSS) and fell into the intermediate-2 risk category. No thrombotic or hemorrhagic event was noted during the follow-up period. There was mild improvement in constitutional symptoms with ruxolitinib, but red cell transfusion requirement gradually increased. Though initial therapy with ruxolitinib is associated with drop in hemoglobin levels, the severe disease manifestations at presentation compels us to consider that homozygous mutations in *CALR* gene might be accountable for an aggressive disease phenotype in PMF.

5. Conclusion

As *CALR* mutation in MPNs is one of the recent advances, its extensive impact on baseline characteristics and clinical behavior of patient, disease outcome, and risks and benefits in long term is yet to be explored. Prospective studies are needed to elucidate the influence of *CALR* mutation in MPNs with extensive focus on the homozygous pattern of mutation.

References

[1] A. Tefferi and A. Pardanani, "CALR mutations and a new diagnostic algorithm for MPN," *Nature Reviews Clinical Oncology*, vol. 11, no. 3, pp. 125-126, 2014.

[2] M. Cazzola and R. Kralovics, "From Janus kinase 2 to calreticulin: the clinically relevant genomic landscape of myeloproliferative neoplasms," *Blood*, vol. 123, no. 24, pp. 3714–3719, 2014.

[3] C. Diaconu, C. Mambet, L. G. Necula et al., "Triple negative myeloproliferative neoplasms - sometimes driver mutations stay low-key in plain sight," *Romanian Biotechnological Letters*, vol. 10, 2017.

[4] A. Tefferi, T. L. Lasho, C. M. Finke et al., "CALR vs JAK2 vs MPL-mutated or triple-negative myelofibrosis: clinical, cytogenetic and molecular comparisons," *Leukemia*, vol. 28, no. 7, pp. 1472–1477, 2014.

[5] E. Rumi, D. Pietra, C. Pascutto et al., "Clinical effect of driver mutations of JAK2, CALR, or MPL in primary myelofibrosis," *Blood*, vol. 124, no. 7, pp. 1062–1069, 2014.

[6] A. Tefferi, "Primary myelofibrosis: 2017 update on diagnosis, risk-stratification, and management," *American Journal of Hematology*, vol. 91, no. 12, pp. 1262–1271, 2016.

[7] T. Klampfl, H. Gisslinger, A. S. Harutyunyan et al., "Somatic mutations of calreticulin in myeloproliferative neoplasms," *New England Journal of Medicine*, vol. 369, no. 25, pp. 2379–2390, 2013.

[8] Z. Wu, Y. Zhang, X. Zhang et al., "A multiplex snapback primer system for the enrichment and detection of JAK2 V617F and MPL W515L/K mutations in Philadelphia- negative myeloproliferative neoplasms," *BioMed Research International*, vol. 2014, Article ID 458457, 11 pages, 2014.

[9] Y. Lin, E. Liu, Q. Sun et al., "The prevalence of JAK2, MPL, and CALR Mutations in Chinese patients WithBCR-ABL1-negative myeloproliferative neoplasms," *American Journal of Clinical Pathology*, vol. 144, no. 1, pp. 165–171, 2015.

[10] J. Chi, M. Manoloukos, C. Pierides et al., "Calreticulin mutations in myeloproliferative neoplasms and new methodology for their detection and monitoring," *Annals of Hematology*, vol. 94, no. 3, pp. 399–408, 2014.

[11] W. Luo and Z. Yu, "Calreticulin (CALR) mutation in myeloproliferative neoplasms (MPNs)," *Stem Cell Investig*, vol. 2, no. 16, 16 pages, 2015.

[12] P. Guglielmelli, J. Nangalia, A. R. Green, and A. M. Vannucchi, "CALRmutations in myeloproliferative neoplasms: hidden behind the reticulum," *American Journal of Hematology*, vol. 89, no. 5, pp. 453–456, 2014.

[13] J. Nangalia, C. E. Massie, E. J. Baxter et al., "Somatic CALR mutations in myeloproliferative neoplasms with nonmutated JAK2," *New England Journal of Medicine*, vol. 369, no. 25, pp. 2391–2405, 2013.

[14] P. T. Alexandre, L. Pontus, K. L. Asvin et al., "Homozygous calreticulin mutations in patients with myelofibrosis lead to acquired myeloperoxidase deficiency," *Blood*, vol. 127, no. 25, pp. 3253–3259, 2016.

[15] X. Cabagnols, J.-M. Cayuela, and W. Vainchenker, "A CALR mutation preceding BCR-ABL1 in an atypical myeloproliferative neoplasm," *New England Journal of Medicine*, vol. 372, no. 7, pp. 688–690, 2015.

[16] M. P. Chao, S. Jaiswal, R. Weissman-Tsukamoto et al., "Calreticulin is the dominant pro-phagocytic signal on multiple human cancers and is counterbalanced by CD47," *Science Translational Medicine*, vol. 2, no. 63, p. 63ra94, 2010.

8

A Rare Cause of Thrombotic Thrombocytopenia Purpura-(TTP-) Like Syndrome, Vitamin B12 Deficiency: Interpretation of Significant Pathological Findings

Morgan Bailey,[1] **Travis Maestas**,[1] **Robert Betancourt**,[1] **Dalia Mikhael**,[2] **and Hani M. Babiker**[3]

[1]*Department of Internal Medicine, University of Arizona, Tucson, AZ, USA*
[2]*Department of Internal Medicine, Banner University Medical Center-Tucson, Tucson, AZ, USA*
[3]*Department of Hematology-Oncology, University of Arizona Cancer Center, Tucson, AZ, USA*

Correspondence should be addressed to Morgan Bailey; mbailey@deptofmed.arizona.edu

Academic Editor: Giuseppe Murdaca

Thrombotic thrombocytopenia purpura (TTP) is a hematological emergency that requires rapid assessment followed by prompt initiation of therapy due to high mortality associated with delayed treatment. TTP has many causes including heritable syndromes, ADAMTS13 deficiency, and drugs-related etiologies. Profound vitamin B12 deficiency can, in rare cases, mimic TTP in presentation, and since plasmapheresis can be of limited benefit, prompt diagnosis is necessary for accurate treatment with B12. Therefore, careful analysis of all clinical signs, symptoms, and labs must be assessed. We report a patient who presented with a diagnosis of TTP, and repeat assessment confirmed a diagnosis of sever vitamin B12 (B12) deficiency with pancytopenia who was appropriately treated with B12.

1. Introduction

TTP is characterized by a microangiopathic hemolytic anemia (MAHA), thrombocytopenia, and end-organ dysfunction which requires accurate diagnosis and plasmapheresis [1]. With an incidence of 4 cases in 100000, TTP can have multiple complications including rapid progression to end-organ dysfunction and death [1, 2]. However, it is not uncommon for other conditions, such as vitamin B12 deficiency, to present in a similar fashion, with thrombocytopenia and microangiopathy. Hence, it is important to keep in mind this rare syndrome in addition to other differential diagnoses including disseminated intravascular coagulation (DIC), hemolytic-uremic syndrome (HUS), and autoimmune hemolysis as they can often be mistaken for TTP [2, 3]. Because the results of ADAMTS13 are not readily available at time of presentation, plasmapheresis is often initiated if there is a suspicion for TTP. The case below illustrates such an example in which the patient presented with pancytopenia and microangiopathy concerning for TTP. Emergent plasmapheresis was initiated, and upon further workup, the patient symptoms were attributable to a severe vitamin B12 deficiency.

2. Case Presentation

A 70-year-old Caucasian woman with no past medical history presented to her local care facility after sustaining a mechanical fall the day prior to presentation. She endorsed progressive fatigue, weakness, and dyspnea on exertion in addition to symmetric, bilateral lower extremity numbness for two months. Per her husband, she had become progressively more confused over the past week in addition to endorsing new onset jaundice and scleral icterus.

On initial presentation, she was confused and dyspneic. Lab work was significant for a severe anemia with a hemoglobin of 5.7 g/dL (12–16 g/dL). She received four units of pRBCs and was subsequently transferred to our care facility for further evaluation. On presentation, temperature was 36.3°C, pulse 70 bpm, blood pressure 105/57 mmHg, respirations 18, and oxygen saturation of 100% on room air. Physical exam findings were significant for mild scleral icterus and palpable splenomegaly. The patient was initially oriented to person only; however, the remainder of the physical exam, including the neurological exam, was unremarkable without motor or sensory deficits on initial presentation. Initial laboratory studies were significant for pancytopenia with WBC of 1.8 K/mm^3 (4.0–11.0 K/mm^3), hemoglobin of 8.3 g/dL (12–16 g/dL), MCV of 103 fL (78–100 fL), RDW 24.7% (11.0–15.0%), haptoglobin of <10 mg/dL (43–212 mg/dL), and platelets of 44 K/mm^3 (130–450 K/mm^3) (Table 1). Direct antiglobulin test was negative. Her chemistry profile was significant for a total bilirubin of 3.7 mg/dL (0.2–1.3 mg/dL) with a direct bilirubin of 1.3 mg/dL (0.1–0.5 mg/dL), and a lactate dehydrogenase of 1908 IU/L. Liver chemistries and serum creatinine were normal. Examination of a repeat peripheral blood smear was significant for hypersegmented neutrophils and moderate ovalocytes (Figure 1). In addition, there was concern for schistocytes on the initial smear prompting concern for TTP. At the time of presentation, ADAMTS13 activity was pending. Initially, the patient underwent plasmapheresis starting on admission, for a total of three days in addition to prednisone. Repeat smear was significant for hypersegmented neutrophils and a macrocytic normochromic anemia without evidence of an increase in schistocytes or microspherocytes to suggest a hemolytic process. Serum B12 level drawn on admission was <150 pg/mL (200–650 pg/L). Serum folate level was normal, and serum methylmalonic acid level was ordered to confirm the diagnosis of B12 deficiency and was significantly elevated at 36090 nmol/L (87–318 nmol/L). Anti-intrinsic factor antibodies were positive. In addition, the patient was found to be hypothyroid with TSH of 13.53 mIU/L (0.4–4.0 mIU/L) and free T4 of 0.58 ng/dL and was started on synthroid at 100 μg daily. The ADAMTS13 result eventually returned within normal limits. Therapy with intramuscular B12 was begun with 1000 μg daily, initiated on the same day as plasmapheresis, for one week followed by 1000 μg weekly for four weeks and then monthly thereafter for life. The patient continued to clinically improve with treatment. Repeat vitamin B12 levels one month after therapy were >2000 pg/mL. CBC values also normalized after therapy (Table 2 and Figure 2). Two months after initial therapy, the patient's confusion had resolved; however, her bilateral lower extremity neuropathy continued to persist until the initiation of gabapentin outpatient.

Table 1: Lab values before and after therapy.

Lab values	On presentation	Three weeks after therapy
Hemoglobin	5.7 g/dL	11.5 g/dL
MCV	103 fL	96 fL
Platelet count	44 K/mm^3	223 K/mm^3
White blood cell count	1.8 K/mm^3	8.4 K/mm^3
Haptoglobin	<10 mg/dL	N/A
Total bilirubin/direct bilirubin	3.7 mg/dL/1.3 mg/dL	1.0 mg/dL/NA
LDH	1908 IU/L	279 IU/L H
Serum B12 level	<150 pg/mL	>2000 pg/mL

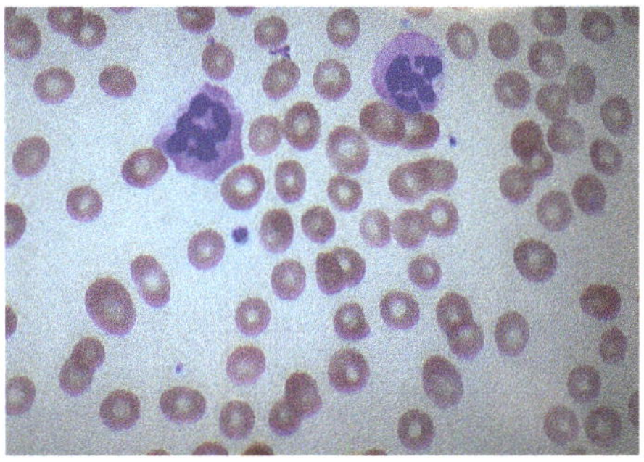

Figure 1: Hypersegmented neutrophils and hypochromic erythrocytes characteristic of a megaloblastic anemia. H&E stain. Magnification: 400x.

3. Discussion

TTP is an emergent diagnosis and necessitates rapid initiation of plasmapheresis if there is suspicion on initial presentation. Due to the high mortality associated with TTP, plasmapheresis is still performed despite ADAMTS13 results not being immediately available. The list of differential diagnoses for hemolytic anemia is broad and can include thrombotic microangiopathies (TMA), autoimmune hemolytic anemia, drug-induced hemolysis (cephalosporins, dapsone, and levodopa), paroxysmal nocturnal hemoglobinuria (PNH), and other hereditary syndromes [13]. Vitamin B12 deficiency is not often associated with hemolytic anemia; however, upon literature review, there have been multiple cases with similar presentations [14] (Table 2). Vitamin B12 deficiency can cause hemolytic anemia most commonly via intramedullary hemolysis of immature reticulocytes; however, thrombotic microangiopathy is rarely seen [15]. Reticulocytopenia in cobalamin deficiency commonly reflects ineffective erythropoiesis in the setting of bone marrow involvement and intramedullary destruction as opposed to peripheral hemolysis as seen with TTP [15, 16]. This mechanism is initiated by premature death via hemolysis of the developing erythrocyte precursors in the bone marrow and is associated with the laboratory findings of hemolysis including elevated LDH, bilirubin, and decreased haptoglobin [16, 17]. However, very few cases of vitamin B12 deficiency have been linked with MAHA, and previous studies indicate that this may arise from acute hyperhomocystinemia which can lead to microangiopathic hemolytic anemia termed pseudothrombotic angiopathy [18]. Therefore, initial laboratory and pathologic findings can often mimic TTP in severe cases of cobalamin deficiency and in rare cases, such as ours, it can present with microangiopathic hemolysis.

4. Conclusion

TTP is a life-threatening microangiopathic hemolytic anemia that can lead to death without timely diagnosis and

Table 2: Case reports of severe vitamin B12 presenting with findings similar to TTP. Cases are organized by age of patient, clinical symptoms at time of presentation, treatment, and outcomes.

Manuscript	Age	Presentation	Treatment	Outcome
Rodrigues et al. [4]	10-month-old F	Two weeks of intermittent vomiting, poor feeding, and decrease in weight percentile from 50% to 5%. Marked pallor, slightly jaundiced appearance, and mild dehydration	Red blood cells transfusion, cyanocobalamin (50 μg subcutaneously, five doses; 100 μg, oral, per day for 1 month), folic acid (5 mg/day), and food diversification	Biochemical and hematologic remission after 1 week and 1 month, respectively. Infant development normalized at 24 months
Tadakamalla et al. [5]	31 yo F	One month of generalized fatigue and bilateral paresthesias of the feet for one week	Plasmapheresis for 4 days followed by IM vitamin B12	B12 def 2/2 pernicious anemia. Complete biochemical response and resolution of symptoms at 4 months
Routh and Koenig [6]	43 yo M	Two-week history of confusion, fever, dyspnea, dizziness, and fatigue associated with diarrhea and hematochezia	3 units FFP, plasmapheresis IM B12	Not reported
Podder et al. [7]	46 yo M	One day history of hematuria and hemoptysis	Plasmapheresis 24 units FFP	Resolution of biochemical parameters. Acquired TTP in the setting of pernicious anemia
Chhabra et al. [8]	52 yo M	Fatigue, loose stools, and weight loss for six months	Intermuscular vitamin B12	Hematological resolution of anemia
Walter et at. [9]	77 yo F	Altered mental status, renal insufficiency, and thrombocytopenia	Plasmapheresis IM vitamin B 12 for life	Resolution of clinical symptoms and anemia 3 weeks after discharge
Merino and Cid [10]	36 yo M	3-4 weeks of asthenia in addition to fatigue and conjunctival pallor	IM vitamin B12 for life	Resolution of clinical and biochemical parameters
Trubin et al. [11]	41 yo F	Two months of fatigue	IM vitamin B12 for 10 days	Resolution of symptoms and correction of anemia
Chapuis et al. [12]	52 yo M	14 days of shortness of breath, general weakness, weight loss, and a sore tongue	2 units pRBCs IM vitamin B12 for life	Resolution of biochemical parameters 9 days after therapy. Resolution of symptoms 6 months after therapy

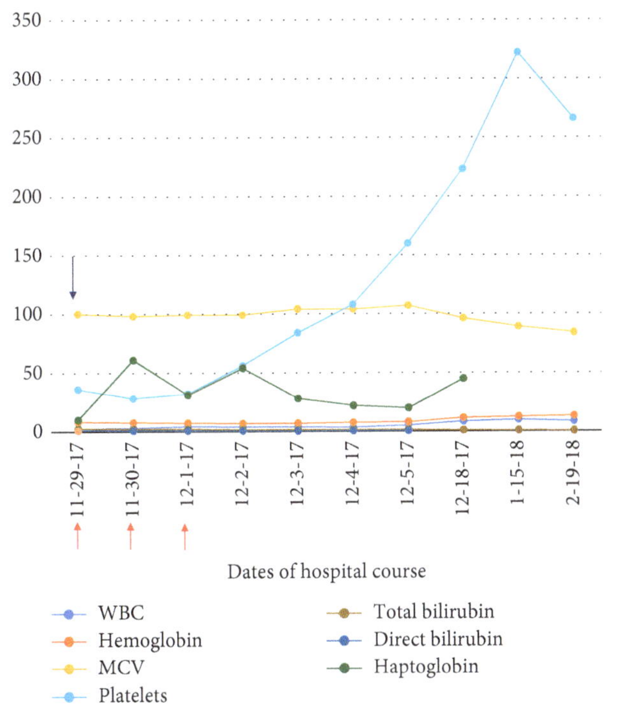

Figure 2: Significant lab values throughout hospital course and three months after initial therapy. Red arrows indicate the dates in which the patient underwent plasmapheresis. The blue arrow indicates the date in which B12 replacement was initiated.

treatment with plasmapheresis. Due to the high mortality associated with TTP, plasmapheresis should be initiated despite pending ADAMTS13 results. As discussed above, TTP can often mimic other common hemolytic anemias; however, there are few cases where severe vitamin B12 deficiency can result in a hemolytic anemia (Table 2). In addition, pathologic findings of severe B12 deficiency can often mimic hemolysis both biochemically and on initial pathology [4, 18, 19]. In the presentation above, the initial working diagnosis was TTP, and thus plasmapheresis was initiated. After further workup and confirmation with normal ADAMTS13 results, the patient was found to be severely deficient in vitamin B12. As discussed, studies have shown that severe vitamin B12 deficiency can present similarly as a hemolytic anemia [1, 4–12] with similar biochemical profiles, thus leading to the initiation of plasmapheresis. This case is important in recognizing this rather unusual presentation of severe vitamin B12 deficiency. Health providers should always act urgently if TTP is suspected, but as this case points out, it is also important to keep other rare causes of hemolytic anemia, such as severe vitamin B12 deficiency.

References

[1] D. W. Abbot, K. D. Friedman, and M. S. Karafin, "Differentiation of pernicious anemia from thrombotic thrombocytopenic purpura: the clinical value of subtle pathologic findings," *Transfusion and Apheresis Science*, vol. 55, no. 3, pp. 318–322, 2016.

[2] F. Yousaf, B. Spinowitz, C. Charytan, and M. Galler, "Pernicious anemia associated cobalamin deficiency and thrombotic microangiopathy: case report and review of the literature," *Case Reports in Medicine*, vol. 2017, Article ID 9410727, 8 pages, 2017.

[3] L. Garderet, E. Maury, M. Lagrange, A. Najman, G. Offenstadt, and B. Guidet, "Schizocytosis in pernicious anemia mimicking thrombotic thrombocytopenic purpura," *The American Journal of Medicine*, vol. 114, no. 5, pp. 423–425, 2003.

[4] V. Rodrigues, A. Dias, M. J. Brito, I. Galvão, and G. C. Ferreira, "Severe megaloblastic anemia in an infant," *BMJ Case Reports*, vol. 2011, Article bcr0220113835, 2011.

[5] A. K. Tadakamalla, S. K. Talluri, and S. Besur, "Pseudo-thrombotic thrombocytopenic purpura: a rare presentation of pernicious anemia," *North American Journal of Medical Sciences*, vol. 3, no. 10, pp. 472–474, 2011.

[6] J. K. Routh and S. C. Koenig, "Severe vitamin B12 deficiency mimicking thrombotic thrombocytopenic purpura," *Blood*, vol. 124, no. 11, p. 1844, 2014.

[7] S. Podder, J. Cervates, and B. R. Dey, "Association of acquired thrombotic thrombocytopaenic purpura in a patient with pernicious anaemia," *BMJ Case Reports*, vol. 2015, Article ID bcr2015211989, 2015.

[8] N. Chhabra, S. Lee, and E. G. Sakalis, "Cobalamin deficiency causing severe hemolytic anemia: a pernicious presentation," *American Journal of Medicine*, vol. 128, no. 10, pp. e5–e6, 2015.

[9] K. Walter, J. Vaughn, and D. Martin, "Therapeutic dilemma in the management of a patient with the clinical picture of TTP and severe B 12 deficiency," *BMC Hematology*, vol. 15, no. 1, p. 16, 2015.

[10] A. Merino and J. Cid, "Very unusual presentation of pernicious anemia with schistocytes in peripheral blood," *Blood*, vol. 122, no. 24, p. 3862, 2013.

[11] P. Trubin, J. Edward, and M. Hand, "Pseudo-thrombotic thrombocytopenic purpura due to severe vitamin B12 deficiency," *Journal of the Louisiana State Medical Society: Official Organ of the Louisiana State Medical Society*, vol. 168, no. 6, pp. 196–200, 2016.

[12] T. M. Chapuis, B. Favrat, and P. Bodenmann, "Cobalamin deficiency resulting in a rare haematological disorder: a case report," *Journal of Medical Case Reports*, vol. 3, no. 1, p. 80, 2009.

[13] S. P. Stabler, "Vitamin B12 deficiency," *New England Journal of Medicine*, vol. 368, no. 2, pp. 149–160, 2013.

[14] N. Noel, G. Maigne, G. Tertian et al., "Hemolysis and schistocytosis in the emergency department: consider pseudothrombotic microangiopathy related to vitamin B12 deficiency," *QJM*, vol. 106, no. 11, pp. 1017–1022, 2013.

[15] E. Andres, S. Affenberger, J. Zimmer et al., "Current hematological findings in cobalamin deficiency. A study of 201 consecutive patients with documented cobalamin deficiency," *Clinical and Laboratory Haematology*, vol. 28, no. 1, pp. 50–56, 2006.

[16] P. N. Tran and M.-H. Tran, "Cobalamin deficiency presenting with thrombotic microangiopathy (TMA) features: a systematic review," *Transfusion and Apheresis Science*, vol. 57, no. 1, pp. 102–106, 2018.

[17] B. S. Joly, P. Coppo, and A. Veyradier, "Thrombotic thrombocytopenic purpura," *Blood*, vol. 129, no. 21, pp. 2836–2846, 2017.

[18] T. Panchabhai, P. Patil, E. Riley, and C. Mitchell, "When the picture is fragmented: vitamin B12deficiency masquerading as

thrombotic thrombocytopenic purpura," *International Journal of Critical Illness and Injury Science*, vol. 6, no. 2, pp. 89–92, 2016.

[19] S. Dalia, C. Milani, J. Castillo, A. Mega, and F. J. Schiffman, "Fooled by the fragments: masquerading microangiopathy," *Medicine and Health, Rhode Island*, vol. 93, no. 1, pp. 25-26, 2010.

9

A Case Study in Process Improvement to Minimize Delays from Obtaining Blood for Red Cell Exchange for a Patient with Sickle Cell Disease and Multiple Red Blood Cell Alloantibodies

Damodaran Narayanan,[1] Noreen B. Hogan,[2] Karen A. Schaser,[2] Patricia Ruegsegger,[1] and William Nicholas Rose[1]

[1]*Department of Pathology, University of Wisconsin Hospital, 600 Highland Ave Madison, WI 53792, Madison, USA*
[2]*Department of Nursing, University of Wisconsin Hospital, 600 Highland Ave Madison, WI 53792, Madison, USA*

Correspondence should be addressed to William Nicholas Rose; wrose@uwhealth.org

Academic Editor: Håkon Reikvam

The process of procuring several units of red blood cells for red cell exchange can sometimes take several hours to days, especially for patients with multiple clinically significant red cell alloantibodies. This can introduce delays, inconveniences, and even health challenges for the patient. For most planned exchanges, these delays are preventable with some foresight and process modifications that are relatively minor yet high leverage. We report a case study of process improvement whereby the apheresis nurse sends an e-mail to the blood bank when the nurse makes the patient's next red cell exchange appointment as the signal to order blood about 6–8 weeks before the exchange.

1. Introduction

Sickle cell disease (SCD) is a common inherited red blood cell (RBC) disorder in the United States, as it affects around 100,000 people and approximately one in 500 African Americans [1, 2]. A common treatment is red cell exchange (RCE), in which about 70% of the patient's blood is replaced by donor RBCs with normal hemoglobin A [1, 2]. One key advantage of RCE over simple transfusion is the prevention of iron overload [1].

In SCD patients, identifying compatible blood products for RCE is important for several reasons. One, SCD patients tend to develop alloantibodies to RBC antigens more frequently (~30%) than do non-SCD patients who are transfused (2–5%) [3, 4].

Two alloimmunized SCD patients who have a delayed hemolytic transfusion reaction (DHTR) may develop the rare but potentially fatal hyperhemolysis syndrome (HHS). HHS includes hemolysis of both transfused and native RBCs for poorly understood reasons [5]. Some cases of HHS also happen independent of alloimmunization [6].

Three, in order to prevent alloantibodies/DHTRs (and, more importantly, the rare complication of HHS that is sometimes associated with a DHTR), extended phenotype matching is often performed [7–9].

In sum, a significant amount of time is often required to obtain RBCs for SCD patients in advance of RCE [10].

2. Case Report

We introduce the patient that was the impetus for our process change. To be clear, we do not claim that the details of the patient alone warrant a case report. Rather, we emphasize that the main purpose of this article is to share the process improvement that was implemented to maximize the quality of care for this patient.

Our patient is a 52-year-old female with hemoglobin SS disease who receives red cell exchanges approximately every 6–8 weeks. She has 5 red cell alloantibodies to the C, E, Fy^a, Fy^3, and Js^a antigens. The anti-Fy^3 is particularly challenging, as essentially 100% of the white population has this antigen.

She also has a warm autoantibody that adds extra time for antibody testing and crossmatching. Finally, she also receives K-negative RBCs to prevent alloimmunization, as this practice of extended phenotype matching is common for patients with SCD. Thus, the patient requires RBC units for RCE that are negative for 6 antigens: C, E, K, Fy^a, Fy^3, and Js^a. About 1% of blood donors in the US are negative for all 6 antigens [11].

Her hematologist informed us that she had multiple experiences with the following type of delay in procuring blood. She would visit our apheresis clinic a day before her scheduled RCE to draw a blood sample for antibody screening and crossmatching of RBC units. This 1-day lead time would often be insufficient. That is, 8–10 suitable units would not be ready the next day because the antibody testing would take at least several hours to a day, and more importantly, the order for several units of RBCs that lacked all 6 of the above antigens could not be routinely fulfilled in just one day.

The patient would show up the next day for her scheduled RCE appointment, and the apheresis nurse would discover that not all of the expected RBC units were available. Thus, the RCE would have to be delayed one or more days. The patient would be told this only after she had arrived for her RCE appointment. In sum, these last-minute cancellations caused inconveniences and treatment delays.

As different people are on apheresis service at different times and, therefore, encountered this particular patient at different times, the apheresis physicians, nurses, and blood bank technologists did not immediately notice these repeated last-minute cancellations for this patient. We credit the hematologist for bringing this problem to our attention.

While we have indicated the main problem and introduced the basics of the process, we will now describe the old process in more detail as well as the changes we made.

3. The Process Challenge and Improvement

3.1. Transfusion of SCD Patients at the UWHC. At the University of Wisconsin Hospital and Clinics (UWHC), approximately 15–20 SCD patients regularly receive outpatient RCEs at an interval of 1 to 4 months between RCEs. Currently, the UWHC blood bank (UWBB) receives its blood products from the American Red Cross (ARC). The blood center does not have access to the UWHC patient information through our electronic medical record. Finally, at the UWHC, we prefer (but do not absolutely require) RBCs that are relatively fresh (<14 days old) for SCD patients to maximize the RBC lifespan in the patient.

3.2. How ARC Maintains Its Inventory. The blood center has implemented several practical guidelines to maintain its inventory of blood products for SCD patients. Every day, based on the demographic information of the donors for that day, ARC identifies units that have a high probability of being used in the future for SCD patients. These include RBC phenotypes that are more common or relatively unique to the black population. These "sickle cell patient units" are stored on separate shelves for ease of access and improved organization.

Unused units are held for a maximum allowable shelf life of 42 days at the ARC. As stated earlier, relatively fresh units are preferred for RCEs for SCD patients at the UWHC. Therefore, once a unit goes past this date, it is usually not used at the UWHC but sent to other ARC branches that may need it.

3.3. Introduction to the Problem. After learning about the repeated delays for this patient with multiple alloantibodies, we investigated the root cause behind these delays and devised a new method to order blood products. We report both the old and new processes.

3.4. Old Process. The process of arranging an outpatient RCE for an SCD patient begins when a physician from the patient's clinical team (usually a hematologist) consults transfusion medicine. The transfusion medicine physician places the RCE order and communicates this to the apheresis nurse. The apheresis nurse makes an appointment for the patient.

The key step we wish to highlight is that the weekday before the RCE, the nurse instructs the UWBB to obtain the required number of compatible units. The UWBB technologist then orders the RBC units from the ARC. An antibody screen is obtained the day of the procedure or the day before, but historical data are used to informally begin the search for units. Thus, in our old process, we typically gave our blood supplier around one day advance notice. This worked well for most SCD patients who had no or few alloantibodies.

As stated earlier, the ARC does not have direct access to UWHC patient information, and therefore, the computerized transfusion appointment made would not be "visible" to the ARC. Therefore, transfusion appointments and the required number of antibody-compatible units had to be communicated separately to the ARC.

The ARC obtains the required number of antibody-compatible units from various locations. First, the ARC identifies relatively fresh compatible units on their "sickle cell shelf." If adequate units are not available from there, our local ARC contacts other ARC branches to obtain additional units.

There were a few disadvantages and inconveniences caused by this method. The main one was that only one day was available to the ARC to identify compatible units. Moreover, due to time limitations, tradeoffs had to be made regarding the freshness of the unit. In some cases, older units had to be used. This is not optimal for the patient because of the shorter RBC lifespan. As we noted, in some instances, RCEs needed to be postponed by a few days to provide more time for the ARC to obtain enough units.

3.5. New Process. Once we identified the pattern in these delays, we resolved to improve our process and decrease these delays. We applied the basic principles of the theory of constraints in the field of systems engineering [12]. We identified that the key constraint was the short time available to the ARC to find units. In other words, this was the rate-limiting step that was causing delays. Thus, our goal was to increase this lead time significantly.

It was not self-evident what the best process would be. Several ideas were generated and considered. Ideally, there would be a wholly automated or computerized solution, but this is not feasible because the blood center cannot access our appointment data directly.

Thus, we devised the following new process. the UWHC and UWBB would communicate with the ARC before the scheduled outpatient RCE appointment with the following details. The process remained the same before and after the apheresis nurse's steps. However, instead of waiting until the day before the RCE, we added a step for the nurse to e-mail the UWBB's senior technologists at the same time that the nurse makes the patient's next RCE appointment. The UWBB senior tech receives this e-mail and uses this as the signal to order RBCs from the blood center about 6–8 weeks before this patient's next RCE. Thus, the order is received by the blood center at least 7 days in advance of the RCE and, in many cases, several weeks in advance.

The processes for the ARC to communicate to the UWBB and for the UWBB to communicate with the clinical teams are "push" processes. If the units are on track to be available, then no signals are sent. However, if a delay is anticipated to affect the availability of blood and the performance of the RCE at the planned time and date, then the ARC pushes this signal via e-mail to UWBB, and the UWBB in turn communicates this via the transfusion medicine resident to the clinical team.

4. Follow-Up

We can report anecdotally of several advantages of this new process. Since implementing this new process, the most important improvement has been that the metric of "delays due to blood procurement for outpatient RCEs" has dropped to zero. In other words, the anecdotally observed number of delays greater than 2 hours went from nonzero in the era before this intervention to zero after this intervention was implemented around 5 years before we write this.

5. Discussion

To our knowledge, a process to ensure the ordering of RBCs at least 7 advance of a scheduled outpatient RCE has not been reported in the medical literature. However, we do not claim that this process is necessarily novel or unique, as colleagues at other institutions may have created similar processes without publishing them.

This may seem like a relatively mundane and trivial change, but sometimes, small modifications can be leveraged to produce large effects. Namely, the lead time for the blood supplier was increased from 1 day to 7 days, and the probability of a treatment delay or last-minute cancellation by us essentially drops to zero. All this is due to a simple e-mail from the apheresis nurse to the blood bank senior technologists. The e-mails between nurses, techs, and blood supplier contacts are HIPAA compliant. Verification emails are sent to confirm receipt and next steps. Moreover, both before and after this process change, the electronic ordering process between the UWBB and the ARC is and remains a manual process.

While this process does not replace the necessary antibody screen that is usually drawn the day before the red cell exchange, the historical phenotyping and antibody specificity results allow the blood center to begin the preliminary search for suitable RBC units. In most cases, the patient's historical antibody data turn out to be the same as the data from the actual sample that is used for the official search.

One tradeoff is that this increased preparedness comes at the expense of an increased risk of wasted effort and, in the worst case of a patient cancellation or no show, potentially wasted RBC units. In other words, because we are finding units farther in advance, we rely more heavily on patient compliance in order to actually use those units for the exchange. In short, increasing the lead time inevitably decreases the window of a "penalty-free" patient cancellation. One practical implication is that this process may not be optimal for a patient who has a proven track record of no shows.

Finally, this process improvement is not directly relevant to emergency or unplanned acute RCEs. An advance notice of weeks or even hours is not feasible for such procedures. We recommend an excellent process analysis for emergency RCEs [10]. However, our key strategy of ordering RBCs as soon as possible to minimize delays from this rate-limiting step still applies to the acute setting. For example, one could create a process that prioritizes the ordering of RBCs as one of the very first steps for an acute RCE. Our literature search did not yield any articles that describe a process similar to our new process specifically for scheduled outpatient RCEs, so we share it here.

6. Conclusions

Despite many variations in operational practices across the world, we believe that our basic idea, maximize the lead time to the blood supplier, may be useful to any service that provides scheduled outpatient red cell exchanges.

Abbreviations

SCD:	Sickle cell disease
RBC:	Red blood cell
RCE:	Red cell exchange
DHTR:	Delayed hemolytic transfusion reaction
HIPAA:	Health Insurance Portability and Accountability Act
HHS:	Hyperhemolysis syndrome
UWHC:	Wisconsin Hospital and Clinics
UWBB:	UWHC blood bank
ARC:	American Red Cross.

References

[1] A. Padmanabhan, L. Connelly-Smith, N. Aqui et al., "Guidelines on the use of therapeutic apheresis in clinical practice - evidence-based approach from the writing committee of the American society for apheresis: the eighth special issue," *Journal of Clinical Apheresis*, vol. 34, no. 3, pp. 171–354, 2019.

[2] S. Wahl and K. C. Quirolo, "Current issues in blood transfusion for sickle cell disease," *Current Opinion in Pediatrics*, vol. 21, no. 1, pp. 15–21, 2009.

[3] B. Aygun, S. Padmanabhan, C. Paley, and V. Chandrasekaran, "Clinical significance of RBC alloantibodies and autoantibodies in sickle cell patients who received transfusions," *Transfusion*, vol. 42, no. 1, pp. 37–43, 2002.

[4] S. A. Campbell-Lee and R. A. Kittles, "Red blood cell alloimmunization in sickle cell disease: listen to your ancestors," *Transfusion Medicine and Hemotherapy*, vol. 41, no. 6, p. 6, 2014.

[5] J.-A. M. Talano, C. A. Hillery, J. L. Gottschall, D. M. Baylerian, and J. P. Scott, "Delayed hemolytic transfusion reaction/hyperhemolysis syndrome in children with sickle cell disease," *Pediatrics*, vol. 111, no. 6, pp. e661–e665, 2003.

[6] L. E. Lee, B. W. Beeler, B. C. Graham, A. P. Cap, N. Win, and F. Chen, "Posttransfusion hyperhemolysis is arrested by targeting macrophage activation with novel use of Tocilizumab," *Transfusion*, vol. 60, no. 1, pp. 30–35, 2020.

[7] S. T. Chou, M. Alsawas, R. M. Fasano et al., "American society of Hematology 2020 guidelines for sickle cell disease: transfusion support," *Blood Advances*, vol. 4, no. 2, pp. 327–355, 2020.

[8] M. R. DeBaun, L. C. Jordan, A. A. King et al., "American Society of Hematology 2020 guidelines for sickle cell disease: prevention, diagnosis, and treatment of cerebrovascular disease in children and adults," *Blood Advances*, vol. 4, no. 8, pp. 1554–1588, 2020.

[9] A. M. Brandow, C. P. Carroll, S. Creary et al., "American Society of Hematology 2020 guidelines for sickle cell disease: management of acute and chronic pain," *Blood Advances*, vol. 4, no. 12, pp. 2656–2701, 2020.

[10] J. A. Smith, J. N. Seheult, J. Sevcik, J. E. Kiss, and A. Kaplan, "Process mapping of the urgent red cell exchange procedure for patients with severe complications of sickle cell disease at a centralized hemapheresis service," *Journal of Clinical Apheresis*, vol. 35, no. 5, pp. 427–434, 2020.

[11] P. D. Issitt and D. J. Anstee, *Applied Blood Group Serology*, Montgomery Scientific Publications, Durham, NC, 1998.

[12] E. M. Goldratt, *Theory of Constraints*, Croton-on-Hudson, North River, 1990.

10

False-Negative Platelet Factor 4 Antibodies and Serotonin Release Assay and the Utility of Repeat Testing in the Diagnosis of Heparin-Induced Thrombocytopenia and Thrombosis

Tarig Omer, Naresh Mullaguri, Pravin George, and Christopher R. Newey

Department of Neurointensive Care, Cerebrovascular Center, Cleveland Clinic Foundation, 9500 Euclid Avenue, Cleveland, Ohio 44195, USA

Correspondence should be addressed to Naresh Mullaguri; mullaguri.nari@gmail.com

Academic Editor: Simon Davidson

Objective. To report a case of false-negative serological tests in the diagnosis of heparin-induced thrombocytopenia (HIT) followed by a brief review of the literature on this topic. *Case Presentation.* A 75-year-old Caucasian female patient was admitted with a traumatic right ankle fracture that required open reduction and internal fixation. Despite postoperative subcutaneous heparin chemoprophylaxis, she developed deep vein thrombosis (DVT) and pulmonary embolism (PE) on day 4 and subsequently started on continuous heparin infusion. On day 5, she suffered a stroke from a complete occlusion of the right common carotid artery with tandem occlusion of the right middle cerebral artery. She underwent successful thrombectomy of both arteries. The proposed stroke mechanism was paradoxical embolism through a patent foramen ovale. Over the next few days, thrombocytopenia was noted, the heparin drip was stopped, and HIT antibodies (antibodies targeting the complex of platelet factor 4 and heparin; PF4-H AB) and serotonin release assay (SRA) tests were sent. Because of the suspicion for HIT, she was started on bivalirudin with subsequent improvement in platelet count. Initial PF4-H AB and SRA tests were negative, bivalirudin was stopped, and heparin was restarted. Subsequently, her platelets trended down, again raising clinical suspicion of HIT. Repeat PF4-H AB and SRA testing resulted positive. *Conclusions.* A positive SRA in the appropriate context is considered for the diagnosis of heparin-induced thrombocytopenia. This case report highlights that false-negative serological evaluation is possible early in the course of the disease. Repeat testing is recommended in patients with high clinical suspicion.

1. Background

Heparin-induced thrombocytopenia (HIT) should be suspected in patients with sudden thrombocytopenia and signs of thrombosis after exposure to unfractionated or low-molecular weight heparin [1, 2]. The pathophysiology of HIT involves endogenous antibodies targeting platelet factor 4 complexed with heparin (PF4-H AB) that causes catastrophic platelet aggregation resulting in predominantly venous and rarely arterial thrombosis and embolism [3]. HIT is considered a rare etiology for ischemic stroke outside of the context of cerebral venous thrombosis [4, 5]. Once HIT is suspected, systemic hypercoagulability should be managed with nonheparin anticoagulants such as bivalirudin or argatroban. Serological evaluation of PF4-H AB antibodies and SRA should be completed before restarting a heparin anticoagulant [1, 3]. The PF4-H AB antibody is considered a very sensitive screening test, and together with a positive SRA in the correct clinical context, it is considered to be virtually diagnostic of heparin-induced thrombocytopenia [6–8]. False-negative PF4-H AB and SRA are reported only early in the course of disease and in patients receiving immunosuppression, massive blood transfusions, or plasmapheresis [8–12]. This manuscript highlights false-negative early serological testing in HIT, stresses the importance of repeat serological testing if there is strong clinical suspicion, and provides a brief review of the pertinent literature.

2. Case Presentation

A 75-year-old Caucasian female with a history of hypertension and well-controlled type 2 diabetes mellitus was admitted after open reduction and internal fixation of an ankle fracture. She was treated with subcutaneous unfractionated heparin (5000 IU three times a day) for deep vein thrombosis (DVT) prophylaxis from day 1. On day 4, a DVT and pulmonary embolism (PE) workup was completed after she developed acute shortness of breath and tachycardia with hypoxemia. DVT and subocclusive saddle-shaped PE were both noted (Figure 1), and she was started on a continuous heparin infusion. The following day she developed sudden onset of left-sided weakness and rightward gaze deviation concerning acute ischemic stroke. CT angiogram of the head and neck and subsequent MRI brain revealed a stroke caused by right-sided common carotid artery occlusion with thrombus extending into the external and internal carotid arteries. A tandem occlusion of inferior branch of the right middle cerebral artery was also noted on cerebral angiography (Figure 1). The patient underwent successful mechanical thrombectomy of the right carotid artery bifurcation thrombus. After the endovascular procedure, thrombocytopenia (153,000/μL to 94,000/μL) was noted. Clinical suspicion was raised for HIT and PF4-H AB, and SRA tests were sent. Heparin infusion was stopped, and she was started on continuous bivalirudin infusion. Transthoracic echocardiogram with bubble study revealed a patent foramen ovale (PFO) with right to left shunting, and the etiology of stroke was presumed a paradoxical embolism. On hospital day 7, PF4-H AB (optical density (OD) < 0.103) and SRA tests resulted negative with uptrending platelet count (105,000/μL) (Figure 2). Bivalirudin was subsequently stopped, and the patient was restarted on therapeutic continuous heparin infusion due to reduced suspicion of HIT as a result of the negative serological tests. From day 8, platelets started to downtrend to 36,000/μL. Clinical re-emergence of HIT was suspected, and heparin infusion was held. Repeat PF4-H AB antibody and SRA tests were sent and resulted positive. The patient was treated with bivalirudin and bridged successfully to warfarin with recovery of platelet count (205,000/μL). She suffered no further thromboembolic events and was eventually discharged to an inpatient rehabilitation facility.

3. Discussion

PF4-H AB and SRA testing can be reported as falsely negative early in the course of the disease in patients with HIT possibly due to low antibody titers [11, 12]. In cases with high clinical suspicion, repeat testing is warranted [8, 12]. DVTs and PE are the most frequent complications of HIT, followed by peripheral arterial thrombosis and stroke [3]. Myocardial infarction is uncommon [13]. The typical onset of thrombocytopenia in HIT occurs 5 to 10 days after the initiation of any heparin therapy [3]. HIT within 24 hours of heparin exposure may be suspected if the patient was exposed to heparin in the previous one to three months and has circulating antibodies [3, 14]. Delayed-onset HIT, in which thrombocytopenia and thrombosis occur after heparin has been withdrawn, is also described; however, the incidence is unknown [14, 15]. Life-threatening thrombosis, amputation, or death is reported if the diagnosis of HIT is missed, characterizing the severity of the disease [1, 3].

There are two types of immunoassays to detect HIT. The first type is an enzyme-linked immunosorbent assay (ELISA) to measure PF4-H AB antibodies quantitatively. The second type is a functional platelet assay called the SRA, which measures the ability of the antibodies from a patient's serum to activate platelets. The PF4-H AB ELISA test is widely available, fast, and straightforward to interpret but has a high incidence of false-positive results [16]. The SRA strongly correlates with the presence of the HIT syndrome and is considered the gold standard with sensitivity and specificity of >95 percent; however, generally it takes a longer time to result and is not widely available [1, 3, 7]. The SRA is generally reserved for those with indeterminate immunoassays (i.e., ELISA with optical density (OD) from 0.40 to 2.00) or those for whom the clinical picture and immunoassay results are discordant [6]. Cases of false-positive and false-negative PF4-H AB ELISA with SRA test have been reported [9–11]. Case reports of the negative serological evaluation of HIT are also described by Jones et al., Patel and Varga early in the disease course [11, 12]. Senzel and Coldren reported false-negative assay after massive blood transfusion, possibly due to dilution of antibodies below the limit of detection [10]. Iluonakhamhe et al. report a case of HIT in the setting of acute intracerebral hemorrhage managed with plasmapheresis. After four cycles, both heparin antibody ELISA and functional assays became negative [17].

In our patient, the false-negative PF4-H AB and SRA may have been secondary to low levels of antibodies early in the disease [11]. It is also possible that there was a lab technical error. It is suggested and highlighted by this report that clinicians be aware of false-negative results when testing for serological markers of HIT. In patients with high clinical suspicion for HIT, even in the presence of negative serological testing, we propose that clinicians closely follow their clinical course and platelet trends and switch to a nonheparin anticoagulant as clinically indicated. Repeat PF4-H AB antibody and SRA testing may help confirm a HIT diagnosis if initial early test results are negative.

4. Conclusions

PF4-H AB ELISA with SRA testing in the appropriate clinical context is considered the gold standard for the diagnosis of HIT; however, false-negative serological evaluation is possible early in the course of the disease. Repeat testing of PF4-H AB ELISA and SRA is recommended in patients with high clinical suspicion who initially test negative.

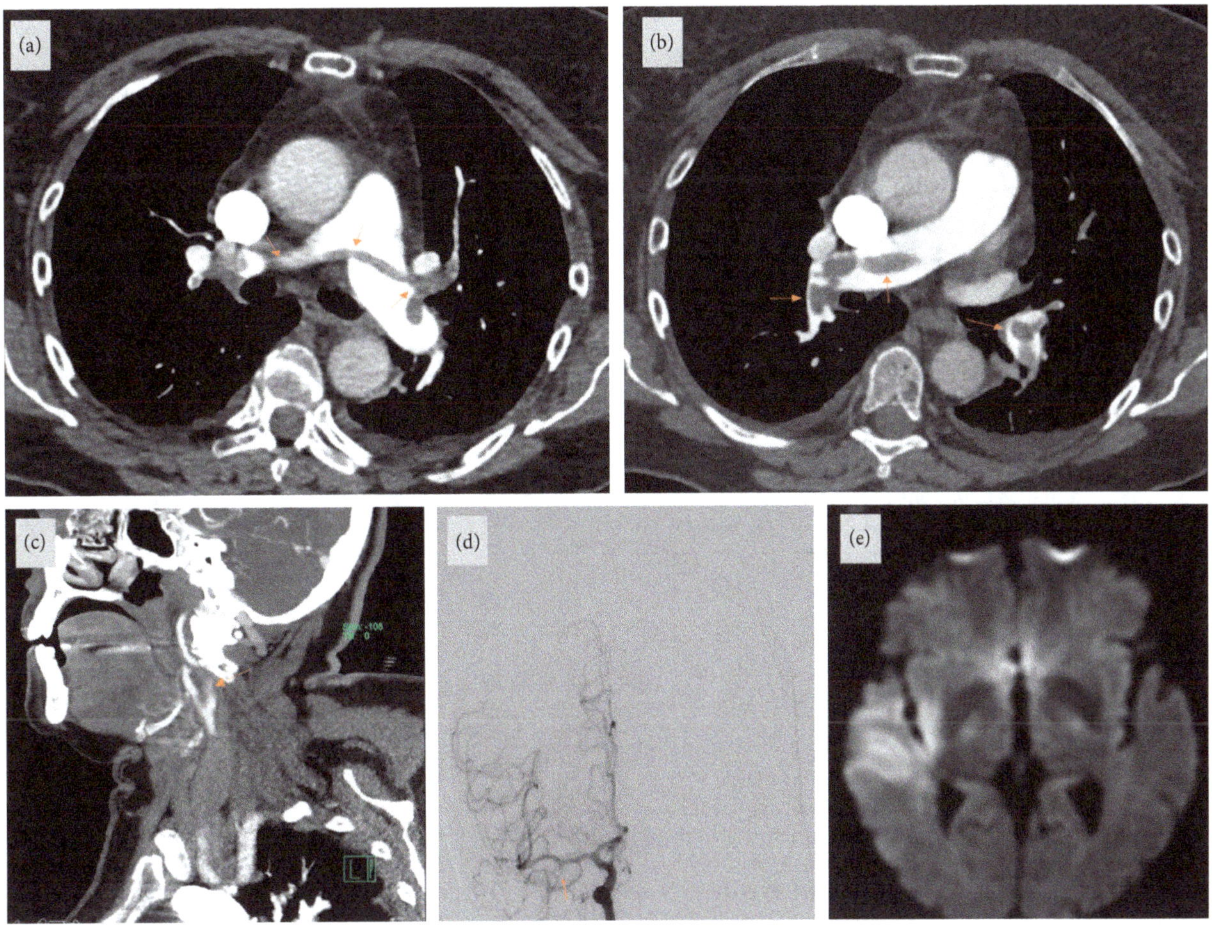

FIGURE 1: (a, b) Computerized tomography angiography of the chest (axial images) showing "saddle" shaped thrombus in the pulmonary artery bifurcation extending into both trunks (arrows); (c) computerized tomography angiography of the neck (sagittal view) showing right common carotid artery bifurcation showing "saddle-shaped" thrombus in the external and internal carotid arteries (arrow); (d) digital subtraction angiography with selective right internal carotid artery injection showing middle cerebral artery inferior division occlusion (arrow); (e) magnetic resonance imaging of the brain diffusion-weighted imaging axial section showing right frontotemporal area infarction corresponding to the middle cerebral artery inferior branch occlusion.

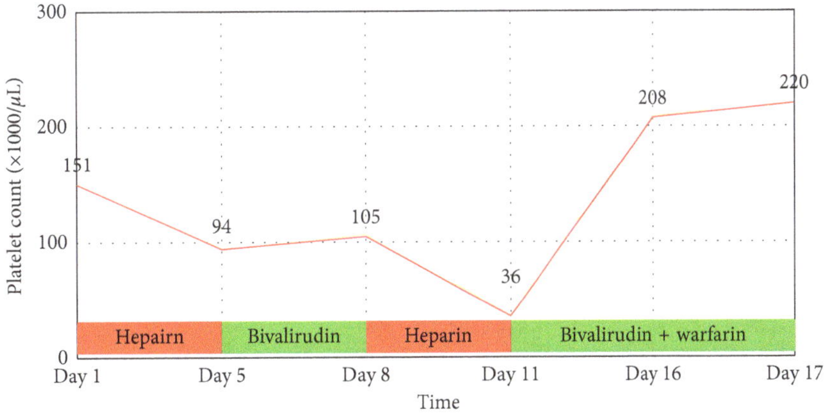

FIGURE 2: Patient's platelet trend during hospitalization while on unfractionated heparin and bivalirudin infusion.

Disclosure

This work was presented as a poster at Cleveland Clinic Neurological Institute Trainee Research Day Meeting 2018 and at the Neurocritical Care Society 16th Annual Meeting.

References

[1] G. M. Lee and G. M. Arepally, "Heparin-induced thrombocytopenia," *Hematology*, vol. 2013, no. 1, pp. 668–674, 2013.

[2] N. Martel, J. Lee, and P. S. Wells, "Risk for heparin-induced thrombocytopenia with unfractionated and low-molecular-weight heparin thromboprophylaxis: a meta-analysis," *Blood*, vol. 106, no. 8, pp. 2710–2715, 2005.

[3] C. G. Solomon and A. Greinacher, "Heparin-induced thrombocytopenia," *New England Journal of Medicine*, vol. 373, no. 3, pp. 252–261, 2015.

[4] C. Pohl, T. Klockgether, A. Greinacher, P. Hanfland, and U. Harbrecht, "Neurological complications in heparin-induced thrombocytopenia," *The Lancet*, vol. 353, no. 9165, pp. 1678-1679, 1999.

[5] M. P. LaMonte, P. M. Brown, and M. J. Hursting, "Stroke in patients with heparin-induced thrombocytopenia and the effect of argatroban therapy," *Critical Care Medicine*, vol. 32, no. 4, pp. 976–980, 2004.

[6] T. E. Warkentin, J. I. Sheppard, J. C. Moore, C. S. Sigouin, and J. G. Kelton, "Quantitative interpretation of optical density measurements using PF4-dependent enzyme-immunoassays," *Journal of Thrombosis and Haemostasis*, vol. 6, no. 8, pp. 1304–1312, 2008.

[7] T. E. Warkentin, D. M. Arnold, I. Nazi, and J. G. Kelton, "The platelet serotonin-release assay," *American Journal of Hematology*, vol. 90, no. 6, pp. 564–572, 2015.

[8] M. Chan, E. Malynn, B. Shaz, and L. Uhl, "Utility of consecutive repeat HIT ELISA testing for heparin-induced thrombocytopenia," *American Journal of Hematology*, vol. 83, no. 3, pp. 212–217, 2008.

[9] T. E. Warkentin, J.-A. I. Sheppard, F. V. Chu, A. Kapoor, M. A. Crowther, and A. Gangji, "Plasma exchange to remove HIT antibodies: dissociation between enzyme-immunoassay and platelet activation test reactivities," *Blood*, vol. 125, no. 1, pp. 195–198, 2014.

[10] L. Senzel and D. Coldren, "Negative heparin-induced thrombocytopenia test result after massive transfusion," *American Journal of Clinical Pathology*, vol. 145, no. 5, pp. 717–719, 2016.

[11] C. G. Jones, S. M. Pechauer, B. R. Curtis et al., "A platelet factor 4-dependent platelet activation assay facilitates early detection of pathogenic heparin-induced thrombocytopenia antibodies," *Chest*, vol. 152, no. 4, pp. e77–e80, 2017.

[12] R. Patel and C. Varga, "Heparin-induced thrombocytopenia in a cardiac surgery patient with early and persistent thrombocytopenia and initial negative immunological and functional assays," *Thrombosis Research*, vol. 169, pp. 93–95, 2018.

[13] A. Greinacher, B. Farner, H. Kroll, T. Kohlmann, T. E. Warkentin, and P. Eichler, "Clinical features of heparin-induced thrombocytopenia including risk factors for thrombosis. A retrospective analysis of 408 patients," *Thromb Haemost*, vol. 94, no. 1, pp. 132–135, 2005.

[14] T. E. Warkentin and R. A. Bernstein, "Delayed-onset heparin-induced thrombocytopenia and cerebral thrombosis after a single administration of unfractionated heparin," *New England Journal of Medicine*, vol. 348, no. 11, pp. 1067–1069, 2003.

[15] M. Refaai, T. Warkentin, M. Axelson, K. Matevosyan, and R. Sarode, "Delayed-onset heparin-induced thrombocytopenia, venous thromboembolism, and cerebral venous thrombosis: a consequence of heparin "flushes"," *Thrombosis and Haemostasis*, vol. 98, no. 5, pp. 1139-1140, 2017.

[16] A. Cuker, P. A. Gimotty, M. A. Crowther, and T. E. Warkentin, "Predictive value of the 4Ts scoring system for heparin-induced thrombocytopenia: a systematic review and meta-analysis," *Blood*, vol. 120, no. 20, pp. 4160–4167, 2012.

[17] E. Iluonakhamhe, O. Ibekwe, S. Samuel, and A. Zakaria, "Plasmapheresis may be an option in urgent management of heparin-induced thrombocytopenia in the setting of acute intracerebral hemorrhage," *Neurocritical Care*, vol. 22, no. 1, pp. 140–145, 2014.

11

Development of Multiple Myeloma of the IgA Type in a Patient with Cold Agglutinin Disease: Transformation or Coincidence?

Øystein Sefland,[1] Ulla Randen,[2] and Sigbjørn Berentsen[3]

[1]*Section of Hematology, Department of Medicine, Haukeland University Hospital, Bergen, Norway*
[2]*Department of Pathology, Akershus University Hospital, Lørenskog, Norway*
[3]*Department of Research and Innovation, Haugesund Hospital, Haugesund, Norway*

Correspondence should be addressed to Sigbjørn Berentsen; sigbjorn.berentsen@haugnett.no

Academic Editor: Masayuki Nagasawa

Cold agglutinin disease (CAD) is an autoimmune hemolytic anemia and a distinct, clonal bone marrow lymphoproliferative disorder, characterized in most cases by a monoclonal IgMκ serum protein. We describe a CAD patient presenting with a monoclonal immunoglobulin of the IgAλ class. For years, she remained asymptomatic apart from the hemolytic anemia until eventually she developed multiple myeloma (MM) of the IgAλ phenotype. Prior to the development of MM, her hemolytic anemia responded to rituximab monotherapy. After she was diagnosed with MM, both conditions responded well to bortezomib-based therapy. We performed further investigations to determine whether her MM represented a progression/transformation of CAD or an independent disease. Flow cytometry and biopsy findings convincingly confirmed two unrelated clonal B-cell disorders. On this background, we also discuss previously published reports on cold agglutinin activity in patients with IgA gammopathy. In conclusion, cold agglutinins of the IgA class do probably not result in CAD. If a monoclonal immunoglobulin other than IgMκ is found in a patient with CAD, the coexistence of two unrelated B-cell clones should be suspected.

1. Introduction

Primary chronic cold agglutinin disease (CAD) is an uncommon type of autoimmune hemolytic anemia (AIHA) and is today considered a specific clonal B-cell lymphoproliferative disorder (LPD) of the bone marrow [1–4]. The involved autoantibodies, known as cold agglutinins (CAs), are monoclonal and directed against the erythrocyte surface carbohydrate antigen termed I [2, 5]. CAs in CAD are almost invariably of the immunoglobulin (Ig) Mk class, whereas descriptions of IgG or IgA immune phenotypes are rare, as it is λ light chain restriction [6–9]. CAD mainly affects elderly or middle-aged people with a median age of 72 years [7].

The underlying bone marrow lymphoproliferation, when demonstrable, is clearly indolent by histology and can hardly be considered a malignant disease in a clinical sense. Median survival has been estimated to be 12.5 years from diagnosis, which does probably not differ much from the general expected survival in this elderly population [7]. Transformation to aggressive lymphoma is an uncommon event, shown to occur in only 3-4% of the patients during a median observation period of more than 10 years [7]. Transformation to, or coexistence with, multiple myeloma (MM) has only been reported in a couple of cases worldwide [9].

Herein, we describe a patient with a stable CAD and an IgAλ monoclonal spike on serum electrophoresis, who for years remained asymptomatic apart from the hemolytic anemia and then developed MM of the IgAλ phenotype. We consider this report highly relevant for colleagues caring for patients with CAD, in particular those who might encounter patients with CAD of apparent non-IgM phenotype.

2. Case Presentation

A woman in her late 60s was transferred in July 2012 from her local hospital because of anemia of at least one and a half year duration. She had no relevant family history, but had been treated for diabetes type 2 and hypertension for decades and paroxysmal atrial fibrillation for a few years. She had suffered from recurrent urinary tract infections, several times with fever and once with verified urosepsis. A concrement had been removed from her right ureter a few months ago.

Her history of anemia started gradually with fatigue in 2010-11. Her hemoglobin (Hb) level was 8.9 g/dL in February 2011, as compared to 13.4 at the last known previous assessment in 2008. She had received an erythrocyte transfusion at her local hospital without any transfusion reaction or other problems, and she had already suffered several exacerbations of anemia during febrile infections. There was no history of acrocyanosis or Raynaud phenomena.

On admission, she was in good general condition and did not present any pathological findings by physical examination. In particular, there was no acrocyanosis, lymphadenopathy, or splenomegaly. Chest radiography and abdominal ultrasonography were unremarkable. Hb was 8.2 g/dL, leukocytes 7.8×10^9/L with normal differential count, platelets 263×10^9/L, mean corpuscular volume (MCV) 99 fL, reticulocytes 88×10^9/L, and C-reactive protein (CRP) 11 mg/L. Serum levels of iron, transferrin, cobalamin, and folic acid as well as transferrin saturation were within the reference range, however, with elevated ferritin at 1257 μg/L. Genetic screening for hemochromatosis showed no HFE gene abnormalities. Concentrations of electrolytes, calcium, creatinine, and liver transaminases were normal. Lactate dehydrogenase (LDH) was elevated at 544 U/L, bilirubin elevated at 43 μmol/L, while haptoglobin was undetectable (less than 0.1 g/L). Her urine was negative for hemoglobin and protein. Serum albumin was 41 g/L with normal immunoglobulin levels (IgG 7.0 g/L, IgA 3.2 g/L, and IgM 0.69 g/L). Serum electrophoresis identified a small spike of monoclonal IgAλ. Free λ chains in serum were slightly elevated at 53 mg/L, however, with a κ/λ ratio within the reference range. The direct antiglobulin test (DAT) was strongly positive for C3d and negative for IgG, IgM, and IgA. CA titer at 4°C was 128. Serum erythropoietin was slightly elevated at 36 IU/L.

Based on these findings, she was diagnosed with CA-mediated AIHA. With a chronic course, no signs of malignancy so far, and no recent specific infection, this AIHA was further classified as primary CAD. A bone marrow trephine biopsy showed erythroid hyperplasia and small lymphocytic infiltrates interpreted as lymphoplasmacytic lymphoma (LPL). Flow cytometry in bone marrow aspirate revealed two small, clonal populations: one of B-lymphocytes that displayed a κ phenotype and the other one of λ positive plasma cells.

The further development in Hb and IgA levels is shown in Figure 1. During the next couple of years, Hb ranged from 9.0 to 10.0 g/dL; she had only mild fatigue and no transfusion requirement. Management consisted of regular follow-up, avoidance of cold exposure, and prompt antibiotic therapy in case of febrile bacterial infection but no CAD-directed pharmacological therapy. By 2014, a second bone marrow biopsy showed erythroid hyperplasia and lymphoid infiltrates, now interpreted as probable CAD-associated LPD [4]. Flow cytometry in bone marrow aspirate again demonstrated 2 pathological clones of κ positive B-lymphocytes (approximately 5%) and λ positive plasma cells (0.7%), respectively.

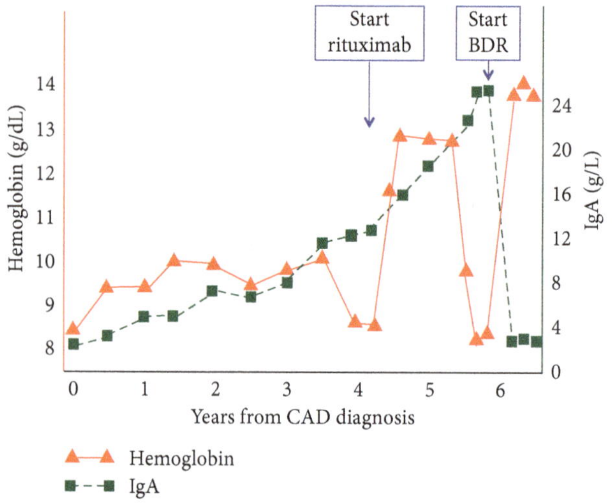

FIGURE 1: Changes in hemoglobin and IgA levels. BDR: bortezomib, dexamethasone, and rituximab combination therapy. CAD: cold agglutinin disease.

Her condition remained stable until late spring 2016, when she deteriorated. Her fatigue worsened, her atrial fibrillation relapsed more frequently, and her Hb level declined to 8.5 g/dL. The reticulocyte count was now elevated at 191×10^9/L, LDH was 303 U/L, bilirubin 96 μmol/L, haptoglobin <0.1 g/L, while IgA had increased to 12.5 g/L and CA titer to 512. The DAT findings were unchanged. We decided to give her rituximab monotherapy [10], four weekly doses of 375 mg/m^2, which she received from August 2016. Hb rose to 12.5 g/dL by December 2016, while bilirubin and LDH normalized. Unexpectedly, however, her IgA level continued to increase from 12.5 g/L immediately before rituximab treatment to 19.6 g/L by January 2017.

From June 2017, Hb started again to decline and IgA continued to increase. In January 2018, she experienced severe lumbar pain after having removed snow from her courtyard, which can be heavy work in Norway. One month later, Hb was 9.5 g/dL, while the absolute reticulocyte count was 153×10^9/L and the levels of LDH, bilirubin, and haptoglobin had not changed significantly. The IgA level was 24.5 g/L and β2-microglobulin 3.5 mg/L. A new trephine biopsy showed hypercellular bone marrow affected by 20% infiltration of monoclonal, λ positive plasma cells, and some small lymphocytic infiltrates. A CT scan showed osteolytic lesions of the skull but no relevant pathological findings in her spine, pelvis, or femora. She was diagnosed with development of MM.

In February 2018, a local visiting hematologist initiated a cycle of melphalan and prednisolone. During the next couple of weeks, Hb declined further to 8.0 g/dL, however, without any neutropenia or thrombocytopenia. Concomitantly, a rise in bilirubin and LDH was observed, and she was diagnosed with an exacerbation of CAD. Melphalan and prednisolone were discontinued after the first cycle.

Hoping to induce remission of both MM and CAD, we decided in March 2018 to offer her bortezomib-based therapy [11] with the addition of dexamethasone and rituximab [10, 12, 13]. She received four cycles at four weeks' interval of bortezomib (1.3 mg/m^2 weekly for 3 weeks), rituximab (375 mg/m^2 once per treatment cycle), and dexamethasone (20 mg on days 1, 2, 8, 9, 15, and 16). She tolerated this combination well; her Hb level increased from 8.0 g/dL to 13.6 g/dL following the first cycle and reached 14.4 g/dL after the second one. Bilirubin and LDH normalized within a couple of weeks, and reticulocyte count declined to the normal range (65×10^9/L). IgA had declined to 3.8 g/L by the start of the second cycle. Her back pain improved. Ten weeks after start of therapy, Hb was 13.2 g/L, bilirubin 7 μmol/L, LDH 247 U/L, haptoglobin 0.24 g/L, and CA titer 64. IgA remained in plateau at 3.9 g/L, while serum electrophoresis did not show any monoclonal spike. DAT was still positive for C3d.

2.1. Bone Marrow Biopsy Data, Revised. The lymphoma pathologist in our group (U.R.) did a centralized, parallel review of all three bone marrow samples based on extensive experience with CAD-associated bone marrow pathology [4]. The 2012 biopsy shows, in addition to erythroid hyperplasia, intraparenchymatous, κ positive B-cell infiltrates consistent with CAD-associated LPD. There are scattered κ positive plasma cells, more of them near the lymphocytic infiltrates, and one distinct infiltrate of λ positive plasma cells. In the 2014 biopsy, the picture has not changed significantly. The trephine biopsy from February 2018 shows an IgAλ positive plasma cell population that has expanded, but IgMκ positive B-cell infiltrates can still be seen. In retrospect, therefore, all three biopsies show two clones; and in the 2018 sample, the CAD-associated IgMκ plasma cell population seems "hidden" among the expanding, myeloma-associated IgAλ plasma cells (Figure 2).

3. Discussion

The patient history raises the question of whether she suffered a transformation of CAD-associated low-grade LPD to an overt B-cell malignancy or had two independent B-cell proliferative diseases. This issue also relates to previously published reports on IgA-mediated CAD.

CAD has been shown by our group and others to be a distinct, low-grade bone marrow LPD, typically different from LPL, marginal zone lymphoma, and other mature B-cell LPDs [4, 14, 15]. An underlying mutated B-cell clone seems present even in patients in whom no LPD or gammopathy is detected by electrophoresis, flow cytometry, or histology [16]. Transformation to aggressive B-cell lymphoma is a rare event, probably occurring in less than 4% of the patients during an observation period of more than 10 years [7]. In the vast majority, a monoclonal serum immunoglobulin can be demonstrated if sensitive techniques are used, most often of the IgMκ class [7, 17, 18]. However, IgA-CAs have been reported in a few cases [8].

Plasma cell neoplasms are classified into three stages: monoclonal gammopathy of undetermined significance (MGUS), smoldering myeloma (SMM), and multiple myeloma (MM), of which the last two are defined as malignant diseases and the MM stage is an indication for therapy [19–21]. With serum monoclonal IgA > 20 g/L, 20% clonal plasma cell infiltration in the bone marrow, skeletal pain, and several cranial osteolytic lesions, our patient had reached the MM stage by the beginning of 2018. MM and SMM are assumed to be preceded by MGUS in all cases [19]. The rate of progression to MM in individuals with IgG- or IgA-MGUS has been estimated to approximately 1% per year, with variations depending on risk factors [20]. MM is of the IgA subtype in approximately 25% of the patients [21].

In our patient, therefore, it was tempting to assume a progression or transformation of a low-grade LPD in CAD, also manifested by a monoclonal IgA gammopathy, to an established B-cell malignancy presenting as MM. Already in 2012, however, there was a discrepancy between the demonstration of a cell clone expressing the λ light chain phenotype, as shown by electrophoresis and histology, and the additional finding of κ positive clonal cells. In retrospect, all three bone marrow examinations provide evidence of two different B-cell clones, one compatible with gammopathy of the IgAλ class, starting with MGUS and progressing to MM, and the other one of the IgMκ phenotype and typical for CAD-associated LPD. The latter did not manifest as a detectable monoclonal gammopathy at any time. For the same reasons, it is highly unlikely that both clones could have evolved from a common early progenitor B-cell.

In patients with CAD responding to B-cell directed therapies, the clinical response with normalization of Hb and parameters of hemolysis is associated with a decrease in the involved monoclonal immunoglobulin and a regression of any morphological signs of LPD [10, 13]. In our patient, however, IgA continued to increase in parallel with the improvement of CAD following rituximab monotherapy. This fits well with the demonstration of two independent clones. The non-IgA nature of the CA in our patient might have been further confirmed by agglutination-elution techniques and electrophoresis of purified CA [17]. In theory, it might also have been possible to further confirm two different clones by molecular studies of cells sorted by flow cytometry-assisted cell sorting [15]. Currently, after achievement of remission with no detectable monoclonal protein and low CA titer, neither of these approaches will be feasible.

The reticulocyte count is usually, but not invariably, increased in patients with AIHA [18]. Based on the normal reticulocyte count at diagnosis, one might speculate whether the coexisting plasma cell clone inhibited the reticulocyte response in some way. However, the later development of reticulocytosis in parallel with the progression of the plasma cell clone excludes this possibility. The reticulocyte count

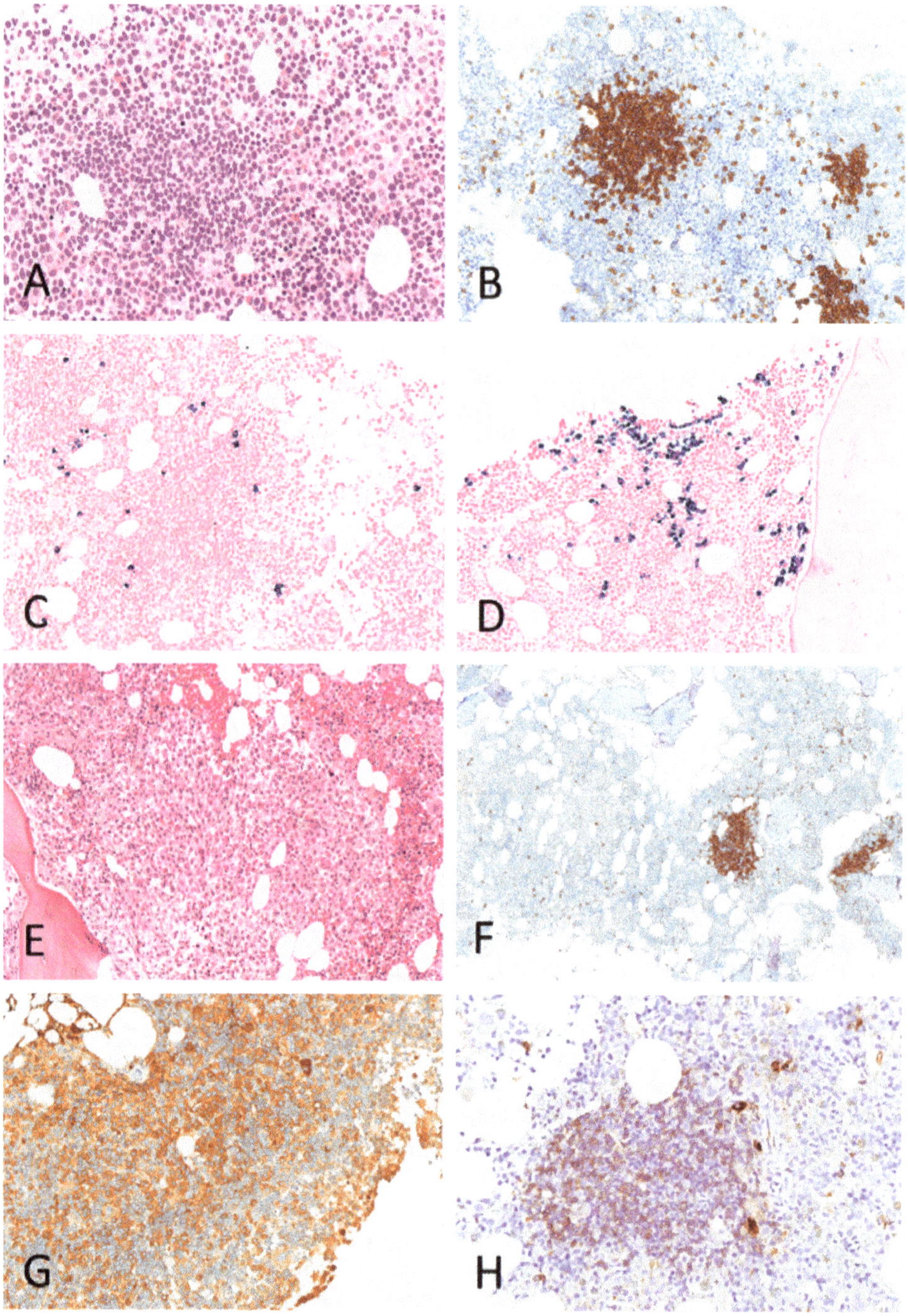

FIGURE 2: Bone marrow trephine biopsies from 2012 (a–d) and 2018 (e–h), respectively. The nodular lymphoid infiltrates (a) are CD20 positive (b) and surrounded by κ positive plasma cells (c), typical for CAD. In other areas, there are small focal aggregates of λ positive plasma cells (d), consistent with MGUS. In the 2018 biopsy, there is extensive plasma cell infiltration (e), consistent with MM. CD20 staining (f) shows remaining CD20 positive CAD infiltrates. The MM is IgA positive (g), whereas the CAD infiltrates are IgM positive (h).

normalized again after achievement of remission with abrogation of hemolysis.

Six case observations have previously been published describing IgA gammopathy in association with the occurrence of CA in serum. The three oldest reports described monoclonal CAs of the IgA class without hemolysis, that is, these individuals did not have CAD [8, 22, 23]. According to a fourth report, an IgA-CA was found to be an early manifestation of MM; this patient had clinical features of CAD, however, with marked symptoms of agglutination and only mild hemolysis [24]. A more recent paper described MM of the IgA type in a patient with CAD, but this report did not include sufficient data to determine whether the patient had one or two cell clones and whether the monoclonal IgA actually was the CA [9]. Römer et al. further characterized an IgA-CA from a subject without clinical CAD and found that this CA was not able to initiate the classical or alternative complement pathway [25]. This is in accordance with a body of evidence showing that erythrocyte-bound IgA does not activate complement

[26–28]. Activation of the classical complement pathway is essential for hemolysis in CAD [28, 29].

In conclusion, our patient who developed MM on a background of CAD did not suffer a progress or transformation of CAD-associated LPD but had two distinct disorders. Both CAD and MM responded well to bortezomib-based combination therapy, which is an established treatment option in MM [21]. The combination therapy seemed to induce a deeper remission of CAD as compared with previous rituximab monotherapy, with full normalization of Hb and haptoglobin levels. Therefore, the addition of bortezomib was probably important for this response. A recently published, small prospective trial of bortezomib therapy for CAD found 3 complete responses and 3 partial responses among 19 patients [11]. These response rates may seem low; however, the patients received only one single cycle of monotherapy. It is logical to hope, therefore, that combination therapy and/or extended treatment duration may yield higher response rates. The efficacy of such a combination therapy should be explored in a prospective trial.

In CAD patients with monoclonal gammopathy other than IgMκ, it should be emphasized that the demonstrable monoclonal serum immunoglobulin may not be identical to the CA. Such patients may have two distinct pathological cell clones and two independent diseases. Although IgA-CAs have been convincingly described, CAD of the IgA type does probably not exist.

Acknowledgments

We thank Lars Helgeland, Department of Pathology, Haukeland University Hospital, for examining two of the bone marrow biopsy samples and providing the blocks. We also thank the patient for permission to publish the case report.

References

[1] M. Michel, "Classification and therapeutic approaches in autoimmune hemolytic anemia: an update," *Expert Review of Hematology*, vol. 4, no. 6, pp. 607–618, 2011.

[2] S. Berentsen, "Cold agglutinin disease," *Hematology American Society of Hematology Education Program*, vol. 2016, no. 1, pp. 226–231, 2016.

[3] S. Berentsen, "How i manage patients with cold agglutinin disease," *British Journal of Haematology*, vol. 181, no. 3, pp. 320–330, 2018.

[4] U. Randen, G. Troen, A. Tierens et al., "Primary cold agglutinin-associated lymphoproliferative disease: a B-cell lymphoma of the bone marrow distinct from lymphoplasmacytic lymphoma," *Haematologica*, vol. 99, no. 3, pp. 497–504, 2014.

[5] E. Ulvestad, S. Berentsen, K. Bø, and F. V. Shammas, "Clinical immunology of chronic cold agglutinin disease," *European Journal of Haematology*, vol. 63, no. 4, pp. 259–266, 1999.

[6] P. L. Swiecicki, L. T. Hegerova, and M. A. Gertz, "Cold agglutinin disease," *Blood*, vol. 122, no. 7, pp. 1114–1121, 2013.

[7] S. Berentsen, E. Ulvestad, R Langholm et al., "Primary chronic cold agglutinin disease: a population based clinical study of 86 patients," *Haematologica*, vol. 91, no. 4, pp. 460–466, 2006.

[8] C. D. Angevine, B. R. Andersen, and E. V. Barnett, "A cold agglutinin of the IgA class," *Journal of Immunology*, vol. 96, no. 4, pp. 578–586, 1966.

[9] C. Chic Acevedo, E. García Torres, and M. Á. Álvarez Rivas, "Enfermedad por crioaglutinina del subtipo IgA como manifestación temprana de mieloma múltiple y resolución tras tratamiento con nuevos fármacos anti-mieloma," *Medicina Clínica*, vol. 147, no. 11, pp. e63–e64, 2016.

[10] S. Berentsen, E. Ulvestad, B. T. Gjertsen et al., "Rituximab for primary chronic cold agglutinin disease: a prospective study of 37 courses of therapy in 27 patients," *Blood*, vol. 103, no. 8, pp. 2925–2928, 2004.

[11] G. Rossi, D. Gramegna, F. Paoloni et al., "Short course of bortezomib in anemic patients with relapsed cold agglutinin disease: a phase 2 prospective GIMEMA study," *Blood*, vol. 132, no. 5, pp. 547–550, 2018.

[12] C. Schöllkopf, L. Kjeldsen, O. W. Bjerrum et al., "Rituximab in chronic cold agglutinin disease: a prospective study of 20 patients," *Leukemia & Lymphoma*, vol. 47, no. 2, pp. 253–260, 2006.

[13] S. Berentsen, U. Randen, M. Oksman et al., "Bendamustine plus rituximab for chronic cold agglutinin disease: results of a nordic prospective multicenter trial," *Blood*, vol. 130, no. 4, pp. 537–541, 2017.

[14] R. de Tute, A. Rawstron, P. Evans, and R. Owen, "Cold agglutinin disease is a phenotypically distinct clonal B-cell disorder," *Clinical Lymphoma Myeloma and Leukemia*, vol. 15, p. e184, 2015.

[15] A. Malecka, G. Trøen, A. Tierens et al., "Frequent somatic mutations of KMT2D (MLL2) and CARD11 genes in primary cold agglutinin disease," *British Journal of Haematology*, vol. 183, no. 5, pp. 838–842, 2018.

[16] C. Arthold, C. Skrabs, G. Mitterbauer-Hohendanner et al., "Cold antibody autoimmune hemolytic anemia and lymphoproliferative disorders: a retrospective study of 20 patients including clinical, hematological, and molecular findings," *Wiener Klinische Wochenschrift*, vol. 126, no. 11-12, pp. 376–382, 2014.

[17] M. Harboe, R. van Furth, H. Schubothe, K. Lind, and R. S. Evans, "Exclusive occurrence of k chains in isolated cold haemagglutinins," *Scandinavian Journal of Haematology*, vol. 2, no. 3, pp. 259–266, 1965.

[18] W. Barcellini, "New insights in the pathogenesis of autoimmune hemolytic anemia," *Transfusion Medicine and Hemotherapy*, vol. 42, no. 5, pp. 287–293, 2015.

[19] O. Landgren, R. A. Kyle, and S. V. Rajkumar, "From myeloma precursor disease to multiple myeloma: new diagnostic concepts and opportunities for early intervention," *Clinical Cancer Research*, vol. 17, no. 6, pp. 1243–1252, 2011.

[20] R. A. Kyle, ""Benign" monoclonal gammopathy-after 20 to 35 years of follow-up," *Mayo Clinic Proceedings*, vol. 68, no. 1, pp. 26–36, 1993.

[21] N. C. Munshi and S. Jagannath, "Plasma cell neoplasms," in *Hematology: Basic Principles and Practice*, R. Hoffman, E. J. Benz, L. E. Silberstein et al.pp. 1381–1418, Elsevier, Philadelphia, PA, USA, 7th edition, 2017.

[22] G. Garratty, L. D. Petz, I. Brodsky, and H. H. Fudenberg, "An IgA high-titer cold agglutinin with an unusual blood group specificity within the Pr complex," *Vox Sanguinis*, vol. 25, no. 1, pp. 32–38, 1973.

[23] H. Tonthat, H. Rochant, A. Henry, M. Leporrier, and B. Dreyfus, "A new case of monoclonal IgA kappa cold ag-

glutinin with anti-Pr(1)d specificity in a patient with persistent HB antigen cirrhosis," *Vox Sanguinis*, vol. 30, no. 6, pp. 464–468, 1976.

[24] A. Pereira, R. Mazzara, L. Escoda, I. Alcorta, B. Nomdedeu, and D. Roelcke, "Anti-Sa cold agglutinin of IgA class requiring plasma-exchange therapy as early manifestation of multiple myeloma," *Annals of Hematology*, vol. 66, no. 6, pp. 315–318, 1993.

[25] W. Römer, U. Rother, and D. Roelcke, "Failure of IgA cold agglutinin to activate C," *Immunobiology*, vol. 157, no. 1, pp. 41–46, 1980.

[26] D. A. Clark, E. N. Dessypris, D. E. Jenkins Jr., and S. B. Krantz, "Acquired immune hemolytic anemia associated with IgA erythrocyte coating: investigation of hemolytic mechanisms," *Blood*, vol. 64, no. 5, pp. 1000–1005, 1984.

[27] P. Chadebech, M. Michel, D. Janvier et al., "IgA-mediated human autoimmune hemolytic anemia as a result of hemagglutination in the spleen, but independent of complement activation and Fc RI," *Blood*, vol. 116, no. 20, pp. 4141–4147, 2010.

[28] S. Berentsen, "Complement activation and inhibition in autoimmune hemolytic anemia: focus on cold agglutinin disease," *Seminars in Hematology*, vol. 55, no. 3, pp. 141–149, 2018.

[29] J. Shi, E. L. Rose, A. Singh et al., "TNT003, an inhibitor of the serine protease C1s, prevents complement activation induced by cold agglutinins," *Blood*, vol. 123, no. 26, pp. 4015–4022, 2014.

12

A Massive Extradural Hematoma in Sickle Cell Disease and the Importance of Rapid Neuroimaging

Per Ole Iversen[1] **Mboka Jacob,**[2] **Jamila Makame,**[3] **Mclean Abisay,**[3] **Mbonea Yonazi,**[3] **Anna Schuh,**[1] **and Julie Makani**[1]

[1]*Department of Haematology and Blood Transfusion, Muhimbili University of Health and Allied Sciences, Dar-es-Salaam, Tanzania*
[2]*Department of Radiology and Imaging, Muhimbili University of Health and Allied Sciences, Dar-es-Salaam, Tanzania*
[3]*Department of Haematology, Muhimbili National Hospital, Dar-es-Salaam, Tanzania*

Correspondence should be addressed to Per Ole Iversen; p.o.iversen@medisin.uio.no

Academic Editor: Marie-Christine Kyrtsonis

Sickle cell disease (SCD) is an inherited hemoglobinopathy leading to several serious organ complications and early death. It is mostly found in equatorial countries like Tanzania. Extradural hematoma (EDH) is a rare, but serious complication to SCD and may have debilitating consequences. Hitherto, there is no report of EDH in SCD where neuroimaging has been available before, during, and after such an event. Here, we describe a young female SCD patient who developed EDH that required surgical evacuation. She had made full recovery after three months. Neuroimaging performed two years prior to this event was unremarkable except for multiple small cerebral infarcts. On admission, neuroimaging revealed a subgaleal hematoma, possibly indicating disruption of the skull cortex due to increased hematopoiesis. Three months after evacuation of the hematoma, neuroimaging showed evidence of brain atrophy and the previously reported cerebral infarcts and multifocal bone infarction, but no vasculopathy. Possibly, disruption of the skull cortex with subsequent bleeding caused the EDH. As the differential diagnoses of neurological complications in SCD are many and some complications are reversible, neuroimaging should be performed without delay.

1. Introduction

Sickle cell disease (SCD) is an autosomal recessive disorder resulting in production of abnormal erythrocytes due to mutation in the gene coding for the beta chain in the hemoglobin (Hb) molecule. SCD is characterized by a range of complications, in particular, anemia, infections, and painful vasoocclusive crisis (VOC) [1]. In addition, silent cerebral infarcts are common in SCD and constitute a risk factor for future cerebral infarcts leading to clinical manifestations [2]. SCD is particularly frequent in Africa and Tanzania which are among the countries with the highest burden of this disease [3].

A severe form of VOC in SCD is extradural hematoma (EDH). Neurological sequelae, impaired cognition, and increased mortality have been reported in SCD patients affected by this complication [4, 5]. The underlying mechanism leading to EDH is not known, but it has been associated with a number of other diseases (e.g., infection, cancer, bleeding disorder, and vasculopathy), as reviewed by Hettige et al. [6]; however, none of them has been convincingly shown to cause EDH. Page et al. suggested that a preexistent bone infarction in SCD could lead to rupture of nearby blood vessels [4]. Alternatively, abnormal skull anatomy in SCD due to increased hematopoiesis with subsequent rupture of the skull cortex could lead to bleeding into the subgaleal and epidural spaces [4, 7]. However, without available neuroimaging data obtained prior to the development of EDH, its cause is difficult to identify.

Due to the rarity, our knowledge of EDH stems from case reports, and in all of them, neuroimaging prior to the bleeding is not available, precluding further examination

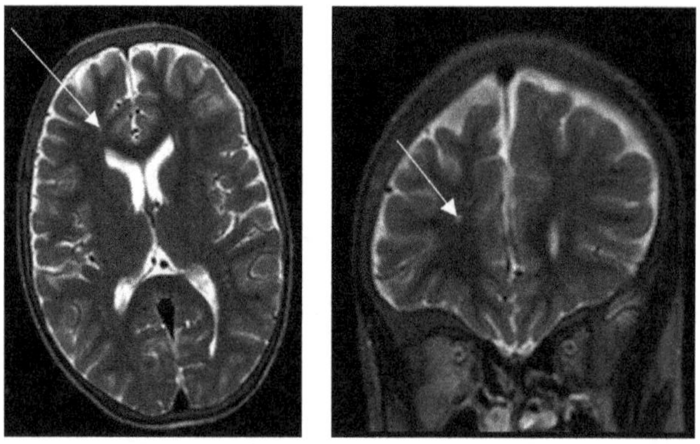

(a) (b)

Figure 1: (a) Axial T2-weighted MRI brain scan demonstrating focal hyperintensity (arrow), probably representing an infarctive lesion on the right frontal lobe deep white matter. (b) The same lesion as seen on the coronal T2-weighted MRI brain scan.

into the possible causes of this often debilitating SCD complication. To the best of our knowledge, this is the first presentation of a SCD patient suffering from an apparent spontaneous form of massive EDH of whom neuroimaging was available prior to and during this event as well as after rehabilitation.

2. Case Presentation

An 18-year-old female from Tanzania was diagnosed with homozygous (HbSS) SCD at one year of age. During childhood and adolescence, she had multiple admissions for painful episodes of bone VOC and infections, but no reported clinical features of affections of the central nervous system. Her steady-state Hb ranged from ~7 to 8 g/dl; HbS from ~70 to 80%, and HbF from ~2 to 11%. She used folic acid (5 mg/day) and intermittently (due to financial constraints) hydroxyurea (0.5–1 g/day).

Two years prior to the current admission, a brain magnetic resonance imaging (MRI) angiography was performed as a screening for cerebral infarctions and vasculopathy as part of a research programme. This showed multiple small cerebral infarcts, and the largest (~3 mm) was located in the right frontal deep white matter (Figures 1(a) and 1(b)). There were no features of skull abnormalities or arteriovenous malformations, and all intracranial arteries were unremarkable.

She was first seen at a local hospital before being transported to Muhimbili National Hospital after one day with loss of consciousness. This was preceded by frontal headache three days prior to hospital admission which increased in severity with time. There was no history of trauma, vomiting, convulsions, or urine/fecal incontinence. One week prior to hospital admission, she had bone pain on and off and low-grade fever, which were relieved by analgesia and antipyretics, respectively.

On arrival at Muhimbili National Hospital, the patient was unconscious with a Glasgow Coma Scale score of 7/15 and febrile (38.9°C), with moderate pallor, but no jaundice. The pupils were dilated and sluggishly reacting to light. In addition, she had developed right-sided hemiparesis. There was no visible evidence of head trauma or signs of meningeal affection.

A computerized tomography (CT) scan of the brain on admission revealed a massive biconvex extradural heterogeneous (predominantly hyperdense) hematoma (4.37 cm in maximum thickness with 1.23 cm of midline shift) overlying the left frontal and parietal lobes (Figures 2(a) and 2(b)). The hematoma compressed the underlying brain matter so that the gyral and sulci pattern was lost and hypodense indicating edema. Moreover, an effaced ipsilateral lateral ventricle and a moderate dilatation of the contralateral lateral ventricle had developed. A subgaleal hematoma overlying the left frontal and parietal bones was also noted (Figures 2(b) and 2(c)). There was no skull lesion or features or signs of osteomyelitis. In addition, we noted two hypodense lesions consistent with bone infarction on the left frontal and right parietal bones (Figure 2(d)).

Her Hb was 5.0 (reference value: 12.0–15.0) g/dl, leukocytes 6.1 (4.0–10.0) × 10^9/l, and platelets 73.0 (150–410) × 10^9/l. The concentration of C-reactive protein was elevated (287; 0–5) mg/l, while screenings for malaria, urinary tract, typhoid, and dengue infections were all negative. Additional blood tests revealed no hypercoagulability or bleeding tendency, including normal INR and APTT.

Due to progressive deterioration of her condition, the patient underwent a left parietal craniotomy and evacuation of the EDH under general anesthesia. She regained consciousness the day after surgery; however, she remained aphasic with right-sided hemiparesis for 3-4 days until her condition started to improve over the next two weeks. She was discharged after 17 days. At the outpatient consultation three months postoperatively, she had no particular complaints and was able to talk normally and walk without support and although not formally tested, there were no apparent language, motor, or cognitive deficits. An MRI brain scan showed (Figures 3(a)–3(d)) (i) no midline shift, marked enlargement of the left lateral ventricle and widening of the sulci on the left frontal, temporal, and parietal lobes and widened left sylvian fissure signifying presence of both subcortical and cortical brain atrophy; (ii) diffuse and focal periventricular white matter hyperintensities along the body and posterior horn of the lateral ventricle which may signify cerebral spinal fluid seepage or reperfusion infarcts; and (iii) left parietal bone signal changes which may be

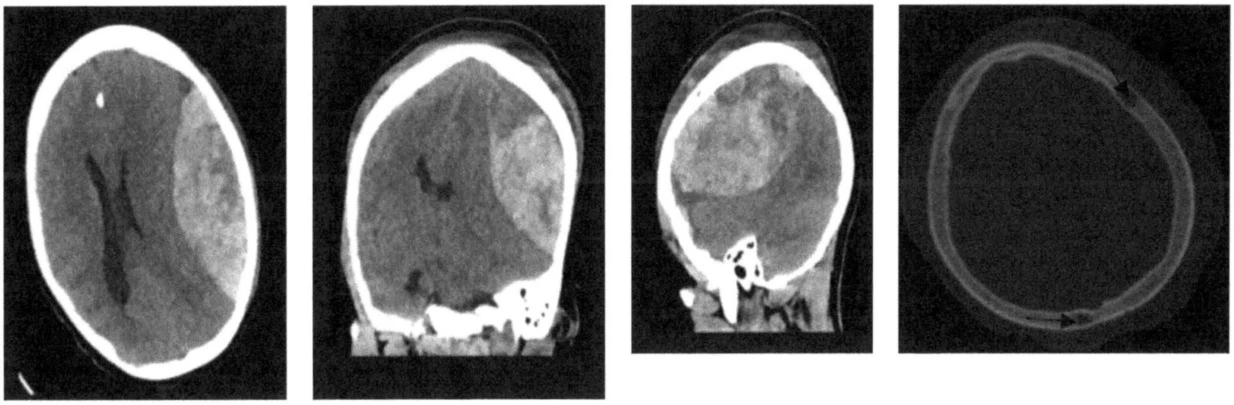

(a) (b) (c) (d)

FIGURE 2: (a) Axial CT brain scan (no contrast) demonstrating left-sided extradural hematoma. (b and c) Coronal and sagittal CT brain scans, respectively, showing the extradural hematoma and subgaleal hemorrhage. (d) The preoperative CT on bone window showed two hypodense lesions (arrows) on the left frontal and right parietal bones.

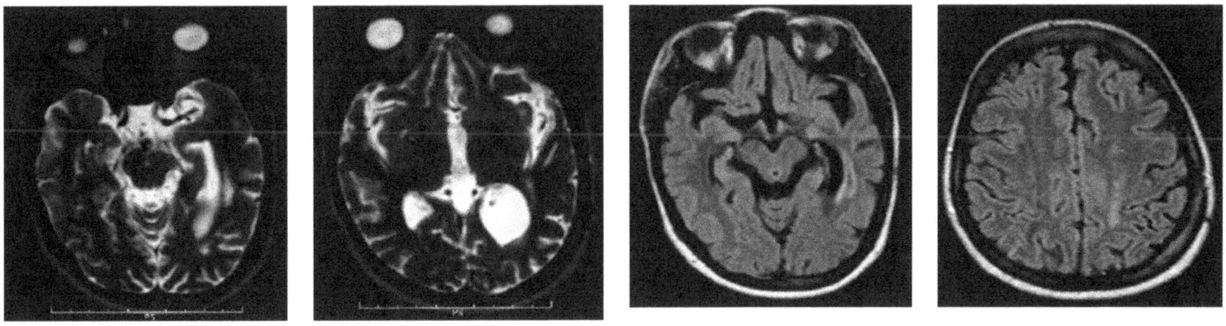

(a) (b) (c) (d)

FIGURE 3: MRI brain scan performed three months after evacuation of the extradural hematoma. (a) Axial T2-weighted MRI scan showing multifocal hyperintensities on the left periventricular area and dilated posterior horn of the left lateral ventricle. (b) Coronal T2-weighted MRI scan and (c) axial "fluid attenuated inversion recovery (FLAIR)-MRI. FLAIR-MRI are used to enhance T2-weighted scans to identify hyperintense lesions by suppressing cerebrospinal fluid. Both images (b and c) show prominent left sylvian fissure and dilated posterior horn of the left lateral ventricle and left temporal lobe atrophy. (d) Axial FLAIR-MRI showing white matter hyperintensity of the left parietal lobe signal changes on the parietal bone.

craniotomy-associated changes or bone infarction. There were no changes of the small cerebral infarcts on the right frontal lobe deep white matter compared to those observed in 2017. MRI angiography was normal with no features of arteriovenous malformations.

3. Discussion

Though silent cerebral infarctions are frequent, EDH in SCD is rare [2, 4, 8]. Based on data from ~4000 SCD patients followed for an average of about 5 years, the Cooperative Study of Sickle Cell Disease found that those with HbSS were more frequently affected compared to other SCD genotypes and that the incidence of hemorrhagic stroke in HbSS patients was the highest among patients aged 20 to 29 years [8].

Here, we present a case of EDH in a SCD patient with previously reported silent cerebral infarction. Although there was no indication of trauma, sexual violence of young females is not uncommon in Tanzania [9]. A gynecological examination was therefore performed and found to be normal. Except for her underlying SCD, our patient had no other risk factors for bleeding or other comorbidities.

In contrast to previous reports of EDH in SCD, we had access to neuroimaging obtained prior to, during, and after the hematoma developed. We found that two years before the current event, small cerebral infarcts were evident. However, neither other forms of vasculopathy, including arteriovenous malformations, nor skull bone abnormalities were detected at that time. Notably, no vasculopathy was noted, either during her current hospital admission or three months after evacuation of the hematoma. The CT brain scan on admission revealed a subgaleal hematoma, possibly indicating a developing skull lesion/expansion due to increased hematopoietic activity leading to disruption of the skull cortex, which could be the cause of the EDH, supporting the notion suggested by Dahdaleh et al. [7]. We also noted the two hypodense lesions in the bone, suggesting that the bone had been affected.

Complications of the central nervous system rank as one of the most serious complications to SCD. Although EDH is rare, its long-term outcome can be debilitating [4, 5] and the associated mortality is high; in their review of 22 young SCD patients with EDH, Hettige et al. found that ~1/3 of them died due to EDH [6]. Therefore, if EDH is suspected in a SCD patient, neuroimaging should be performed without delay, which is feasible also in low-resource settings such as ours [10].

References

[1] F. B. Piel, M. H. Steinberg, and D. C. Rees, "Sickle cell disease," *New England Journal of Medicine*, vol. 376, no. 16, pp. 1561–1573, 2017.

[2] L. C. Jordan, A. A. Kassim, M. J. Donahue et al., "Silent infarct is a risk factor for infarct recurrence in adults with sickle cell anemia," *Neurology*, vol. 91, no. 8, pp. e781–e784, 2018.

[3] J. Makani, S. E. Cox, D. Soka et al., "Mortality in sickle cell anemia in Africa: a prospective cohort study in Tanzania," *PLoS One*, vol. 6, no. 2, Article ID e14699, 2011.

[4] C. Page, K. Gardner, S. Height, D. C. Rees, T. Hampton, and S. Lay Thein, "Nontraumatic extradural hematoma in sickle cell anemia: a rare neurological complication not to be missed," *American Journal of Hematology*, vol. 89, no. 2, pp. 225–227, 2014.

[5] J. Hamm, N. Rathore, P. Lee et al., "Cranial epidural hematomas: a case series and literature review of this rare complication associated with sickle cell disease," *Pediatric Blood & Cancer*, vol. 64, no. 3, Article ID e26237, 2017.

[6] S. Hettige, A. Sofela, S. Bassi, and C. Chandler, "A review of spontaneous intracranial extradural hematoma in sickle-cell disease," *Acta Neurochirurgica*, vol. 157, no. 11, pp. 2025–2029, 2015.

[7] N. S. Dahdaleh, T. E. Lindley, P. A. Kirby, H. Oya, and M. A. Howard, "A "neurosurgical crisis" of sickle cell disease," *Journal of Neurosurgery: Pediatrics*, vol. 4, no. 6, pp. 532–535, 2009.

[8] K. Ohene-Frempong, S. J. Weiner, L. A. Sleeper et al., "Cerebrovascular accidents in sickle cell disease: rates and risk factors," *Blood*, vol. 91, no. 1, pp. 288–294, 1998.

[9] K. J. Vagi, K. A. Brookmeyer, R. M. Gladden et al., "Sexual violence against female and male children in the United Republic of Tanzania," *Violence against Women*, vol. 22, no. 14, pp. 1788–1807, 2016.

[10] M. Jacob, D. E. Saunders, J. M. Kawadler et al., "Neuroimaging in patients with sickle cell anemia: capacity building in Africa," *Blood Advances*, vol. 2, no. 1, pp. 26–29, 2018.

13

Highly Aggressive CD4-Positive Mast Cell Leukaemia (Leukaemic Variant) Associated with Isolated Trisomy 19 and Hemophagocytosis by Neoplastic Mast Cells: A Case Report with Challenging Experience and Review

Dina Sameh Soliman,[1,2,3] Ahmad Al-Sabbagh,[1] Feryal Ibrahim,[1] Amna Gameil,[4] Mohamed Yassin,[4] and Halima El-Omri[4]

[1]*Department of Laboratory Medicine and Pathology, National Center for Cancer Care and Research, Hamad Medical Corporation, Doha, Qatar*
[2]*Clinical Pathology Department, National Cancer Institute, Cairo University, Cairo, Egypt*
[3]*Clinical Pathology and Laboratory Medicine, Weill-Cornell Medicine, Doha, Qatar*
[4]*Department of Hematology and Medical Oncology, National Center for Cancer Care and Research, Hamad Medical Corporation, Doha, Qatar*

Correspondence should be addressed to Dina Sameh Soliman; dsoliman@hamad.qa

Academic Editor: Sudhir Tauro

Background. Mast cell leukaemia is a unique disease among hematopoietic neoplasms, being one of the rarest leukaemia subtypes. In addition, its prompt diagnosis is usually challenging. This is due to its heterogeneity in clinical presentations and cytomorphological and immunophenotypical features together with potential associations with other hematologic neoplasms which can complicate the condition and delay accurate diagnosis. To the best of our knowledge, this is the first case report of CD4-positive mast cell leukaemia. *Case Presentation.* A 39-year-old male presented with acute onset of fever, abdominal pain, and generalized body aches of two-week duration. Peripheral blood smear showed circulating blasts (13%) with coarsely basophilic granulation. Bone marrow (BM) aspirate showed extensive infiltration with immature mast cells of blast-like morphology with trilineage dysplasia and evident hemophagocytic activity exhibited by histiocytes and neoplastic mast cells. BM biopsy was diffusely infiltrated with many atypical mast cells positive for CD45, CD117, mast cell tryptase, CD25, and CD4 with partial positivity for CD7 and CD30. Cytogenetics showed an abnormal karyotype: 47, XY, +1947, XY, +19[13]/46, XY[9]. Molecular analysis revealed a *KIT* D816V mutation consistent with a diagnosis of systemic mastocytosis, mast cell leukaemia. *Conclusion.* The expression of T-cell associated markers by abnormal mast cells is well documented; however, CD4 and CD7 expression have not previously been described in association with mast cell leukaemia. Coexpression of CD2, CD4, CD7, and CD30 by the mast cells particularly in skin lesions may provoke misinterpretation as a cutaneous T-cell neoplasm. To the best of our knowledge, this is the first report of CD4-positive mast cell leukaemia. Moreover, hemophagocytic mast cell leukaemia is a very rare morphologic variant, and possible correlation between this finding and expression of CD4 by neoplastic mast cells is a topic for further investigation.

1. Background

Mast cell leukaemia (MCL) is a very rare form of aggressive systemic mastocytosis (SM) accounting for <0.5% of all mastocytosis patients in the French Reference Center for Mastocytosis (CEREMAST), representing one of the rarest leukaemia subtypes. It is characterized by the leukaemic spread of mast cells (MCs), with frequent multiorgan involvement. The prognosis is exceedingly poor, and therapy usually fails with a median survival of less than 6 months.

According to the 2008 WHO and the most recently revised WHO classification (2016), MCL diagnosis is based on the presence of >20% atypical/immature MCs in the BM smears and/or >10% in the blood in addition to fulfilment of the WHO diagnostic criteria of SM [1].

The case described here showed a unique pathologic feature with exceptional immunophenotypic profile being a de novo leukaemic variant with atypical expression of CD4, CD7, and mast cells exhibiting erythrophagocytosis.

Although high suspicion index based on morphologic characteristics was the clue to the diagnosis, the main diagnostic challenges were the nonspecific clinical and pathological features, absence of symptoms of mast cell activation, scarcity of circulating neoplastic cells at initial presentation, and expression of T-cell-associated markers on neoplastic MCs (CD25, CD4, CD7, and CD30).

2. Case Presentation

A 39-year-old male, with a past medical history of treated tuberculosis, presented to the emergency department complaining of fever, generalized weakness, vague abdominal pain, vomiting, headache, and generalized body aches of two-week duration with a history of nasal bleeding of moderate severity. Upon examination, there was submandibular lymphadenopathy (2×1 cm) and palpable liver (7 cm below the costal margin) and no gastrointestinal manifestations and skin lesions.

Laboratory workup revealed high urea level at 18.84 mmol/L (3.2–7.4), serum creatinine at 141 μmol/l (64–110), lipase at 182 U/L (8–78), myoglobin at 108 ng/ml (1–78), and normal liver function tests.

Further investigations revealed very high ferritin level >40000 mcg/L (24–336), low serum B12 level (<111 pmol/L), normal fibrinogen level at 4.77 gm/L (1.8–3.5), and normal triglyceride level at 0.6 mmol/L (normal: <1.7 mmol/L). Viral serology for hepatitis B and C and HIV was negative.

His complete blood count showed pancytopenia, with hemoglobin of 6.4 gm/dL (13.0–17.0), total white blood count (WBC) of $1.7 \times 10^3/\mu l$ (4.0–10.0), absolute neutrophil count (ANC) $0.9 \times 10^3/\mu l$, and platelet count of $2 \times 10^3/\mu l$ (150–400). BM failure was suspected, and the patient was admitted for further workup.

Sepsis workup was requested, and the patient was started on antimicrobials and vitamin B12 replacement.

Computerized tomography (CT) scan of the head showed bilateral subdural haemorrhage with no midline shift, and the patient was managed conservatively with transfusion support. Whole body CT scan showed bilateral pleural effusion, extensive pulmonary consolidation, thrombosis of the celiac artery and its branches with splenic infarction, mild hepatomegaly, and massive splenomegaly. The spleen showed poor heterogeneous enhancement suggestive of infarction.

First, peripheral blood smear (PS) was inconclusive as it showed very few circulating atypical cells. Subsequent PS (Figure 1) showed marked leukopenia with some circulating abnormal blastoid cells (13%) of medium size with fine nuclear chromatin and unevenly distributed deeply basophilic/metachromatic coarse granules. Few blasts showed nuclear bilobation.

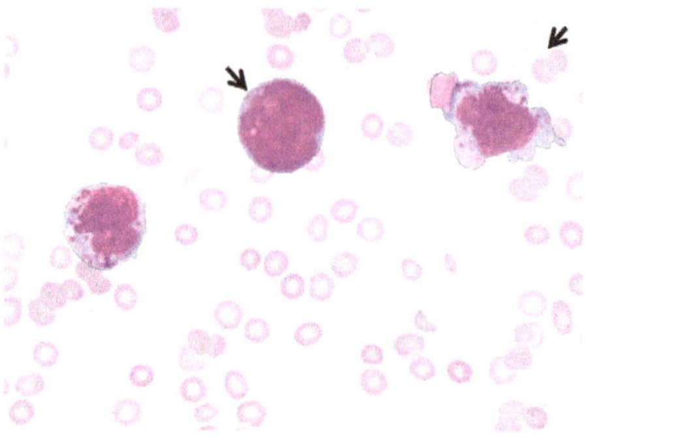

FIGURE 1: Peripheral smear showing immature cells with blast morphology (arrows) and atypical mast cells.

Bone marrow (BM) aspirate was infiltrated with numerous atypical and immature MCs of blast-like morphology (26%) showing fine nuclear chromatin and few prominent nucleoli. The majority of blasts showed eccentric nuclei with abundant cytoplasm and coarse giant metachromatic/basophilic granules (metachromatic blasts) (Figure 2(a)). Few blasts were agranular with high nucleocytoplasmic ratio and few were spindle-shaped. The majority of neoplastic MCs exhibited marked atypia and pronounced pleomorphism (Figures 2(b) and 2(c)) of (Type I) (Figure 2(b), A–I) with eccentric round/oval nuclei, uneven granules distribution/hypogranulation, and spindle-shaped mast cells with elongated cytoplasmic projections. Neoplastic MCs Type II (promastocytes) (Figure 2(c), A–H), with indented, bilobed nuclei and abundant degranulated/hypogranulated cytoplasm or with coalescent granules and uneven distribution were frequent.

There was trilineage dysplasia with prominent megaloblastic changes mostly in the form of giant granulocytes, megakaryocytes with multilobulation, and some megaloblastic erythroid precursors (composite, Figure 2(d)) with some mitotic figures noted (Figure 2(e)). There was an evident hemophagocytic activity (predominantly erythrophagocytosis) exhibited by histiocytes and neoplastic mast cells (Figure 2(f)).

On H&E, BM biopsy was markedly hypercellular, largely replaced by sheets of neoplastic mast cells showing abundant clear cytoplasm with round/indented nuclei (including many forms with immature nuclear chromatin), and admixed with a reactive background composed of fibroblasts, eosinophils, small lymphocytes, and polyclonal plasma cells (Figure 3(a) and 3(b)). There was a mild increase in reticulin fibres (MF 0-1). By immunohistochemistry (IHC)(Figure 3), the neoplastic MCs were positive for CD45, CD117, mast cell tryptase, CD25, CD43, CD4, and partially positive for CD30 and CD7 while negative for CD2. Histiocytes/macrophages were prominent with evident hemophagocytic activity. Toluidine blue and Giemsa stain highlighted the metachromatic granules of the more differentiated MCs while the majority was negative. Megakaryocytes appeared focally increased with some small

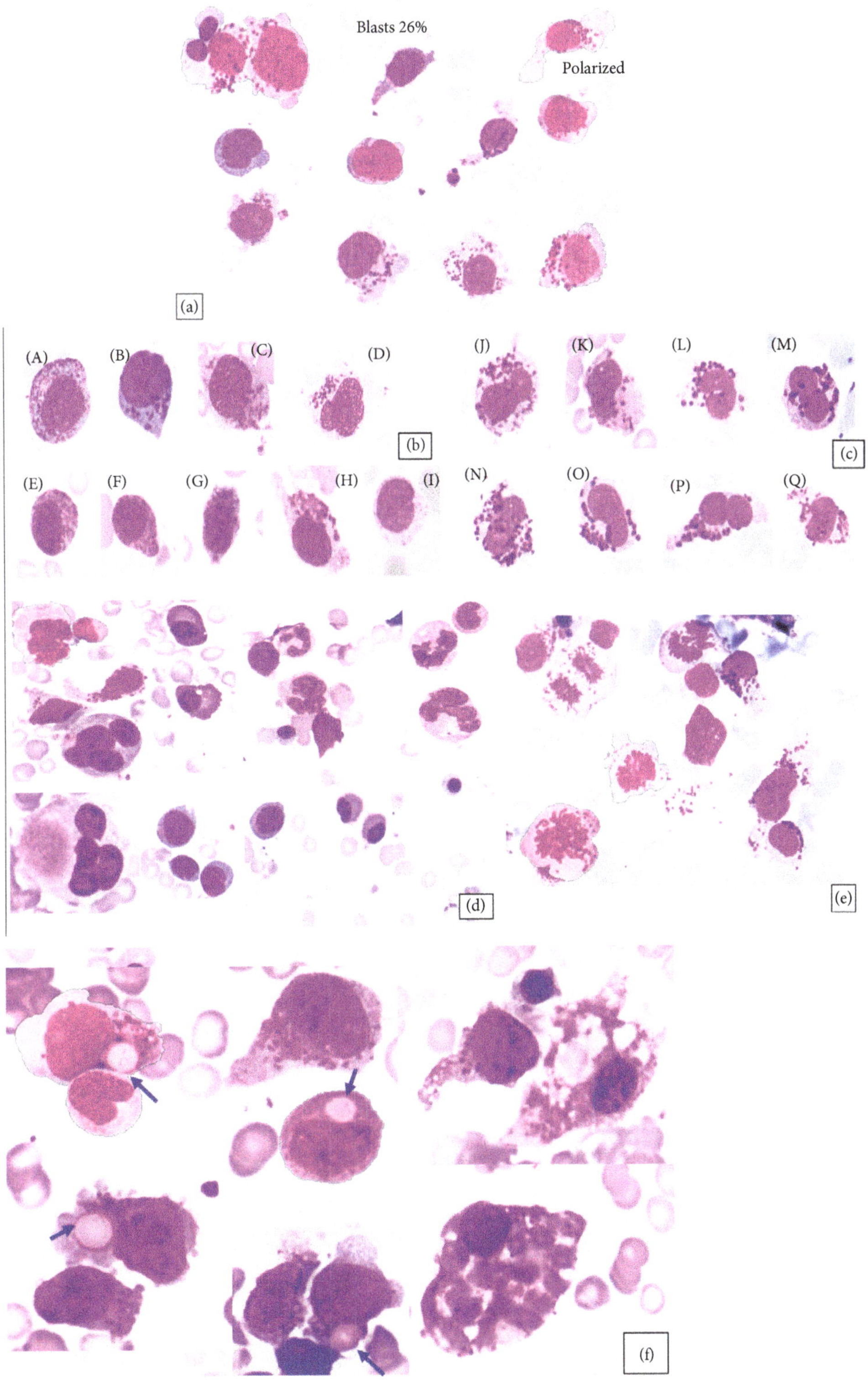

FIGURE 2: BM aspirate smear (100x) showing a variety of neoplastic MCs. The majority of blasts show abundant cytoplasm and coarse giant metachromatic blasts (a). Neoplastic MCs (Type I) (A–I) with eccentric round/oval nuclei, uneven granule distribution/hypogranulation, and spindle-shaped MCs with elongated cytoplasmic projections (b). Neoplastic MCs Type II (promastocytes) (A–H) with indented, bilobed nuclei, abundant hypogranulated cytoplasm, or with coalescent granules with uneven distribution (c). There is trilineage dysplasia with macronormoblasts, giant neutrophils, and dysplastic nuclear lobulation in megakaryocytes (arrows) (d). Increased mitotic figures (e). Prominent erythrophagocytosis exhibited by neoplastic mast cells (blue arrow) and histiocytes (f).

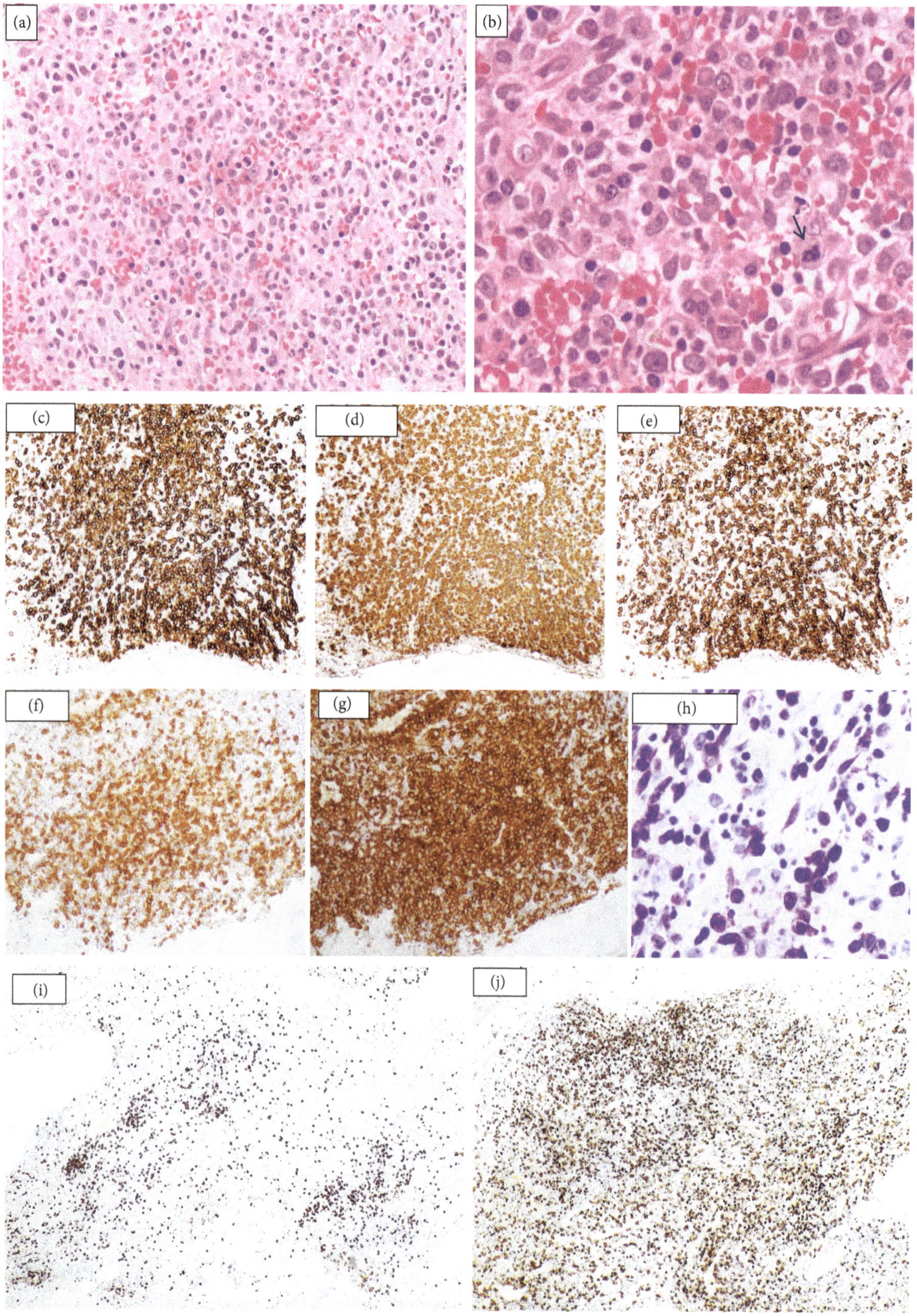

FIGURE 3: BM biopsy (H&E) showing diffuse infiltration by atypical mast cells 20x (a). 50x magnification of BM biopsy showing increased mitotic figures (arrow) and evident erythrophagocytosis (b). Immunohistochemistry on BM biopsy: the neoplastic mast cells are positive for (c) CD117, (d) tryptase, (e) CD25, and (g) CD4 and show partial positivity for (j) CD7 and (f) CD30. (i) CD3 immunostain was included to show the normal CD3-positive T cells. (h) Toluidine blue highlighted the more differentiated MCs.

hypolobated forms and some degree of morphologic atypia. Serum tryptase level revealed very a high level at 434.00 mcg/L (negative < 11 mcg/L).

Flow cytometry on BM (Figure 4) showed an abnormal population of cells in the blast gate comprising 25%, expressing CD45 (moderate), CD117 (bright), CD33, and HLA-DR with partial aberrant CD25 expression. The neoplastic cells showed aberrant expression of CD4, aberrant partial expression of CD7, and partial expression of CD36. In addition, the analysis showed a small population of cells (~4%) with low side and forward light scatter expressing CD33 and CD4 with a minor subpopulation expressing CD117, CD64, and CD14, possibly representing dysplastic myeloid/hypogranular mast cells. The neoplastic mast cells are negative for cMPO, CD64, CD14, CD19, CD20, cCD3, sCD3, CD5, CD2, CD11c, and CD11b.

Cytogenetic studies showed an abnormal karyotype with isolated trisomy 19 (47, XY, +19[13]).

Molecular analysis of blood confirmed a *KIT* D816V mutation with negative *BCR/ABL-1*, consistent with a diagnosis of systemic mastocytosis, mast cell leukaemia.

The patient developed acute kidney injury with progressive deterioration in renal function (serum creatinine at 245 μmol/L) and disseminated intravascular coagulopathy (DIC). Echocardiography showed severe pulmonary hypertension with normal systolic left ventricular function (ejection fraction of 60%).

On the 3rd day after hospitalization, he developed respiratory distress and was started on noninvasive pressure ventilation (NIPV), diuretics, and broad-spectrum antibacterial, antifungal therapy with steroid along with supportive measures after bone marrow results.

The patient developed septic shock with multiorgan failure, so he underwent hemodialysis and was started on prednisone but unfortunately developed cardiac arrest (asystole) and died two weeks after admission.

3. Discussion and Conclusion

Since 1950, there are fewer than 70 well-documented cases of MCL reported to date; 51 MCL cases were summarized in the largest review published in *Blood* in 2013 [2]. MCL shares more clinical and biologic features with aggressive systemic mastocytosis (ASM) than with acute myeloid leukaemia (AML) [3].

When considering a diagnosis of MCL; it is important to distinguish the following subvariants of MCL : 1, primary (de novo) MCL versus secondary MCL, the latter is preceded by another subtype of mastocytosis, commonly evolution form ASM and 2, "Pure" MCL versus MCL associated with hematological neoplasm (MCL-AHN). The majority of MCL cases are de novo (73%), i.e., not preceded by chronic mastocytosis and not associated with hematologic neoplasms. More recently, MCL has been divided into a chronic form without obvious organ damage (no C-findings present) and a more aggressive (acute) variant, termed acute MCL where organ damage (C-findings) is present [4].

No difference was found in overall survival between de novo MCL vs. secondary MCL ($P = 0.9$) or MCL-AHN vs. MCL ($P = 0.2$) [5].

"Aleukaemic variant" of MCL (with circulating MCs <10%) is the most frequently described form accounting up to 62% of 52 cases reported by Georgin-Lavialle et al. [2]. MCL with more than 10% circulating MCs "leukaemic variant" (as reported here) is a rare presentation, reported in 2 out of 28 cases of MCL (7%) [5].

3.1. Challenging Diagnosis and Differential Diagnosis. This case fulfilled the diagnostic criteria for SM with the presence of multifocal dense infiltrates of MCs (>15 MCs in aggregates) detected in BM sections (a major criterion for SM) in addition to all 4 minor criteria: (a) >25% of the MCs in the BM infiltrate has atypical morphology and >25% of all MCs in BM aspirate smears is immature or atypical, (b) detection of an activating point mutation at codon 816 of *KIT* in the blood, (c) the aberrant expression of CD25 in addition to normal MC markers, and (d) very high serum total tryptase (>20 ng/ml) in absence of an associated myeloid neoplasm. We classified the case as de novo MCL; a leukaemic variant with acute onset, as there was no previous history of mast cell disease or other hematologic neoplasms, no history of skin manifestations, and no history of long-standing cytopenias.

The major differential diagnosis included the following: acute basophilic leukaemia, tryptase-positive AML, and blastic plasmacytoid dendritic neoplasms (CD4/CD56-positive). However, the characteristic morphology, very bright CD117 and negativity for CD34, excludes AML. Immunophenotypic detection of abnormal MCs expressing very bright CD117, mast cell tryptase, and CD25 distinguish MCL from acute basophilic leukaemia and blastic plasmacytoid dendritic neoplasms.

This case did not show any of the mediator release symptoms caused by mast cell activation/degranulation that include severe hypotension, syncope, anaphylaxis, flushing, headache, purities, or gastrointestinal symptoms. This is in line with what was reported by Georgin-Lavialle et al. [2], who concluded that symptoms of MC activation are more frequent among MCL patients without *KIT* D816V mutation than those in the group with this mutation. Skin involvement that is usually seen in patients with indolent SM is less frequently detected in ASM and is rarely seen in MCL [4].

The diagnosis of MCL is usually challenging because of heterogeneous clinical and morphological features. In general terms, MCs are not readily recognized on BM sections and commonly confused with a variety of other cells that include fibroblasts, histiocytes, hairy cells, and monocytes. Besides, the lack of a specific MC marker also hampers prompt identification and characterization of MCs in BM.

In our case, the presence of circulating atypical cells with the characteristic coarse metachromatic granules was the first clue in making the diagnosis. Morphologically, the neoplastic MCs were so pleomorphic and showed a spectrum of maturation; however, with many metachromatic blasts mixed with numerous more differentiated neoplastic MCs (Type I and Type II) and few well-differentiated MCs. Mitotic figures were frequently seen reflecting a high proliferative index. Mitoses are rarely seen in mast cell

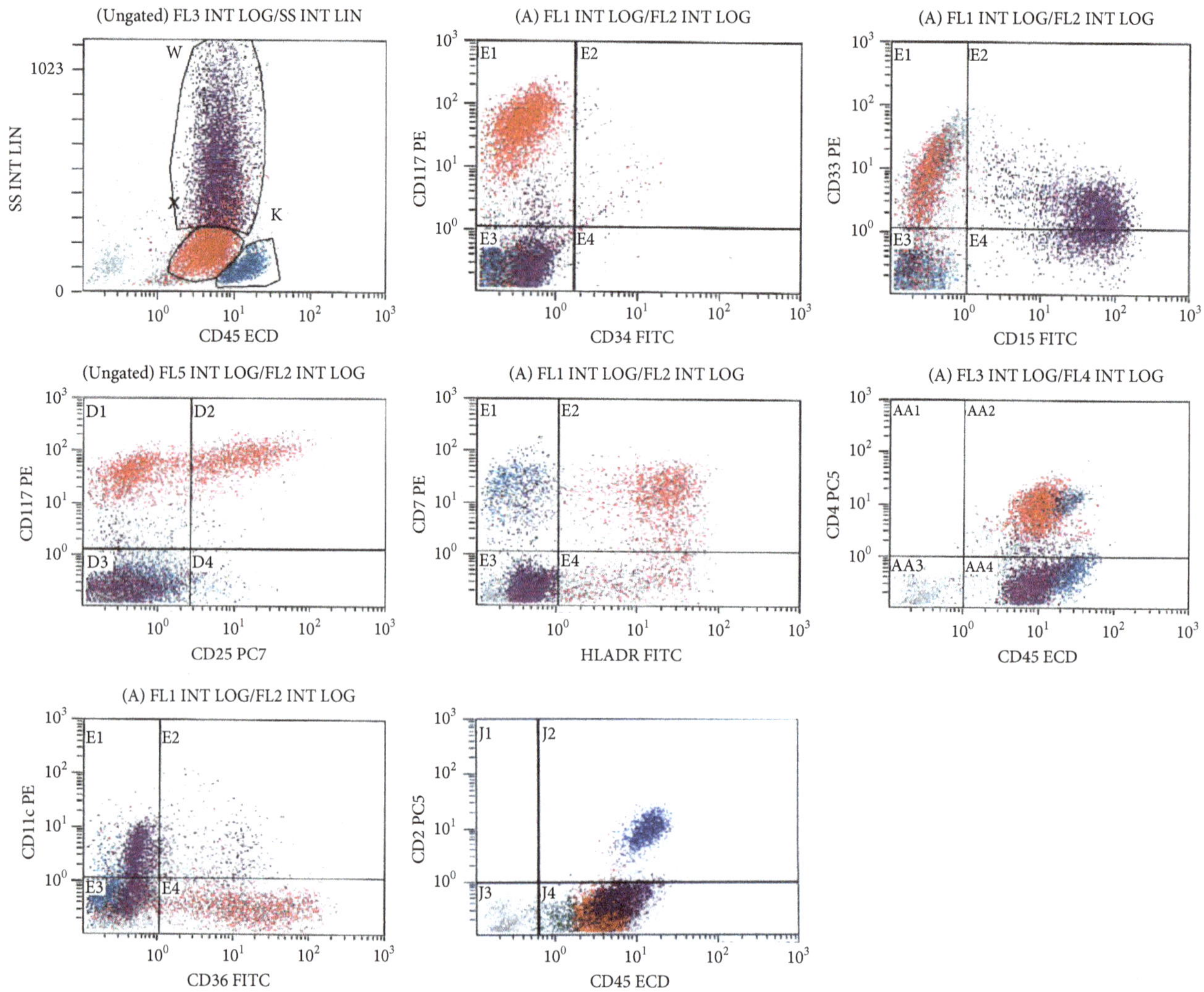

FIGURE 4: FCM shows an abnormal population of mast cells (red) in the blast gate; approximately 26% (of the total cells) expressing bright CD117, and the majority is positive for CD33 and HLADR with partial aberrant CD25 on a subpopulation (~11% of total). The cells show aberrant expression of CD7 and CD4, partial expression for CD36, and negative for CD2.

neoplasms even in aggressive forms of mastocytosis, except in patients with MCL [5]. Interestingly; some MCs exhibited pronounced hemophagocytosis, a unique and extremely rare finding described in MCL in which highly atypical mast cells exhibit erythrophagocytosis. "Hemophagocytic" MCL is not, however, regarded as a distinct subtype of MCL [6, 7].

The significance of this morphology and its relation to disease aggressiveness are unknown.

3.2. Immunophenotype of MCs and MCL. Immunophenotypically, it is widely accepted that normal and neoplastic MCs express mast cell tryptase, CD117 (bright), CD45, CD33, CD11c, CD43, and CD68, but lack the expression of the myeloid markers (CD14, CD15, and myeloperoxidase) and B-cell-related antigens [1].

The neoplastic MCs usually show high light side scatter and almost always express tryptase and CD117 (bright). Other frequently expressed markers on abnormal MCs include CD25, CD2, and CD30. Flow cytometry is quite sensitive in detecting MCs even in a low percentage as they usually have a very bright CD117 expression. Because of the low frequency of MCs in BM samples, most data about the normal maturation patterns of MCs are based on in vitro differentiation studies [8].

Recent reports suggest that the combined use of only two markers (CD117 and CD45) would be sufficient to identify MCs appropriately in BM (CD117high/CD45low) [9].

Although expression of CD2 and/or CD25 is the most common immunophenotypic aberrancies on MCs and is acknowledged as a minor criterion for the diagnosis of mastocytosis, about one-third of MCL cases reported in the literature had a double-negative CD2/CD25 immunophenotype [2]. Normal well-differentiated MCs usually do not express CD2 or CD25 [10].

The association between *KIT* D816 mutation and dual expression of CD2/CD25 on MCs in SM is very frequent; dual coexpression of CD2 and CD25 was found in 66% of *KIT* D816-positive MCL patients compared with those who were *KIT* D816 negative (25%) [2].

CD25+/CD2− MCs seen in our case are a rare occurrence in MCL and are reported in 13% of MCL cases reviewed by Georgin-Lavialle et al.; CD25 and CD2 expressions varied; 13% were CD25+/CD2−; 54% of patients were double positive (CD25+/CD2+); 38% were CD25−/CD2− double negative; and 4% were showing CD25−/CD2+ phenotype [2].

Compared to patients with indolent SM, the number of "CD2-positive" MCL patients is low, and if detected, the levels are usually lower than those found on MCs in indolent SM [11].

It has been recently proposed that aggressive forms of mastocytosis, including MCL, exhibit an immature phenotype reflected by the expression of immaturity markers such as CD123, CD34, and HLA-DR and reduced expression of CD117 and FceRI [12]. In our case, although many MCs were morphologically immature (blastoid) looking, they did not express any of the latter immaturity markers (apart from FceRI which is not included in our panel), in addition to a very bright expression of CD117.

Recently, CD30 expression is becoming a widely accepted marker for neoplastic MCs and reported in many cases of MCL (up to 57%). This could have the potential to be a possible therapeutic target for anti-CD30 immunotherapy. Interestingly, CD30 also served as a marker to differentiate neoplastic from benign MCs after allogeneic bone marrow transplantation [13, 14].

3.3. CD4 Expression on Neoplastic Mast Cells and Its Suggested Role. CD4 is a marker of T-helper cells. It is also expressed on monocytes, macrophages, and dendritic cells. CD4 expression on normal and neoplastic MCs is not well addressed in the literature, as it had been reported very occasionally on normal MCs mainly in the context of HIV infection [15]. However, several studies have proposed that normal MCs are negative for CD4 [16–18]. Few studies have analyzed CD4 expression in mastocytosis. Although Mirowski et al. [16] reported CD4 expression in frozen sections in cases with cutaneous mastocytosis, Escribano et al. [11] concluded a lack of CD4 expression on MCs. Soilleux and his group had studied CD4 expression on 6 cases of mastocytosis (one SM and 5 cutaneous) after they had encountered a challenging case of CD4-positive cutaneous mastocytosis and found that all the other six cases showed positive mast cell immunostaining for CD4, albeit at slightly lesser staining intensity than small lymphocytes [19].

The actual characterization of CD4 expression on abnormal MCs (particularly in cases of SM) is not well documented and is probably underreported as the previously reported cases rather incidentally detected particularly in cases of cutaneous mastocytosis when CD4 immunostain was performed as part of the panel done to exclude T-cell neoplasms.

It seems reasonable to suggest that a direct cross-talk between T cells and MC populations exists, as recent in vitro studies indicated that MCs may be triggered to degranulate and release cytokines upon heterotypic adhesion to activated T cells [20].

Activated MCs release several cytokines that attract and activate CD4+ T cells to differentiate into Th2 cells, inducing humoral immunity [20, 21]. Histamine (produced by MCs) may stimulate T-cytotoxic cells to produce interleukin 16 (IL-16) which is chemotactic for MCs and CD4-positive T cells [22–24]. As CD4 has recently been shown to serve as an IL-16 receptor, thus, it was intriguing to speculate that IL-16 (acting via CD4) plays a pivotal role in the recruitment, activation, and differentiation of MCs in mastocytosis as well as recruitment of T lymphocytes in mast cell lesions [19]. No sufficient data regarding IL-16 in mastocytosis are currently available. A suggested cross-talk between mast cells and T cells is shown in Figure 5.

The role of the CD4 molecule in human monocyte/macrophage function and development is not known. Scott et al. have identified a new function for the CD4 molecule on human peripheral monocytes in triggering the differentiation of these cells into mature functional macrophages, following their interaction with HLA II [25].

Erythrophagocytosis by leukaemic blasts, a poor prognostic feature, is mostly seen in AML with monocytic differentiation particularly those associated with cytogenetic abnormalities involving [8, 16] *t* (p11; p13) and AML with *t* (16; 21) (p11; q22) which is seen in various subtypes of AML. Upon the literature review, we have noticed that CD4 expression on leukaemic blasts had been reported frequently in cases that showed pronounced erythrophagocytosis. Most of these cases are monocytic leukaemias, particularly the rare category of AML with *t* (8; 16). However, it was also reported in T-ALL and in AML with the BCR-ABL1 fusion gene [26–28]. Correlation between CD4 expression (a marker for monocytes/macrophages) on neoplastic MCs and the evident erythrophagocytosis seen in this case needs to be explored further.

3.4. Cytogenetic Findings in MCL. No recurrent cytogenetic abnormality was detected in MCL, and a normal cytogenetic profile was found in the majority of cases. In a study performed on 342 consecutive adult patients with SM conducted at the Mayo Clinic between 1976 and 2007 including only 4 patients with MCL showed that the recurrent chromosomal abnormalities in mastocytosis generally included trisomy 8, monosomy 7, del(13q), del(5q), trisomy 10, del(20q), trisomy 6, trisomy 19, and trisomy X, but none of these were detected in MCL [29].

Isolated trisomy 19 detected in our case was previously reported to be strongly associated with myeloid malignancies [30]. A compilation of previously published hematologic neoplasms with trisomy 19 as the sole chromosomal abnormality revealed that the great majority of cases had been myelodysplastic syndromes (MDS) (25 of 31 cases) and fewer cases of myelodysplastic/myeloproliferative neoplasms (MDS/MPN) and AML. Among reported cases of AML with isolated trisomy 19(14 cases), only four cases have had raised on top of MDS, with the trisomy 19 accruing during the time of leukaemic transformation [30]. Up to our best knowledge, trisomy 19 has never been reported in association with MCL. Of note, our case exhibited a background of myelodysplasia; however, mostly, as megaloblastic changes attributed to an

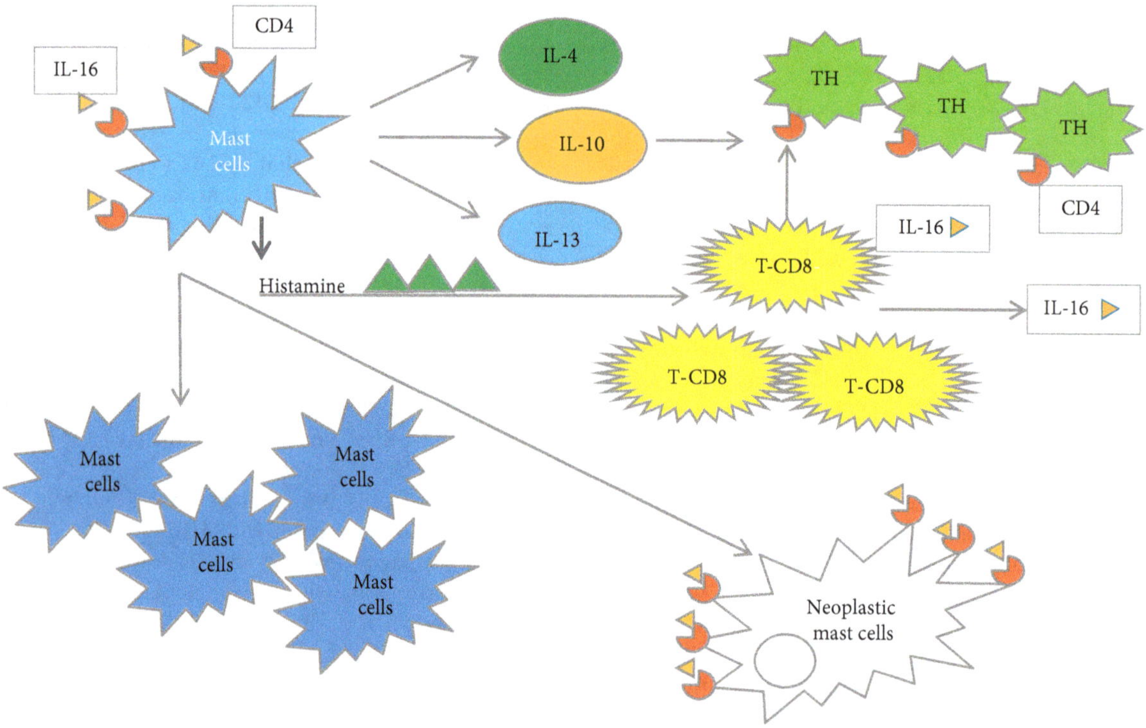

FIGURE 5: A proposed cartoon showing possible interaction between mast cells and T cells and the role of CD4 molecules. Activated MCs release several cytokines that attract and activate $CD4^+$ T cells to become Th2 cells. Histamine may stimulate T-cytotoxic cells to produce interleukin 16 (IL-16), a chemotactic for MCs and CD4-positive T cells. IL-16 acting via CD4 may play a pivotal role in the recruitment, activation, and differentiation of MCs in mastocytosis as well as recruitment of T lymphocytes in mast cell lesions.

associated vitamin B12 deficiency, the possibility of associated MDS cannot be entirely excluded.

4. Conclusion

This a report of an extraordinary rare variant of aggressive MCL, with an interesting morphologic, immunophenotypic, and cytogenetic features including hemophagocytosis by neoplastic MCs in addition to the expression of CD4 and CD7 (partially) and trisomy 19. To the best of our knowledge, this is the first case report of CD4-positive MCL. The expression of CD2 and CD25 by abnormal MCs is well documented in the literature; however; expression of other T-cell-associated markers such as CD4 and CD7 was not reported before in ASM or MCL. It is not unexpected given their common lineage that MCs may express some T-cell-associated antigens. Coexpression of CD2, CD4, CD7, and CD30 by the MCs particularly in skin lesions may provoke misinterpretation as a cutaneous T-cell neoplasm.

Currently, insufficient data on CD4 expression in MCL are available in the literature; therefore, the true incidence and significance of its expression remains unknown and requires further investigation. A possible correlation between CD4 expression (a marker for monocytes/macrophages) on neoplastic MCs and the associated erythrophagocytosis seen in this case is probable [31].

Acknowledgments

Thanks are due to Dr. Susanna Akiki who kindly revised the final manuscript. Flow cytometry, cytogenetics, and molecular genetics laboratory staff in Hamad Medical Corporation are acknowledged for their great support.

References

[1] S. H. Swerdlow, E. Campo, N. L. Harris et al., *WHO Classification of Tumours of Haematopoietic and Lymphoid Tissues*, IARC Press, Lyon, France, Revised 4th edition, 2017.

[2] S. Georgin-Lavialle, L. Lhermitte, P. Dubreuil, M.-O. Chandesris, O. Hermine, and G. Damaj, "Mast cell leukemia," *Blood*, vol. 121, no. 8, 2013.

[3] C. G. Valentini, M. Rondoni, E. M. Pogliani et al., "Mast cell leukemia: a report of ten cases," *Annals of Hematology*, vol. 87, no. 6, pp. 505–508, 2008.

[4] P. Valent, K. Sotlar, W. R. Sperr et al., "Refined diagnostic criteria and classification of mast cell leukemia (MCL) and myelomastocytic leukemia (MML): a consensus proposal," *Annals of Oncology*, vol. 25, no. 9, pp. 1691–1700, 2014.

[5] D. D. Metcalfe, "Mast cells and mastocytosis," *Blood*, vol. 112, no. 4, 2008.

[6] M. Jawhar, J. Schwaab, M. Meggendorfer et al., "The clinical and molecular diversity of mast cell leukemia with or without associated hematologic neoplasm," *Haematologica*, vol. 102, no. 6, pp. 1035–1043, 2017.

[7] H. Hans-Peter, K. Sotlar, G. Metzgeroth et al., "Mastocytosis and the updated WHO classification (2016, 2017): what is really new?," *Annals of Hematology & Oncology*, vol. 5, no. 2, p. 1194, 2018.

[8] N. Tedla, C.-W. Lee, L. Borges, C. L. Geczy, and J. P. Arm, "Differential expression of leukocyte immunoglobulin-like receptors on cord blood-derived human mast cell progenitors and mature mast cells," *Journal of Leukocyte Biology*, vol. 83, no. 2, pp. 334–343, 2008.

[9] C. Teodosio, A. C. García-Montero, M. Jara-Acevedo et al., "Mast cells from different molecular and prognostic subtypes of systemic mastocytosis display distinct immunophenotypes," *Journal of Allergy and Clinical Immunology*, vol. 125, no. 3, pp. 719.e4–726.e4, 2010.

[10] T. I. George, K. Sotlar, P. Valent et al., "Mastocytosis," in *Hematopathology*, E. S. Jaffe, D. A. Arber, E. Campo, N. L. Harris, and L. Quintanilla-Martinez, Eds., pp. 911–930, Elsevier, Amsterdam, Netherlands, 2nd edition, 2017.

[11] L. Escribano, A. Orfao, J. S. Villarrubia et al., "Sequential immunophenotypic analysis of mast cells in a case of systemic mast cell disease evolving to a mast cell leukemia," *Cytometry*, vol. 30, no. 2, pp. 98–102, 1997.

[12] C. Teodosio, A. C. García-Montero, M. Jara-Acevedo et al., "An immature immunophenotype of bone marrow mast cells predicts for multilineage D816V KIT mutation in systemic mastocytosis," *Leukemia*, vol. 26, no. 5, pp. 951–958, 2012.

[13] P. Valent, K. Sotlar, and H.-P. Horny, "Aberrant expression of CD30 in aggressive systemic mastocytosis and mast cell leukemia: a differential diagnosis to consider in aggressive hematopoietic CD30-positive neoplasms," *Leukemia & Lymphoma*, vol. 52, no. 5, pp. 740–744, 2011.

[14] K. Sotlar, S. Cerny-Reiterer, K. Petat-Dutter et al., "Aberrant expression of CD30 in neoplastic mast cells in high-grade mastocytosis," *Modern Pathology*, vol. 24, no. 4, pp. 585–595, 2011.

[15] D. D. Taub, J. A. Mikovits, G. Nilsson et al., "Alterations in mast cell function and survival following in vitro infection with human immunodeficiency viruses-1 through CXCR4," *Cellular Immunology*, vol. 230, no. 2, pp. 65–80, 2004.

[16] G. Mirowski, K. F. Austen, L. Chiang et al., "Characterization of cellular dermal infiltrates in human cutaneous mastocytosis," *Laboratory Investigation*, vol. 63, pp. 52–62, 1990.

[17] M.-T. Krauth, Y. Majlesi, S. Florian et al., "Cell surface membrane antigen phenotype of human gastrointestinal mast cells," *International Archives of Allergy and Immunology*, vol. 138, no. 2, pp. 111–120, 2005.

[18] W. R. Sperr, H. C. Bankl, G. Mundigler et al., "The human cardiac mast cell: localization, isolation, phenotype, and functional characterization," *Blood*, vol. 84, no. 11, pp. 3876–3884, 1994.

[19] E. J. Soilleux, J. Bowling, and K. Hollowood, "CD4 expression by mast cells in mastocytosis: a case report," *Journal of Clinical Pathology*, vol. 62, no. 6, pp. 564–566, 2009.

[20] P. Salamon, N. G. Shoham, I. Puxeddu, Y. Paitan, F. Levi-Schaffer, and Y. A. Mekori, "Human mast cells release oncostatin M on contact with activated T cells: possible biologic relevance," *Journal of Allergy and Clinical Immunology*, vol. 121, no. 2, pp. 448.e5–455.e5, 2008.

[21] E. Stelekati, Z. Orinska, and S. Bulfone-Paus, "Mast cells in allergy: innate instructors of adaptive responses," *Immunobiology*, vol. 212, no. 6, pp. 505–519, 2007.

[22] P. H. Hart, "Regulation of the inflammatory response in asthma by mast cell products," *Immunology and Cell Biology*, vol. 79, no. 2, pp. 149–153, 2001.

[23] J. C. Qi, R. L. Stevens, R. Wadley et al., "IL-16 regulation of human mast cells/basophils and their susceptibility to HIV-1," *The Journal of Immunology*, vol. 168, no. 8, pp. 4127–4134, 2002.

[24] W. W. Cruikshank, H. Kornfeld, and D. M. Center, "Interleukin-16," *Journal of Leukocyte Biology*, vol. 67, no. 6, pp. 757–766, 2000.

[25] K. Scott, S. Krutzik, B. Levin, V. Rezek et al., "Ligation of CD4 on human blood monocytes triggers macrophage differentiation," *Journal of Immunology*, vol. 186, no. 1, p. 158, 2011.

[26] A. Montewis and M. Eveillard, "Acute myeloid leukemia with erythrophagocytosis indicative of KAT6A rearrangement," *Blood*, vol. 128, no. 2, p. 314, 2016.

[27] A. Watanabe, K. Akahane, S. Somazu et al., "Erythrophagocytosis in T-cell type acute lymphoblastic leukaemia with near-tetraploidy," *Journal of Clinical Pathology*, vol. 69, no. 12, pp. 1129–1132, 2016.

[28] H. Murayama, H. Matsushita, Y. Obayashi, and K. Ando, "Erythrophagocytosis by blasts in acute myeloid leukaemia harbouring theBCR-ABL1fusion gene," *British Journal of Haematology*, vol. 167, no. 5, p. 586, 2014.

[29] K.-H. Lim, T. Ayalew, T. L. Lasho et al., "Systemic mastocytosis in 342 consecutive adults: survival studies and prognostic factors," *Blood*, vol. 113, no. 23, pp. 5727–5736, 2009.

[30] B. Johasson, R. Billström, N. Mauritzson, and F. Mitelman, "Trisomy 19 as the sole chromosomal anomaly in hematologic neoplasms," *Cancer Genetics and Cytogenetics*, vol. 74, no. 1, pp. 62–65, 1994.

[31] "Highly aggressive CD4-positive mast cell leukemia (leukaemic variant) associated with hemophagocytosis," in *Proceedings of the Thirty First International Symposium on Technical Innovations in Laboratory Hematology*, Brussels, Belgium, May 2012.

14

Two Consecutive Episodes of Severe Delayed Hemolytic Transfusion Reaction in a Sickle Cell Disease Patient

Clarisse Mpinganzima,[1] Alf Haaland,[1] Anne Guro Vreim Holm,[2] Swee Lay Thein,[3] Geir Erland Tjønnfjord,[1,4] and Per Ole Iversen[1,5,6]

[1]*Department of Haematology, Oslo University Hospital, Oslo, Norway*
[2]*Department of Orthopedic Surgery, Oslo University Hospital, Oslo, Norway*
[3]*Sickle Cell Branch, National Heart Lung and Blood Institute, National Institutes of Health, Bethesda, MD, USA*
[4]*Institute of Clinical Medicine, University of Oslo, Oslo, Norway*
[5]*Department of Nutrition, Institute of Basic Medical Sciences, University of Oslo, Oslo, Norway*
[6]*Division of Human Nutrition, Stellenbosch University, Tygerberg, South Africa*

Correspondence should be addressed to Per Ole Iversen; p.o.iversen@medisin.uio.no

Academic Editor: Kostas Konstantopoulos

Patients with sickle cell disease (SCD) suffer from anemia and painful vaso-occlusive crisis (VOC) and sometimes need blood transfusions. Delayed hemolytic transfusion reaction (DHTR) is a rare life-threatening complication observed in SCD and mimics VOC. We describe a female SCD patient undergoing three surgical procedures during which DHTR developed following the first two. Prior to a planned tonsillectomy, she received transfusion and three days after surgery developed severe hemolysis as well as pain and respiratory symptoms. On suspicion of VOC, she received additional transfusions and became hemodynamically unstable, and her hemolytic anemia worsened. Gradually, she recovered and could be discharged after two weeks; DHTR was not suspected. Sixteen months later, an arthroplasty was performed due to avascular necrosis, and again she was transfused preoperatively. Similar to the initial surgery, she developed symptoms and signs of VOC after three days, but this time, DHTR was suspected and further transfusions were withheld. Although immunosuppressive medication did not alleviate the condition, she improved on combined treatment with darbepoietin, rituximab, and eculizumab. Six months later, a second arthroplasty was performed uneventfully after prophylaxis with rituximab and without transfusion. DHTR should be considered in the presence of severe, unexplained hemolysis following a recent transfusion, and additional transfusions in this setting should be given only on vital indication.

1. Introduction

Sickle cell disease (SCD) is an inherited hemoglobinopathy prevalent in equatorial regions such as sub-Saharan Africa. This is partly because carriers (heterozygotes) of the mutated sickle cell gene are protected against fatal complications of severe malaria [1]. The disease is characterized by hemolytic anemia, infections, and vaso-occlusive crisis (VOC) with acute as well as chronic pain, leading to significant lifelong morbidity and increased mortality.

In case of severe anemia, blood transfusions may be indicated in SCD. Repeated transfusions often result in the formation of anti-red blood cell (RBC) alloantibodies, and alloimmunization occurs more frequently in SCD patients than in other heavily transfused patient groups [2]. The prevalence of alloimmunization in SCD patients is reportedly between 30% and 50% [2, 3]. Delayed hemolytic transfusion reaction (DHTR) is a life-threatening complication due to alloimmunization. Generally, DHTR is rare, but it has been typically described among SCD patients, possibly due to mismatch between donor-RBC antigens

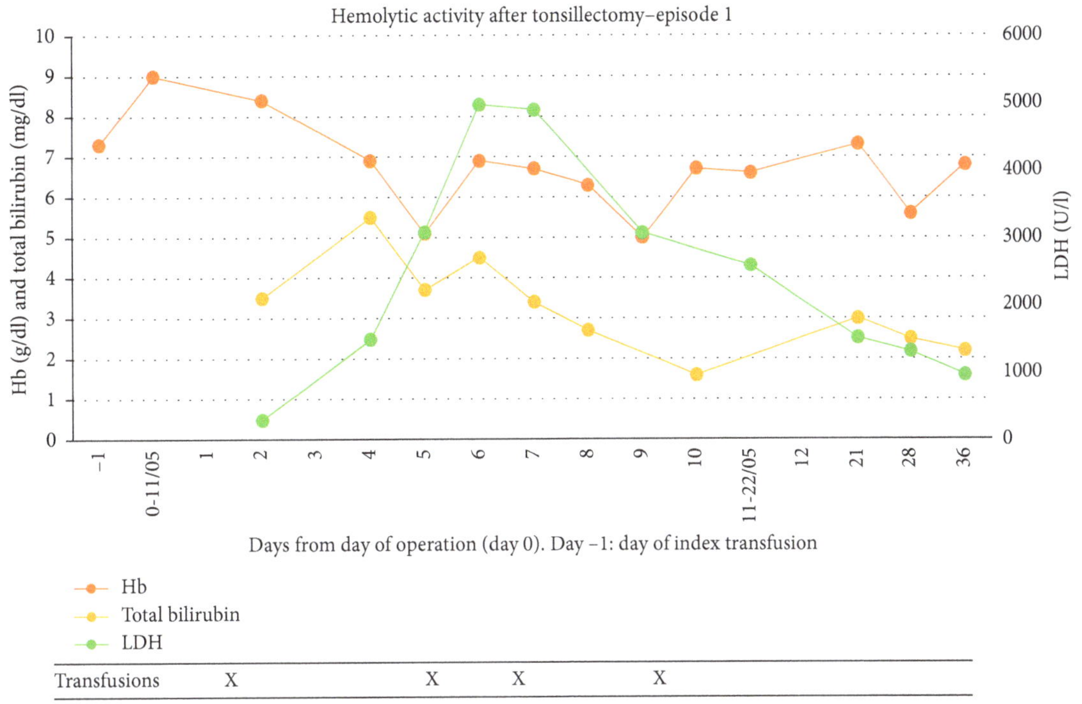

Figure 1: Time course of blood values obtained during and after the first episode. Reference ranges: Hb (11.7–15.3 g/dl); bilirubin (0.3–1.5 mg/dl); LDH (105–205 U/l).

(mainly Caucasian) and SCD-recipients (mainly Africans) [4]. There is to date no consensus definition of DHTR, but it is characterized by unequivocal evidence of severe hemolysis leading to a marked drop in hemoglobin levels below pre-fusion level, with or without detectable alloantibodies, and often appearing within 24 hours to 3 weeks after transfusion [5]. The true prevalence of DHTR among SCD patients is difficult to assess since this condition is probably often undiagnosed, but a prevalence ranging from 4% to 8% of transfused adult SCD patients has been reported with those receiving acute transfusions being at highest risk compared to those receiving chronic transfusions [6, 7].

Our knowledge about DHTR stems from case reports and case series usually involving only one DHTR event per patient. We here present an unusual case of repeated DHTRs without documented alloimmunization in a SCD patient treated at our unit on three different occasions where we suspect DHTR as the major underlying mechanism of the severe complications observed during the first two admissions. Consequently, a different approach to the third admission led to an uneventful clinical course.

2. Case Presentation

A 28-year-old Nigerian female with homozygous SCD became a regular outpatient at our department in 2013 after an uneventful (without any blood transfusion) pregnancy and birth in the USA. As a child, she had received several transfusions, apparently with no complications. She had the following blood type profile: 0; D+; C-; E-; c+; e+; K-; S-; in addition to anti-C and anti-E antibodies. She had never used any medication except folic acid.

2.1. Episode 1. In May 2017, she underwent an elective tonsillectomy at our hospital (a tertiary reference center in Norway; day 0). Except for routine pre-transfusion screening, neither extended screening for new alloantibodies nor a direct antiglobulin test was performed. On day −1, she received a scheduled transfusion of two cross-matched units of RBC with hemoglobin (Hb) increasing from a baseline value of 7 to 9.0 g/dl. After an uncomplicated procedure, she was transferred to a local hospital with an uneventful clinical course until day +4 when she developed generalized skeletal pain and fever, but no chest or respiratory symptoms. As Figure 1 shows, her Hb declined till day +5. There were concurrent signs of increased hemolysis with total bilirubin increasing to 5.5 mg/dl and lactate dehydrogenase (LDH) more than tripled in the same time period. On suspicion of VOC, she was on day +4 treated with analgesics, fluids, low-molecular-weight heparin, and antibiotics according to our guidelines. Her condition deteriorated within the next 24 hours, and she became increasingly respiratory distressed. A CT scan showed bilateral pulmonary infiltrates. Acute chest syndrome was suspected, and she received partial exchange transfusion with two cross-matched units of RBC, resulting in a transient Hb rise. Two additional units of RBC were administered, and the patient was transferred to the intensive care unit on day +6. Hb was then 6.9 g/dl, which over the next 6 hours fell to 5.1 g/dl. LDH peaked at 4,974 U/l, whereas haptoglobin was not detectable. Retrospectively, we noted a relative reticulocytopenia with a maximum value of 120×10^9/l. She became hemodynamically unstable, and vasopressor support and two more units of RBC were given before she was intubated. She was extubated the following day, and over the next few days, her condition stabilized; the

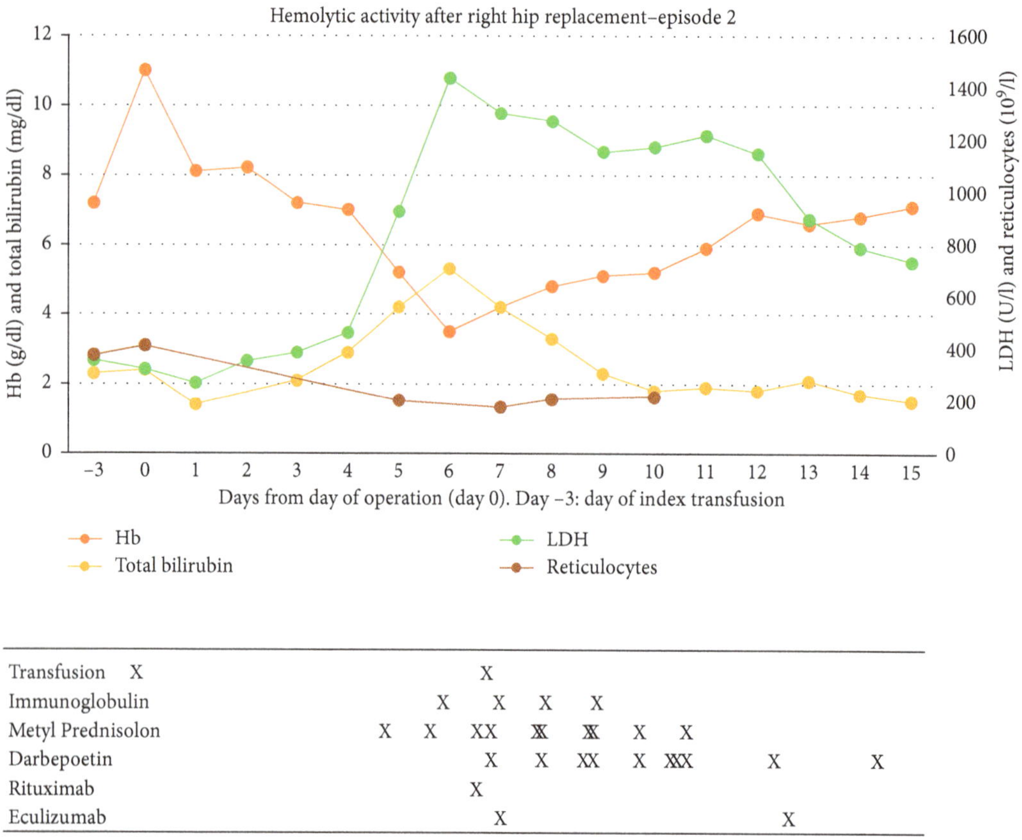

Figure 2: Time course of blood values obtained during and after the second episode. Reference range: reticulocytes (20–100 × 10^9/l).

hemolytic parameters were markedly reduced by day +9, and she was discharged on day +13 with subsequent visits as an outpatient. All bacterial cultures from this admission were negative. Notably, during this first episode, DHTR was never suspected.

2.2. Episode 2. Due to avascular necrosis of her right hip, the patient underwent an arthroplasty in September 2018. On day −3 prior to surgery, she received a planned transfusion with three cross-matched units of RBC, raising her Hb to 11.0 g/dl. Her pre-transfusion screening revealed no new alloantibodies. After an uncomplicated orthopedic procedure on day 0, she was transferred to our department. On day +3, she developed skeletal pain but no symptoms related to the newly operated hip. On suspicion of VOC, treatment was initiated with fluids, analgesics, and antibiotics. As illustrated in Figure 2, her Hb fell gradually towards her baseline level without any obvious signs of bleeding or accelerated hemolysis during days 0 to +3. However, on day +5, she developed rapid and marked hemolysis with hemoglobinuria, Hb fell to 5.3 g/dl, and LDH rose to above 1,000 U/l. As noted in the first episode, there was a lack of adequate reticulocyte response with values falling from 413 to 177 × 10^9/l. We suspected DHTR, and further transfusions were avoided. Intravenous immunoglobulin therapy (30 g daily) was initiated for 4 days. On day +6, Hb plummeted to 3.5 g/dl, and LDH and total bilirubin peaked at 1470 U/l and 5.3 mg/dl, respectively, and intravenous methylprednisolone (500 mg per day for 5 days) was administered. Screening for new alloantibodies and a direct antiglobulin test were both negative. Her HbA-fraction declined from 33.5% at day 0 to 12.3% on day +6. Using the nomogram proposed by Mekontso Dessap et al. [8], the likelihood of DHTR was considered as high. Because of the critically low Hb, she received one cross-matched unit of RBC on day +6. Rituximab (an anti-CD20 antibody, 1000 mg i.v.) was given together with the transfusion. Two single doses of eculizumab (an anti-complement factor 5 antibody, 900 mg i.v.) were administered on days +6 and +12, whereas the erythropoietin analogue darbepoietin (200 mg s.c.) was given every second day from day +6 for a week. Over the next days, hemolysis declined, and her Hb stabilized. On day +4, complement factor C1q was 170 (reference 70–150) mg/l, increasing to 357 mg/l on day +6, whereas after the administration of eculizumab, markers of the classical, the lectin, and the alternative pathways for complement activation were all reduced towards undetectable levels. Despite signs of significant intravascular hemolysis, no serious organ dysfunction was recorded. She was discharged on day +15. On follow-up, she received pneumococcal and meningococcal vaccines. She had a full recovery and was thereafter not admitted for VOC, infections or transfusions.

2.3. Episode 3. Due to progressive avascular necrosis of the contralateral hip, an arthroplasty was performed in March 2019. Screening for new alloantibodies and a direct antiglobulin test were both negative. As a preoperative strategy

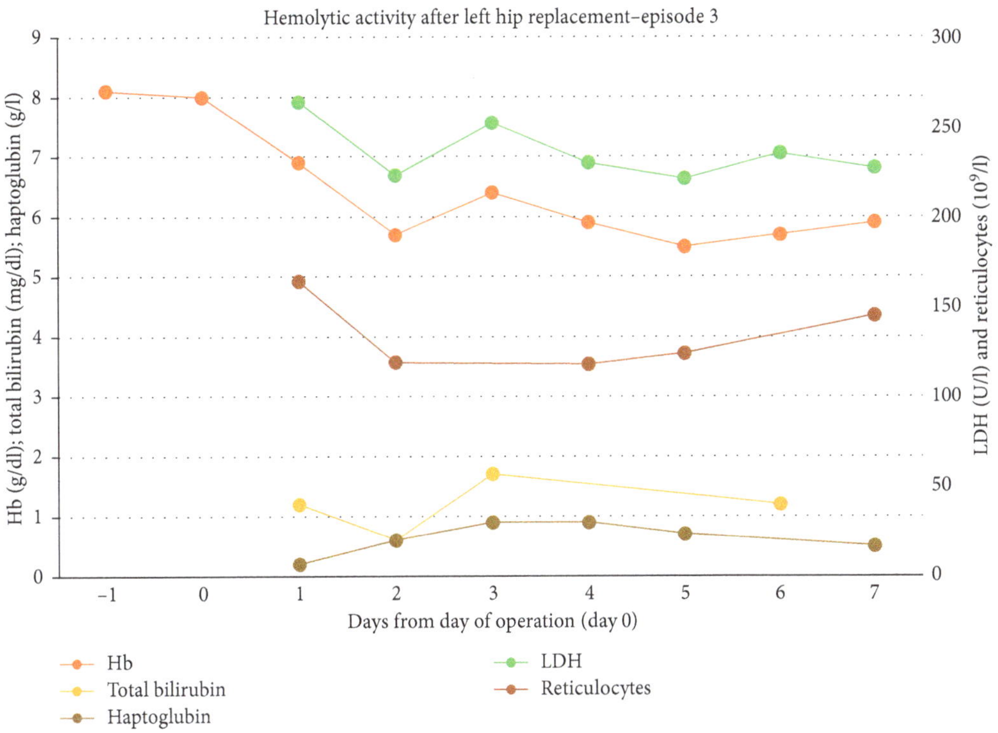

FIGURE 3: Time course of blood values obtained during and after the third episode. Reference range: haptoglobin (0.4–2.1 g/dl).

to optimize erythropoiesis, she received darbepoietin for two months as well as hydroxyurea, but no prophylactic transfusions. She maintained a preoperative Hb of about 8 g/dl, and she was also given one prophylactic dose of rituximab (1000 mg i.v.) 2.5 weeks before surgery. Both the surgery and the postoperative stay in hospital were uneventful and with no signs of hemolysis (Figure 3). She was discharged one week later. Regular follow-up visits at the outpatient clinic until December 2019 revealed no complications.

3. Discussion

We here present a SCD patient who received preoperative blood transfusions during two consecutive hospital admissions which were most likely complicated by DHTR. Although DHTR was not suspected during the first admission, we were alert to this complication during the second admission. Hence, we were able to provide her with adequate prophylactic treatment and avoided DHTR during her third admission.

Retrospectively, we believe the symptoms she presented during her postoperative hospital admission in 2017 represented the start of DHTR. A main challenge in identifying DHTR in SCD patients is that the symptoms often mimic VOC. In a large French observational study of about 3,000 SCD patients, the most common presenting symptoms and signs were hemoglobinuria (94%), pain (89%), fever (64%), and severe anemia (44%) [7]. Suppression of erythropoiesis reflected in reticulocytopenia ($<150 \times 10^9/l$) was observed in 40% of the patients. Progression to acute chest syndrome or even multi-organ failure was not uncommon in the most severe cases with an overall mortality of 6% [4]. Since transfusions are sometimes indicated in VOC, such treatment may further exacerbate hemolysis if DHTR is present [4–6].

Hyperhemolysis refers to the destruction of allogenic and autologous erythrocytes, potentially leading to severe and fatal hemolysis [6,7]. In line with this, our patient had a steep decline in Hb and spiking LDH on days +5 and +6 during the first and second episode, respectively. Alloantibody and direct antiglobulin screenings are imperative since it can aid in early identification of "missed" or evanescent antibodies. This is important also because patients may be treated at different institutions over the course of a lifetime, and without universal medical records, they may receive transfusions of blood with antibodies "lost to follow-up". Moreover, follow-up screenings at regular intervals following a diagnosed DHTR will increase the likelihood of detecting new alloantibodies [9].

No new alloantibodies were detected in the acute setting during the second episode, and a direct antiglobulin test was negative. However, no repeated screenings were done between the first two episodes or after the second episode. Neither did we perform extended antibody screening for low-frequency antigens. Notably, hyperhemolysis may occur without newly formed alloantibodies and has been described in up to 1/3 of SCD patients [5, 8]. The pathophysiology of antibody negative DHTR is not fully understood, but may involve macrophage activation and/or heme involvement leading to endothelial damage and subsequent activation of the alternative complement pathway [10, 11].

There is little evidence-based data for the therapeutic approach to patients with suspected DHTR, and current treatment modalities are mainly based on expert recommendations [12]. Immunoglobulins or high-dose steroids are the recommended first-line therapy. Our patient received both agents as her hemolysis spiked, however, Hb still plummeted to 3.4 g/dl. We therefore chose to give a single transfusion at this critical anemia. We gave rituximab prior to transfusion to prevent new alloantibodies [13]. Relative reticulocytopenia secondary to suppressed erythropoiesis is a feature of DHTR, and it was observed in our patient during both episodes 1 and 2. To stimulate endogenous blood production, we administered an erythropoietin analogue. Eculizumab has been used in the management of patients with severe DHTR and severe hemolysis [14]. Our patient had elevated C1q indicating increased complement activation and thus received eculizumab along with rituximab. We do not know which agent contributed most to the resolution of the hemolysis, so we can only speculate that eculizumab was the most effective drug since it is known to result in rapid reduction of hemolysis [15].

DHTR is a rare life-threatening complication to transfusions in SCD patients. Our patient illustrates the dilemma that DHTR can be misdiagnosed as VOC, a complication of SCD that is much more common than DHTR. Hence, a DHTR diagnosis should always be considered in the presence of an unexplained increase in hemolysis following a recent transfusion, and further transfusions should be avoided unless life-threatening anemia is present.

References

[1] F. B. Piel, A. P. Patil, R. E. Howes et al., "Global distribution of the sickle cell gene and geographical confirmation of the malaria hypothesis," *Nature Communications*, vol. 1, p. 104, 2010.

[2] R. Balbuena-Merle and J. E. Hendrickson, "Red blood cell alloimmunization and delayed hemolytic transfusion reactions in patients with sickle cell disease," *Transfusion Clinique et Biologique*, vol. 26, no. 2, pp. 112–115, 2019.

[3] K. Yazdanbakhsh, B. H. Shaz, and C. D. Hillyer, "Immune regulation of sickle cell alloimmunization," *ISBT Science Series*, vol. 12, no. 1, pp. 248–253, 2017.

[4] R. M. Fasano, M. J. Miller, S. Chonat, and S. R. Stowell, "Clinical presentation of delayed hemolytic transfusion reactions and hyperhemolysis in sickle cell disease," *Transfusion Clinique et Biologique*, vol. 26, no. 2, pp. 94–98, 2019.

[5] K. Stowell, R. E. Ware, and F. Noizat-Pirenne, "Red blood cell alloimmunization in sickle cell disease: pathophysiology, risk factors, and transfusion management," *Blood*, vol. 120, no. 3, pp. 528–537, 2012.

[6] D. Narbey, A. Habibi, P. Chadebech et al., "Incidence and predictive score for delayed hemolytic transfusion reaction in adult patients with sickle cell disease," *American Journal of Hematology*, vol. 92, no. 12, pp. 1340–1348, 2017.

[7] A. Habibi, A. Mekontso-Dessap, C. Guillaud et al., "Delayed hemolytic transfusion reaction in adult sickle-cell disease: presentations, outcomes, and treatments of 99 referral center episodes," *American Journal of Hematology*, vol. 91, no. 10, pp. 989–994, 2016.

[8] A. Mekontso Dessap, F. Pirenne, K. Razazi et al., "A diagnostic nomogram for delayed hemolytic transfusion reaction in sickle cell disease," *American Journal of Hematology*, vol. 91, no. 12, pp. 1181–1184, 2016.

[9] F. Pirenne and K. Yazdanbakhsh, "How I safely transfuse patients with sickle-cell disease and manage delayed hemolytic transfusion reactions," *Blood*, vol. 131, no. 25, pp. 2773–2781, 2028.

[10] C. Rieux, E. De Meyer, and K. Boudjedir, "Les hémolyses retardées post-transfusionnelles chez les patients drépanocytaires: un nouveau défi pour le réseau d'hémovigilance," *Transfusion Clinique et Biologique*, vol. 22, no. 1, pp. 37–41, 2015.

[11] S. Chonat, M.-O. Quarmyne, C. M. Bennett et al., "Contribution of alternative complement pathway to delayed hemolytic transfusion reaction in sickle cell disease," *Haematologica*, vol. 103, no. 10, pp. e483–e485, 2018.

[12] K. Gardner, C. Hoppe, A. Mijovic, and S. L. Thein, "How we treat delayed haemolytic transfusion reactions in patients with sickle cell disease," *British Journal of Haematology*, vol. 170, no. 6, pp. 745–756, 2015.

[13] F. Thein, A. Habibi, A. Mekontso-Dessap et al., "The use of rituximab to prevent severe delayed haemolytic transfusion reaction in immunized patients with sickle cell disease," *Vox Sanguinis*, vol. 108, no. 3, pp. 262–267, 2015.

[14] G. Dumas, A. Habibi, T. Onimus et al., "Eculizumab salvage therapy for delayed hemolysis transfusion reaction in sickle cell disease patients," *Blood*, vol. 127, no. 8, pp. 1062–1064, 2016.

[15] R. A. Brodsky, N. S. Young, E. Antonioli et al., "Multicenter phase 3 study of the complement inhibitor eculizumab for the treatment of patients with paroxysmal nocturnal hemoglobinuria," *Blood*, vol. 111, no. 4, pp. 1840–1847, 2008.

15

Severe Late-Onset Drug-Induced Immune Thrombocytopenia Following IFN β-1a Treatment: A Case Report of a 52-Year-Old Woman with Relapse-Remitting Multiple Sclerosis

Christophe Cisarovsky,[1] **Marie Théaudin**,[2] **Pierre-Alexandre Bart**,[1] **Grégoire Stalder**,[3] **and Lorenzo Alberio**[3]

[1]*Division of Internal Medicine, Department of Medicine, Lausanne University Hospital and University of Lausanne, Rue du Bugnon 46, CH-1011 Lausanne, Switzerland*
[2]*Division of Neurology, Department of Clinical Neurosciences, Lausanne University Hospital and University of Lausanne, Rue du Bugnon 46, CH-1011 Lausanne, Switzerland*
[3]*Service and Central Laboratory of Hematology, Department of Oncology and Department, Laboratories and Pathology, Lausanne University Hospital and University of Lausanne, Rue du Bugnon 46, CH-1011 Lausanne, Switzerland*

Correspondence should be addressed to Christophe Cisarovsky; christophe.cisarovsky@gmail.com

Academic Editor: Kostas Konstantopoulos

Interferon β-1a (IFNβ1a) is considered safe in relapsing-remitting multiple sclerosis (RRMS). Drug-induced thrombocytopenia (DITP) is a rare but underreported adverse event that is often confused with other causes of thrombocytopenia. We report the case of a 52-year-old woman who developed limb and oral mucosa petechiae and hematochezia, 10 years after beginning IFNβ1a. Blood work showed an isolated severe thrombocytopenia and ruled out other autoimmune diseases, viral infections, intravascular hemolysis, and renal impairment. Oral corticosteroids and tranexamic acid were initiated with a favorable platelet response. IFNβ1a was resumed, leading to recurrence of thrombocytopenia. Platelets came back to normal after intravenous immunoglobulins and IFNβ1a was definitively discontinued. To our knowledge, this is the first case of drug-induced immune thrombocytopenia (DITP) associated with IFNβ1a.

1. Introduction

Interferons (IFN) β-1a and 1b were the first effective treatment for relapsing-remitting multiple sclerosis (RRMS) and are still used as first-line therapies [1]. They are less efficient than most of the recent disease-modifying drugs but have the advantage of an excellent safety profile. However, around 5% of the patients experience hematologic toxicity including mild anemia or thrombocytopenia, which rarely requires dose adjustment or treatment discontinuation [2]. Suggested mechanisms are decreased megakaryocytes proliferation and maturation, and impaired production of platelets [3, 4]. Thrombocytopenia <75 G/L is very uncommon and should prompt further investigations.

Drug-induced thrombocytopenia (DITP) is often not initially recognized and has an estimated incidence rate of 1 case per 100 000 inhabitants per year [5]. This incidence might be substantially higher in hospitalized patients, elderly persons, or those on specific medications. IFNβ are not listed in the comprehensive database of all substances that can cause thrombocytopenia (http://www.ouhsc.edu/platelets), and immune thrombocytopenia (ITP) is not a side effect that is described by the European Medicines Agency [6]. Of note, cases of thrombotic microangiopathies (hemolytic uremic syndrome and thrombotic thrombocytopenic purpura), which associate thrombocytopenia with anemia and multiorgan failure, have been previously described and are treated differently [7]. Very recently, a further case of

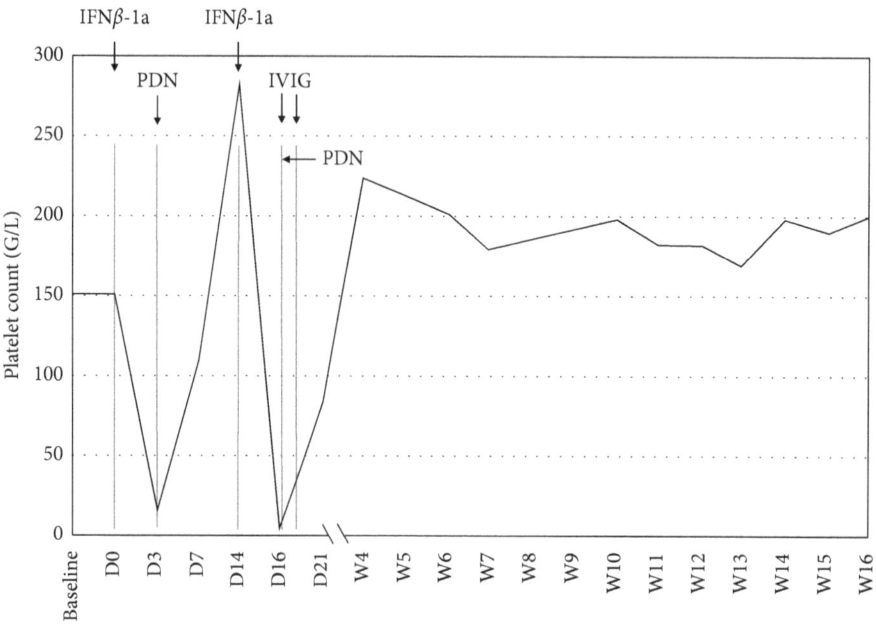

FIGURE 1: Platelet count at baseline (2 months before), since the last interferon β-1a injection before the occurrence of petechial lesions (IFNβ-1a, D0) and upon rechallenge (D14), and their evolution with subsequent treatments. Prednisone (PDN) is only shown when 1 mg/kg has been initiated. Two administrations of intravenous immunoglobulins (IVIG, 2 g/kg total dose) were performed.

thrombotic thrombocytopenic purpura in a woman with relapse-remitting multiple sclerosis treated with IFNβ-1a was published [8].

Here, we report the first case to our knowledge of a patient with severe relapsing thrombocytopenia following repetitive IFNβ-1a (Avonex®, Biogen, Switzerland AG) treatment and successfully managed with tranexamic acid, oral corticosteroids, intravenous immunoglobulins, and definitive drug withdrawal. We highlight the unusual appearance of this side effect after a 10-year period of treatment tolerance.

2. Clinical Case

A 52-year-old woman presented to the emergency department with unexplained bruises, petechial lesions on the four limbs and in the mouth, and hematochezia. She was diagnosed with RRMS at age 32 and had been treated for the last ten years with IFNβ-1a (30 μg) once weekly, without any relapse over the previous 6 years. The last IFNβ-1a injection was three days before the onset of symptoms (Figure 1, D0, platelet count 152 G/L). Except for a low body mass index (BMI 18 kg/m^2), no other comorbidities were known and she did not take any medication but clonazepam, calcium, and vitamin D supplementation. Physical examination was otherwise normal, notably regarding fever. Blood examination showed severe thrombocytopenia (13 G/L; reference range: 150–350 G/L). Other blood parameters were normal and included blood smear, coagulation tests, hemolysis parameters, liver and renal functions, proteinuria and urinary sediment, HIV/viral hepatitis B and C/CMV/EBV/*H. pylori* serologies, serum immunofixation, autoantibodies (antinuclear, anti-neutrophil cytoplasmic antibodies, anti-nucleosome, anti-nucleoproteins), direct and indirect antiglobulin tests, and vitamins dosage (B9 and B12). Abdominal echography was normal. We first made a working diagnosis of ITP and the initial treatment consisted of oral tranexamic acid (1 g tid), corticosteroids (prednisone 1 mg/kg/day), and advice to IFNβ-1a discontinuation. After 24 hours, the platelet count rose to 57 G/L (Figure 1) and progressive platelet normalization allowed the patient to be discharged after six days. Eleven days after symptom onset, prednisone was tapered from 40 mg/d to 30 mg/d and IFNβ-1a injections resumed. Two days later, the patient noticed hemorrhagic blistering on her lips. Platelet count dropped to 1 G/L, requiring intravenous immunoglobulins (IVIG, 1 g/kg for 2 days) and a new oral corticosteroids at 1 mg/kg/day. *Fundus oculi* examination was normal. Brain magnetic resonance imaging showed no sign of RRMS activity. Platelet kinetic was rapidly favorable and we then made the diagnosis of immune DITP following IFNβ-1a treatment. Lifelong drug discontinuation was advised to her neurologist. Unfortunately, between 6 and 10 months after, thrombocytopenia relapsed in the context of a viral infection and of unknown origin, suggesting ITP. Given the high immunogenic status of the patient, she is currently considered for rituximab or ocrelizumab treatment, which are both effective in multiple sclerosis and other immune-mediated disorders, such as ITP [9].

3. Discussion

We report the first case of severe immune-mediated DITP following long-term IFNβ-1a treatment. The causal relationship between the drug and thrombocytopenia was confirmed by a positive drug rechallenge [10].

Table 1: Left panel: differential diagnosis of thrombocytopenia. Middle panel: drugs with drug-platelet antibodies involved in drug-induced thrombocytopenia (Adapted from https://www.ouhsc.edu/platelets). Right panel: mechanisms of immune-mediated drug-induced thrombocytopenia (adapted from 10).

Differential diagnosis of thrombocytopenia	Drugs implicated in drug-induced thrombocytopenia (immune-mediated platelet destruction)	Mechanisms of drug-dependent antibodies
(i) Pseudothrombocytopenia (ii) Medications (immune-mediated platelet destruction and non-immune suppression of platelet production) (iii) Herbal preparation, food (walnut and sesame seeds), and beverages (tonic water and cranberry juice) (iv) Infectious diseases (CMV, EBV, Parvovirus B19, HIV, VHB, VHC, *H. pylori*, *M. tuberculosis*, and *M. pneumoniae*) (v) Vaccines (measles, influenza, and VHB) (vi) Hematological and solid cancers (vii) Hemolysis and DIC (viii) Hypersplenism (ix) Autoimmune diseases (SLE, scleroderma, Sjögren's disease, and MCTD) (x) Vitamin deficiencies (B9 and B12) or copper deficiency (xi) Thrombotic microangiopathy (TTP and HSU) (xii) Iodinated contrast product	(i) NSAIDs (naproxen, diclofenac, and ibuprofen) (ii) Antibiotics (rifampicin, penicillins, trimethoprim-sulfamethoxazole, and vancomycin) (iii) Antiepileptics (carbamazepine, phenytoin, and valproic acid) (iv) Quinine and quinidine (v) H2-receptor antagonists (ranitidine and cimetidine) (vi) Chlorothiazide and hydrochlorthiazide (vii) Chemotherapy (oxaliplatin and gold) (viii) Glycoprotein IIb/IIIa receptor antagonists (tirofiban, abciximab, and eptifibatide) (ix) Interferon α	(i) Classic drug-dependent antibodies targeted to neoepitope created by noncovalent binding of the drug to platelet glycoproteins (ii) Hapten-induced antibodies created by covalent binding of drug to platelet proteins (iii) Specific fiban- and Fab-binding antibodies (glycoprotein IIb/IIIa receptor antagonists) (iv) Autoantibody production in response to a given drug (gold and alemtuzumab) (v) Platelet-localizing immune complexes leading to their activation and clearance

Abbreviations: CMV: cytomegalovirus; DIC: disseminated intravascular coagulation; EBV: Epstein–Barr virus; HIV: human immunodeficiency virus; HUS: hemolytic uremic syndrome; MCTD: mixed connective tissue disease; NSAIDs: Nonsteroidal anti-inflammatory drugs; SLE: systemic lupus erythematosus; TTP: thrombotic thrombocytopenic purpura; VHB/VHC: viral hepatitis B/C.

Thrombocytopenia in DITP usually occurs within 5–10 days after initiation of a new drug or within hours of subsequent exposure [10]. In our case, thrombocytopenia occurred 3 days after the last IFNβ-1a injection and 1–2 days upon rechallenge. DITP is generally severe (<20 G/L) with concomitant bleeding symptoms and signs (petechial lesions, bruising, and epistaxis) and deaths have been reported. The primary treatment for DITP is to discontinue the suspected causative agent, with an expected platelet count rise within 1–10 days. Patients experiencing mucous blistering or life-threatening bleeding may benefit from IVIG therapy, plasmapheresis, or platelet transfusion. Corticosteroids seem inefficient in the treatment of DITP, unless the patient is at high risk for, or is actively bleeding [10]. Co-occurrence of corticosteroid dose decrease and IFNβ-1a injection before thrombocytopenia relapse prompted us to continue the steroids for three months. We did not test for the presence of specific drug antibodies. Of note, results would not have led to treatment modification since the detection of drug-platelet antibodies lacks validation and standardization among the variety of techniques and drugs involved in DITP [10].

No such antibodies were previously described for IFNβ-1a [10]. Clonazepam treatment was never discontinued and therefore an unlikely cause of DITP. Patient's low BMI might have had a possible role in a dose-related toxicity, even though IFNβ-1a had been well tolerated for 10 years.

DITP can be immune-mediated (drug-dependent antibodies) or non-immune-mediated (bone marrow suppression). Major drugs with known evidence of immune-mediated thrombocytopenia and mechanisms of the development of drug-dependent antibodies are listed in Table 1. Non-immune-mediated thrombocytopenia involves direct myelosuppression through impairment of megakaryocyte survival, proliferation, and maturation (e.g., valganciclovir, IFNα/β, and chemotherapy).

Thrombocytopenia occurs in a wide variety of contexts that are summarized in Table 1 [11]. Thrombocytopenia and cases of ITP in multiple sclerosis have been described, however, at a lower frequency than potentially fatal thrombotic microangiopathies (uremic hemolytic syndrome and thrombotic thrombocytopenic purpura) [7]. Unlike IFNα, IFNβ has never been associated with immune-mediated DITP.

We reported this serious adverse effect of IFNβ-1a to the *swiss pharmacovigilance* (*Swissmedic*). Criteria used to establish the relationship with drug-induced thrombocytopenic purpura were all met [12]. Indeed, therapy with the candidate drug preceded the thrombocytopenic event and recovery from thrombocytopenia was complete and sustained after discontinuation of the drug. Other causes of thrombocytopenia were ruled out, except for the possible role of the autoimmune status of multiple sclerosis, which manifested months later as ITP. Finally, a positive drug rechallenge was performed, being considered as a diagnostic criterion.

4. Conclusion

This case highlights an unknown but potentially lethal side effect of IFNβ-1a treatment: immune-mediated DITP. Remarkably, immune-mediated DITP occurred years after treatment initiation. Treatment consists of long-term drug withdrawal and IVIG in case of severe thrombocytopenia with bleeding manifestations. Other forms of severe thrombocytopenia associated with anemia and multiorgan failure have been associated with IFNβ-1a treatment (thrombotic microangiopathies); however, they present and are treated differently. Immune-mediated DITP has also been described with other disease-modifying therapies for multiple sclerosis (fingolimod, natalizumab, and alemtuzumab), highlighting the importance for neurologists of knowing of this category of possible side effects.

Consent

Written consent has been obtained from the patient.

References

[1] C. H. Goldschmidt and L. H. Hua, "Re-evaluating the use of IFN-β and relapsing multiple sclerosis: safety, efficacy and place in therapy," *Degenerative Neurological and Neuromuscular Disease*, vol. 10, pp. 29–38, 2020.

[2] P. Rieckmann, P. O'Connor, G. S. Francis, G. Wetherill, and E. Alteri, "Haematological effects of interferon-β-1a (Rebif®) therapy in multiple sclerosis," *Drug Safety*, vol. 27, no. 10, pp. 745–756, 2004.

[3] S. Negrotto, C. J. De Giusti, M. J. Lapponi et al., "Expression and functionality of type I interferon receptor in the megakaryocytic lineage," *Journal of Thrombosis and Haemostasis*, vol. 9, no. 12, pp. 2477–2485, 2011.

[4] A. Yamane, T. Nakamura, H. Suzuki et al., "Interferon-α2b—induced thrombocytopenia is caused by inhibition of platelet production but not proliferation and endomitosis in human megakaryocytes," *Blood*, vol. 112, no. 3, pp. 542–550, 2008.

[5] P. M. L. A. van den Bemt, R. H. B. Meyboom, and A. C. G. Egberts, "Drug-induced immune thrombocytopenia," *Drug Safety*, vol. 27, no. 15, pp. 1243–1252, 2004.

[6] Avonex. Summary of Product Characteristics, 2022, https://www.ema.europa.eu/en/docu-ments/product-information/avonex-epar-product-information_en.pdf.

[7] A. F. Ben-Amor, A. Trochanov, and T. Z. Fischer, "Cumulative review of thrombotic microangiopathy, thrombotic thrombocytopenic purpura, and hemolytic uremic syndrome reports with subcutaneous interferon β-1a," *Advances in Therapy*, vol. 32, no. 5, pp. 445–454, 2015.

[8] C. F. Plesa, D. M. Chitimus, C. A. Sirbu et al., "Thrombotic thrombocytopenic purpura in interferon beta-1a-treated patient diagnosed with relapsing-remitting multiple sclerosis: a case report," *Life*, vol. 12, no. 1, pp. 80–85, 2022.

[9] C. Kaegi, B. Wuest, C. Crowley, and O. Boyman, "Systematic review of safety and efficacy of second- and third-generation CD20-targeting biologics in treating immune-mediated disorders," *Frontiers in Immunology*, vol. 12, Article ID 788830, 2021.

[10] I. Marini, G. Uzun, K. Jamal, and T. Bakchoul, "Treatment of drug-induced immune thrombocytopenias," *Haematologica*, vol. 107, no. 6, pp. 1264–1277, 2022.

[11] L. Alberio, "My patient is thrombocytopenic! Is (s)he? Why? And what shall I do?: a practical approach to thrombocytopenia," *Hämostaseologie*, vol. 33, no. 2, pp. 83–94, 2013.
[12] J. N. George, G. E. Raskob, S. R. Shah, M. A. Rizvi, S. A. Hamilton, and S. Osborne, "Drug-induced thrombocytopenia: a systematic review of published case reports," *Annals of Internal Medicine*, vol. 129, no. 11_Part_1, pp. 886–890, 1998.

16

ETV6: A Candidate Gene for Predisposition to "Blend Pedigrees"?A Case Report from the NEXT-Famly Clinical Trial

Simona Bernardi,[1,2] **Mirko Farina**,[1] **Camilla Zanaglio**,[1,2] **Federica Cattina**,[1] **Nicola Polverelli**,[1] **Francesca Schieppati**,[3] **Federica Re**,[1,2] **Chiara Foroni**,[1,2] **Michele Malagola**,[1] **Andrew J. Dunbar**,[4] **and Domenico Russo**[1]

[1]*Chair of Hematology, Unit of Blood Diseases and Stem Cell Transplantation, Department of Clinical and Experimental Sciences, University of Brescia, ASST Spedali Civili di Brescia, 25123 Brescia, Italy*
[2]*CREA Laboratory (Centro di Ricerca Emato-Oncologica AIL), ASST Spedali Civili di Brescia, 25123 Brescia, Italy*
[3]*Unit of Transfusion Medicine, ASST Papa Giovanni XXIII, 24127 Bergamo, Italy*
[4]*Department of Medicine, Leukemia Service, Memorial Sloan Kettering Cancer Center, New York, NY, USA*

Correspondence should be addressed to Simona Bernardi; simonabernardi86@gmail.com

Academic Editor: Stephen E. Langabeer

Background. The identification of germline mutations in familial leukemia predisposition genes by next generation sequencing is of pivotal importance. Lately, some "blend pedigrees" characterized by both solid and hematologic malignancies have been described. Some genes were recognized as related to this double predisposition, while the involvement of others is still a matter of debate. *ETV6* was associated with hematologic malignancies, in particular myeloid malignancies, and recently described as mutated also in oncologic patients. No clear evidences in its involvement in blend pedigrees are known. *Case Presentation.* We present our recent experience in the identification of an *ETV6*-mutated "blend pedigree," suggesting the involvement of *ETV6* in the predisposition to both solid and hematologic neoplasia. The pedigree recognition started with a MDS case enrolled in the NEXT-Famly protocol. The patient presented 9 relatives affected by solid tumors and hematological malignancies. Following the clinical trial protocol, the patient underwent NGS analysis, which confirmed the presence of a mutation on the noncoding region of *ETV6* both on tumor and on germline DNA. The mutation resulted was shared by the still alive affected relatives. *Conclusion.* This evidence supports the involvement of *ETV6* in the predisposition to both solid and hematologic neoplasia and the importance of the investigation of the noncoding regions of the genes as recently suggested by different expert groups.

1. Introduction

Acute myeloid leukemias (AML) and myelodysplastic syndromes (MDS) are clonal disorders of hematopoietic stem cells. With the advent of next-generation sequencing (NGS) technology, significant progress has been made in furthering our understanding of the molecular pathophysiology and complexity of these diseases [1]. NGS has also led to an increasing clinical awareness of inheritable leukemia syndromes and the genes involved. It is well established that several inheritable single-gene syndromes are associated with AML and MDS, including bone marrow failure syndromes (BMFS), Li-Fraumeni syndrome, and Down syndrome [2], which tend to affect individuals at a younger age. Widespread incorporation of a detailed medical and family history into the clinical care of every patient with unexplained cytopenias, aplastic anemia, or MDS/AML will continue to identify an increasing number of individuals with these disorders.

Family pedigrees of inheritable MDS/AML have been previously reported [3–5]. Detailed genetic investigations of these pedigrees have led to the identification of a number of individual genes that predispose to the development of AML and/or MDS [6]. Other data suggest these genes, when comutated with acquired somatic alterations, ultimately lead to the development of overt myeloid disease. The identification of additional potential candidate genes have been recently published in limited reports, including *SRP72* [7].

The clinical relevance of these syndromes is highlighted by the updated World Health Organization (WHO) classification of myeloid neoplasia, which now recognizes "Myeloid Neoplasm with Germline Predisposition" as a separate entity [8]. These syndromes are often associated with inherited mutations often affecting genes critical to hematopoiesis [9], including *RUNX1*, *CEBPα*, and *ETV6*. The WHO (Table 1) classifies three general categories of germline myeloid neoplasms: "pure" familial MDS and AML with no significant nonhematopoietic pathology, MDS/AML-susceptibility mutations with concomitant platelet abnormalities, and MDS/AML occurring in the setting of an underlying clinical genetic syndrome, including those characterized by BMFS (Table 2). For all these disorders, MDS and AML are often the predominant hematopoietic malignancies; however, lymphoid neoplasia as well as solid tumors can also occur [10–14].

NGS has been essential to the identification of novel molecular alterations in familial MDS/AML, and it has contributed to further understanding of inherited leukemia syndromes, and improved identification of inherited AML predisposition alleles. This has opened the opportunity to carry out a personalized management approach to affected patients [15–17]. For example, because long-term outcomes of MDS secondary to BMFS and familial MDS/AML are historically poor, hematopoietic stem cell transplantation should be considered sooner in the disease course, with exception for patients with germline mutations in *CEBPα* [18]. Nevertheless, a diagnosis of familial MDS/AML adds several considerations to pretransplant planning, namely, in the choice of the conditioning regimen and the selection of the hematopoietic stem cell donor [19–21].

The cases of MDS/AML with germline predisposition also differ from typical sporadic MDS and AML in that they are frequently associated with unique nonhematopoietic manifestations, requiring more dedicated disease surveillance [18].

In order to better recognize patients who may have an inherited predisposition to leukemia and MDS, clinicians must take a complete family history and be familiar with the characteristics of familial MDS/AML syndromes. In this scenario, evaluation of the family pedigree often reveals multiple family members affected by both hematologic and solid tumors. Moreover, other genes conventionally associated with solid tumors inheritance, such as *BRCA1* and *BRCA2*, have also been more recently been implicated in both pediatric and adult MDS/AML cases [22, 23].

In parallel with these well-established evidences, there is a group of four genes still considered as associated with a "possible tumor risk" that must be confirmed. *PTPN11* is not included in the ones recognized by the WHO classification, while *DDX41*, *GATA2*, and *ETV6* have been already linked with defined familial MDS/AML [24].

ETV6 is located at chromosome 12p13 and encodes a hematopoietic transcription factor involved in early embryonic and adult hematopoiesis as well as in the regulation of differentiation and maturation of erythropoietic and megakaryopoietic cell lineages [25, 26].

Alterations of *ETV6* have been shown to be important players in leukemogenesis since its recognition as a *PDGFB* translocation partner in chronic myelomonocytic leukemia [27]. *ETV6* is also frequently found to be partnered in numerous other variant translocations across hematologic malignancies which affect *ETV6* transcription and gene regulation [28]. Moreover, deletions [29] and somatic mutations in *ETV6* have also been reported in myeloid disease, including in MDS [30–32] and AML [33] as well as in CML [34], and are generally associated with poor outcomes [29].

More recently, germline mutations of *ETV6* have been identified in a small number of family pedigrees. Germline mutations involving the *ETV6* gene are often missense and inherited in an autosomal dominant fashion (Table 3), even if the penetrance of hematologic neoplasia depends both on the different mutated locus and between families affected by the same *ETV6* variant [26]. Patients often have variable thrombocytopenia with mild-to-moderate bleeding tendency and are predisposed to develop both myeloid and lymphoid malignancies. In particular, *ETV6* is suggested to be mostly predisposing to acute lymphoblastic leukemia rather than to myeloid malignancies [35], even if it was not reported in the conventional WHO classification.

Notably, additional nonhematological malignancies in *ETV6*-mutant carriers have also been documented [36–41]. With the paucity of germline-mutated *ETV6* cases published, additional mutations are still being discovered. Given this, we describe herein a novel mutation of *ETV6* found in an individual family pedigree linked to both hematologic and solid tumor malignancy.

2. Case Presentation

We analyzed a 70-year-old woman who presented with progressive thrombocytopenia that has been present for 8 years, and monocytosis in June 2014. The bone marrow biopsy performed at that time showed a MDS with multilineage dysplasia according to WHO classification [8], with a bone marrow blast count percentage totaled <5%. Cytogenetics revealed a translocation (3; 21). Therefore the patient falls within the intermediate 1 risk group, according to IPSS. She was started on danazole 400 mg/day which was eventually increased to 600 mg/day, with a low response in platelets count (30–40,000/mmc). The treatment was well tolerated, and no major bleeding was observed. After two years on therapy, she again developed worsening thrombocytopenia (10,000/mmc). Repeat bone marrow evaluation revealed MDS with excess blasts type 1 (MDS-EB 1). She was subsequently treated with 5-azacitidine at a dose 75 mg (sqm)/day x 7 days monthly for 15 cycles, for which she achieved a complete hematological response after 4 cycles. The treatment was discontinued in November 2017 for hematological toxicity and evolution of the disease to MDS-EB type 2 (IPSS intermediate 2). The patient subsequently evolved to AML and died due to

Table 1: WHO-defined myeloid neoplasm with germline predisposition.

Myeloid neoplasm with germline predisposition without preexisting disorder or organ dysfunction (i) *CEBPA* mutation (ii) *DDX41* mutation
Myeloid neoplasm with germline predisposition and preexisting platelet disorders (i) *RUNX1* mutation (ii) *ANKRD26* mutation (iii) *ETV6* mutation
Myeloid neoplasm with germline predisposition and other organ dysfunction (i) *GATA2* mutations (ii) Telomere biology disorders (iii) Bone marrow failure syndrome (Fanconi anemia, dyskeratosis congenita, severe congenital neutropenia, Swachman–Diamond syndrome, and Blackan-Diamond syndrome)

Table 2: Characteristics of AML/MDS predisposition syndromes.

Disease	Clinical characteristics	Mutated gene	Pattern of inheritance	Penetrance
Familial AML with mutated *CEBPA*	AML	*CEBPA*	AD	≈100%
Myeloid neoplasm with germline *DDX41* mutation	MDS/AML	*DDX41*	AD	Unknown
Familial platelet disorder/AML	MDS/AML/T cell ALL, lifelong thrombocytopenia, bleeding propensity	*RUNX1*	AD	40%
Thrombocytopenia and predisposition to myeloid malignancies	Thrombocytopenia, platelet dysfunction, MDS/AML	*ANKRD26*	AD	Unknown
Myeloid neoplasm with germline *ETV6* mutation	Thrombocytopenia, platelet dysfunction, MDS/AML	*ETV6*	AD	≈100%
Familial MDS/AML with mutated *GATA2*	MDS/AML, MonoMAC syndrome, Emberger syndrome	*GATA2*	AD	70%
Telomere biology disorders	MDS/AML, macrocytosis, mild to moderate single or multiple cytopenias, aplastic anemia	*TERT*, *TERC*	AD	Variable
Bone marrow failure associated with *SRP72* mutations	Aplastic anemia, MDS	*SRP72*	AD	Unknown

AML = acute myeloid leukemia; MDS = myelodisplastic syndrome; AD = autosomic dominant.

Table 3: Main hotspot mutations in the *ETV6* gene and their impact on the protein.

Mutation	Domain	Effect
P214L	Central regulatory domain	(i) Repression of DNA binding by the ETS domain (ii) Defective proplatelet formation and megakaryocyte maturation (iii) Alteration of proplatelet spreading (iv) Down regulation of several cytoskeletal proteins (v) *ETV6* delocalization
N385Vfs	ETS	(i) Reduction in repressive activity (ii) Targeted proteins downregulation
Y401N	ETS	(i) Impaired interaction with corepressor (ii) Defective proplatelet formation and megakaryocyte maturation
R369W/R369Q	ETS	(i) Reduction in repressive activity (ii) Targeted protein downregulation (iii) *ETV6* delocalization

ETS = highly conserved C-teminal DNA-binding domain.

disease progression. Her family history revealed several cases of hematological disease (2 cases of AML diagnosed at 62 and 48 years, 1 case of MDS diagnosed at 60 years associated with history of thrombocytopenia, and 2 cases of thrombocytopenia diagnosed at 49 and 57 years). In addition, several solid neoplasms distributed over 4 generations were also present (2 cases of gastric cancer diagnosed at 58 and 42 years, 1 pulmonary adenocarcinoma associated with history of thrombocytopenia diagnosed at 52 years, and 1 undetermined) (see Figure 1). Due to these

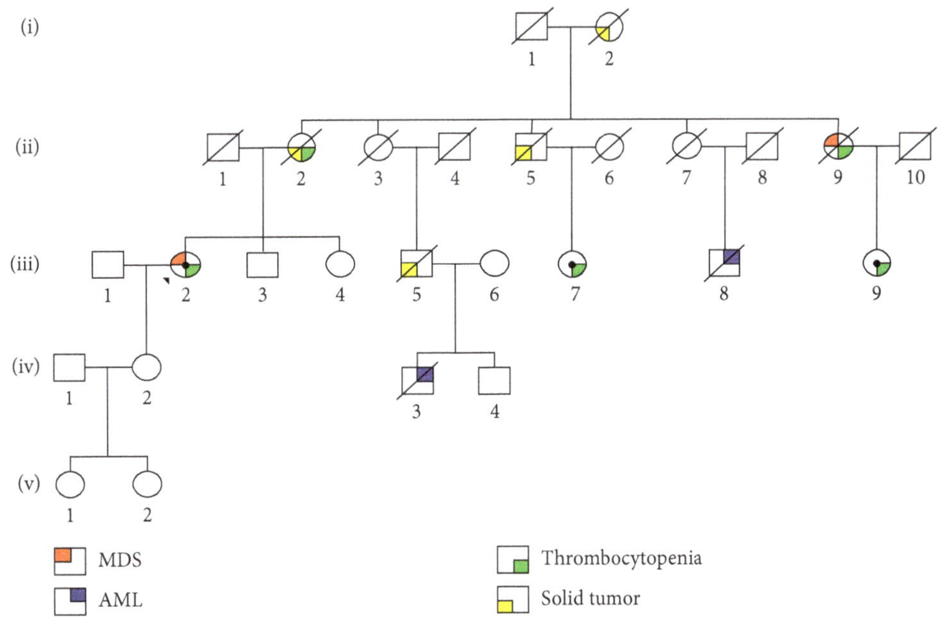

FIGURE 1: Case index pedigree (black arrow indicates the case index; black dot indicates subject presenting mutation; MDS = myelodisplastic syndrome; AML = acute myeloid leukemia).

evidences, the patient provided written informed consent in accordance with the Declaration of Helsinki and she was enrolled in the Next-Famly Italian Multicentric Study (NCT03058588). The written informed consent was attached to the patient's medical record as recommended by the Good Glinical Practice (ICH) guidelines [42]. As part of the study, a gene panel deep sequencing (GPDS) was performed on isolated peripheral blood mononuclear cells (PBMCs) at time of diagnosis. Tumor DNA was first screened by using the MiSeq Illumina NGS platform for mutations in the following 25 genes: *ASXL1, BCOR, NRAS, TP53, RUNX1, CEBPA, FLT3, EZH2, IDH1, IDH2, NPM1, DNMT3A, TET2, CBL, KRAS, ETV6, SF3B1, SRSF2, U2AF1, ZRSR2, GATA2, TERT, TERC, SRP72,* and *ANKRD26*. The sequencing focused only on exons and/or regulatory domains of each gene. The library preparation was conducted following the manufacturer's instructions, and DNAs were sequenced by MiSeq Illumina NGS platform using 2 × 150 sequencing (V2 kit, TruSeq). The coverage considered as acceptable for the consistence of the results was fixed at 1500x. The data analysis was performed using Web Annovar. During bioinformatics analysis, polymorphisms were discarded by comparison with NCBI, dbSNP, 1000 genomes, and EXAC, automatically investigated by using Web Annovar. However, since these databases contain known disease-associated mutations, all detected variants were compared with gene-specific mutation databases, ClinVar, and COSMIC. The ranking of unknown mutations was performed using Sift, Polyphen2, Mutation tester, FATHMM, ProVean, MetaSVM, M-CAP.

Review of NGS in this patient revealed a novel point mutation in *ETV6* at c.514 C>*T* in the 3′UTR locus not present in the interrogated database.

Since a suspected mutation was found, germline DNA from epithelial buccal cells was sequenced using traditional Sanger methods (SS). Germline DNA was extracted from buccal epithelial cells collected using the Isohelix SK-2 DNA Buccal Swab Collection Kit [43].

SS confirmed the presence of the variant c.514C>*T* of *ETV6* on the germline DNA of the index case (Figure 2). Considering the presence of a germline mutation, affected relatives still living at time of analysis were enrolled in the study and tested for the presence of the identified mutation. The germline mutation was confirmed in two enrolled cousins. Unfortunately, DNA was not available for additional testing on family members affected by solid tumors as they had already deceased.

miRANDA (microRNA.org) and PolymiRST Database Version 3.0 analysis suggested that the affected *ETV6* 3′UTR sequence serves as an miRNA-binding site, specifically the regulatory microRNA hsa-miR5092. Notably, the mutated one was predicted to bind microRNAs, hsa-miR4717-3p and hsa-miR942-3p. microRNAs have a known role in gene regulation. In order to assess the potential effect of the mutation on *ETV6* transcription in the index case, *ETV6* mRNA was isolated from PBMCs and quantified on the QuantStudio 3D digital PCR system (ThermoFisher Scientific) using the Hs01045747_m1 Taqman Gene probe (ThermoFisher Scientific) with Hs039290997_g1 Taqman *GAPDH* probe (ThermoFisher Scientific) as a housekeeper gene. Ten AML cases presenting with wild-type *ETV6* as well as 3 healthy individuals served as controls. The results of the quantification of *ETV6*, normalized for *GAPDH* transcript, are reported in Figure 3. Notably, affected relatives as well as the index case harboring the *514C>*T* mutation demonstrated a significant down regulation of *ETV6* gene expression in

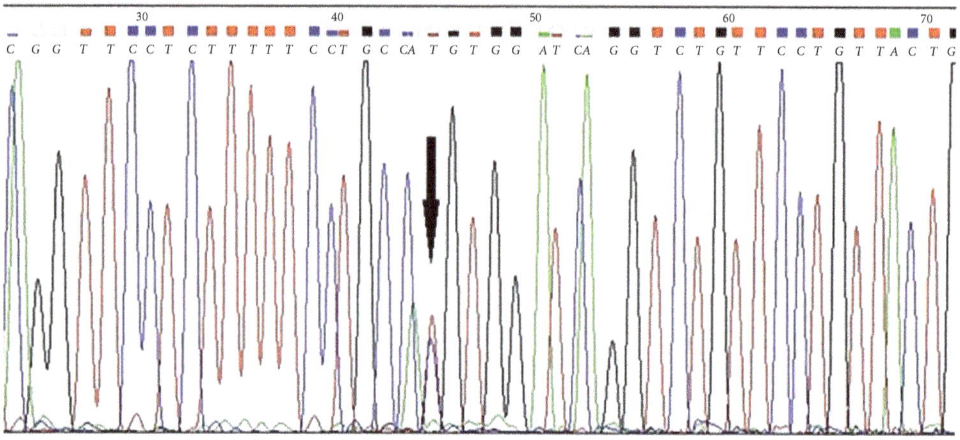

FIGURE 2: Electropherogram of the locus containing the mutation revealed by Sanger sequencing. The black arrow indicates the point mutation.

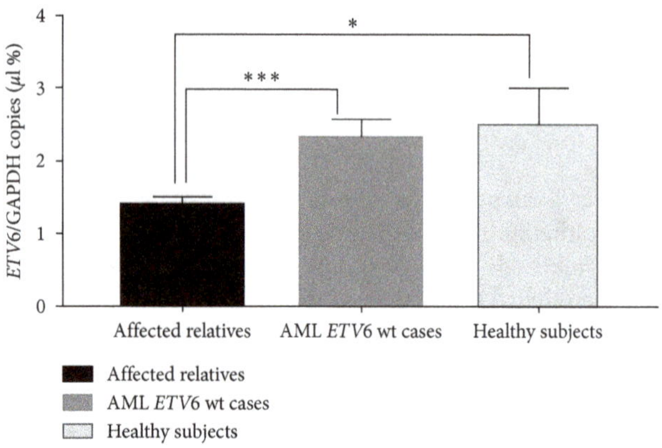

FIGURE 3: Quantification of *ETV6* transcripts by dPCR. The quantification was performed on PBMCs RNA. *ETV6* transcript levels were normalized for *GAPDH* transcript levels and expressed as ratio. Black block: affected relatives; Dark grey block: AML wt-*ETV6* cases; Light grey block: healthy subjects. Affected relatives presenting *514C>*T* variants resulted with *ETV6* statistically down regulated in comparison with AML cases presenting wild-type *ETV6* (****P* = 0.0004) and healthy controls (**P* = 0.02). PBMCs = peripheral blood mononuclear cells; AML = acute myeloid leukemia.

comparison to AML *ETV6* wild-type ($P = 0.0004$) and healthy controls ($P = 0.02$).

3. Discussion

The identification of some genes involved in inheritance of hematological malignancies allowed to recognition of an independent entity in last revision of WHO classification and also represents a further step toward the precision and personalized therapy [15, 24].

Moreover, the study of some pedigrees highlights the possible involvement of some genes in both tumorigenesis and leukemogenesis [44]. The definition of intermediate phenotype typically defined as "blend pedigree" leading to a high prevalence of both solid and hematological neoplasia is mandatory to clarify both the biological processes involved in the development of these different malignancies and for the establishment of an efficient treatment strategy and clinical survival.

Some "blend pedigrees" have already been reported in the literature and some genes have been linked to this condition. The implication of some of them in the pathogenesis of genetic predisposition to neoplasia is still a matter of debate. Recent evidences highlighted the importance of sequencing by NGS in these patients and also of investigating the regulatory and intragenic portions instead of the only coding regions which are conventionally queried [17, 24]. This approach is still mandatory for the study of *ANKRD26* since the known mutations associated with MDS/AML pedigrees affect the 5′UTR of the gene [45].

The family presented in this paper has been recognized thanks to the investigation of the noncoding sequences of all the genes included in our panel. The mutation was detected in 3′UTR of *ETV6* and no variants in this locus has been described before as causative of MDS/AML familiarity.

ETV6 is conventionally associated to hematological diseases both of lymphoid and myeloid lineages [35, 45], but more recently it has been implicated in both liquid and solid tumor malignancies (so-called "blend families"). The lack of acute lymphoblastic leukemia cases in the described family is uncommon and it might be due to the mutated locus, never described before. The mutation is associated with a down-regulation of *ETV6* transcript, while the previously reported mutations modify the *ETV6* protein structure. This different pathogenetic mechanism may affect lesser the lymphoid lineage than the myeloid one. Moreover, *ETV6* *514C>*T* seems to be associated with double predisposition to both hematologic and solid tumor malignancies and not to the conventional predisposition to hematologic disorder described in the literature [8, 37, 40, 41]. The pedigree we studied and reported was strongly suspected to be a "blend pedigree" in that the *ETV6* mutation–identified mutation might have led to both hematological and solid tumor malignancies. Recent studies reinforce this hypothesis since *ETV6* has been reported as a tumor suppressor also in primary cutaneous mammary analog secretory carcinoma [46], of pediatric papillary thyroid cancers [47], and in gastric cancer [48]. In particular, this last paper is particularly interesting due to the presence of 2 cases of gastric cancers in the described family. Unfortunately, due to the lack of the deceased patients' permission for further investigation, it was not possible to analyze the presence of the *ETV6* mutation in relatives affected by solid tumors.

Another important perspective that could be investigated in the future is the relationship between the t(3; 21), detected in the reported case, and *ETV6* 3′ UTR mutations. A possible cooperation of *ETV6* *514C>*T* with this or other lesions may be evaluated. In fact, in absence of WGS analysis, we cannot be sure that *514C>*T* in *ETV6* is the only causative mutation of the high susceptibility of the described family's members, but considering the evidences in the scientific literature, the reduction of the *ETV6* expression and the presence of the mutation in all alive affected family members, we may assess that the described mutation is strongly suspected to predispose to hematologic and solid malignancies. Nevertheless, further investigation on cell and animal models will give us pivotal data among the leukemogenesis process, since no evidences concerning this aspect have been reported.

Since the role of this variant in leukemogenesis and tumorigenesis has to be confirmed, we suggest to always carry out a careful family history because many pedigrees, strongly suspected to be "blend pedigree," could be misunderstood.

Our experience adds an indication of a possible involvement of *ETV6* in the "blend pedigrees" field, but new studies have to be conducted to investigate familiar predisposition to malignancies with a special focus on these entities, which are still an unexplored scenario.

Abbreviations

AML: Acute myeloid leukemia
MDS: Myelodysplastic syndrome
NGS: Next-generation sequencing
BMFS: Bone marrow failure syndromes
WHO: World Health Organization
IPSS: International Prognostic Scoring System
MDS-EB: Myelodysplastic syndrome with excess of blasts
SS: Sanger sequencing
GPDS: Gene panel deep sequencing.

References

[1] E. Liew and C. Owen, "Familial myelodysplastic syndromes: a review of the literature," *Haematologica*, vol. 96, no. 10, pp. 1536–1542, 2011.

[2] C. Owen, M. Barnett, and J. Fitzgibbon, "Familial myelodysplasia and acute myeloid leukaemia—a review," *British Journal of Haematology*, vol. 140, no. 2, pp. 123–132, 2007.

[3] R. C. Anderson, R. Lorenz, S. Nedumgottil et al., "Familial leukemia; a report of leukemia in five siblings, with a brief review of the genetic aspects of this disease," *Archives of Pediatrics & Adolescent Medicine*, vol. 81, no. 3, pp. 313–322, 1951.

[4] M. Horwitz, D. E. Sabath, W. A. Smithson, and J. Radich, "A family inheriting different subtypes of acute myelogenous leukemia," *International Journal of Hematology*, vol. 52, no. 4, pp. 295–304, 1996.

[5] C. W. Heath and W. C. Moloney, "Familial Leukemia," *New England Journal of Medicine*, vol. 272, no. 17, pp. 882–887, 1965.

[6] D. V. Babushok, M. Bessler, and T. S. Olson, "Genetic predisposition to myelodysplastic syndrome and acute myeloid leukemia in children and young adults," *Leukemia & Lymphoma*, vol. 57, no. 3, pp. 520–536, 2016.

[7] A. H. West, L. A. Godley, and J. E. Churpek, "Familial myelodysplastic syndrome/acute leukemia syndromes: a review and utility for translational investigations," *Annals of the New York Academy of Sciences*, vol. 1310, no. 1, pp. 111–118, 2014.

[8] D. A. Arber, A. Orazi, R. Hasserjian et al., "The 2016 revision to the World Health Organization classification of myeloid neoplasms and acute leukemia," *Blood*, vol. 127, no. 20, pp. 2391–2405, 2016.

[9] J. E. Churpek, R. Lorenz, S. Nedumgottil et al., "Proposal for the clinical detection and management of patients and their family members with familial myelodysplastic syndrome/ acute leukemia predisposition syndromes," *Leukemia & Lymphoma*, vol. 54, no. 1, pp. 28–35, 2013.

[10] N. Nishimoto, Y. Imai, K. Ueda et al., "T cell acute lymphoblastic leukemia arising from familial platelet disorder," *International Journal of Hematology*, vol. 92, no. 1, pp. 194–197, 2010.

[11] M. Stelljes, A. Corbacioglu, R. F. Schlenk et al., "Allogeneic stem cell transplant to eliminate germline mutations in the gene for CCAAT-enhancer-binding protein α from hematopoietic cells in a family with AML," *Leukemia*, vol. 25, no. 7, pp. 1209-1210, 2011.

[12] P. G. N. J. Mutsaers, A. A. van de Loosdrecht, K. Tawana, C. Bödör, J. Fitzgibbon, and F. H. Menko, "Highly variable clinical manifestations in a large family with a novel GATA2 mutation," *Leukemia*, vol. 27, no. 11, pp. 2247-2248, 2013.

[13] C. N. Hahn, C. L. Toze, A. Koochin et al., "Heritable GATA2 mutations associated with familial myelodysplastic syndrome and acute myeloid leukemia," *Nature Genetics*, vol. 43, no. 10, pp. 1012–1017, 2011.

[14] M. Lewinsohn, A. L. Brown, L. M. Weinel et al., "Novel germ line DDX41 mutations define families with a lower age of MDS/AML onset and lymphoid malignancies," *Blood*, vol. 127, no. 8, pp. 1017–1023, 2016.

[15] C. M. Niemeyer and C. Mecucci, "Practical considerations for diagnosis and management of patients and carriers," *Seminars in Hematology*, vol. 54, no. 2, pp. 69–74, 2017.

[16] N. Rusk and V. Kiermer, "Primer: sequencing--the next generation," *Nature methods*, vol. 5, no. 1, p. 15, 2008.

[17] C. D. DiNardo, A. Valentin, P. Ulz et al., "Improving the detection of patients with inherited predispositions to hematologic malignancies using next-generation sequencing-based leukemia prognostication panels," *Cancer*, vol. 124, no. 13, pp. 2704–2713, 2018.

[18] E. M. Nickels, J. Soodalter, J. E. Churpek, and L. A. Godley, "Recognizing familial myeloid leukemia in adults," *Therapeutic Advances in Hematology*, vol. 4, no. 4, pp. 254–269, 2013.

[19] C. J. Owen, C. L. Toze, A. Koochin et al., "Five new pedigrees with inherited RUNX1 mutations causing familial platelet disorder with propensity to myeloid malignancy," *Blood*, vol. 112, no. 12, pp. 4639–4645, 2008.

[20] P. F. Fogarty, H. Yamaguchi, A. Wiestner et al., "Late presentation of dyskeratosis congenita as apparently acquired aplastic anaemia due to mutations in telomerase RNA," *The Lancet*, vol. 362, no. 9396, pp. 1628–1630, 2003.

[21] A. Buijs, P. Poddighe, R. van Wijk et al., "A novel CBFA2 single-nucleotide mutation in familial platelet disorder with propensity to develop myeloid malignancies," *Blood*, vol. 98, no. 9, pp. 2856–2858, 2001.

[22] J. Zhang, M. F. Walsh, G. Wu et al., "Germline mutations in predisposition genes in pediatric cancer," *New England Journal of Medicine*, vol. 373, no. 24, pp. 2336–2346, 2015.

[23] E. Schulz, A. Valentin, P. Ulz et al., "Germline mutations in the DNA damage response genes BRCA1, BRCA2, BARD1 and TP53 in patients with therapy related myeloid neoplasms," *Journal of Medical Genetics*, vol. 49, no. 7, pp. 422–428, 2012.

[24] K. Tawana, M. W. Drazer, and J. E. Churpek, "Universal genetic testing for inherited susceptibility in children and adults with myelodysplastic syndrome and acute myeloid leukemia: are we there yet?," *Leukemia*, vol. 32, no. 7, pp. 1482–1492, 2018.

[25] T. Yamagata, K. Maki, K. Waga, and K. Mitani, "TEL/ETV6 induces apoptosis in 32D cells through p53-dependent pathways," *Biochemical and Biophysical Research Communications*, vol. 347, no. 2, pp. 517–526, 2006.

[26] S. Feurstein and L. A. Godley, "Germline ETV6 mutations and predisposition to hematological malignancies," *International Journal of Hematology*, vol. 106, no. 2, pp. 189–195, 2017.

[27] T. R. Golub, G. F. Barker, M. Lovett, and D. G. Gilliland, "Fusion of PDGF receptor β to a novel ets-like gene, tel, in chronic myelomonocytic leukemia with *t*(5;12) chromosomal translocation," *Cell*, vol. 77, no. 2, pp. 307–316, 1994.

[28] E. De Braekeleer, N. Douet-Guilbert, F. Morel, M.-J. Le Bris, A. Basinko, and M. De Braekeleer, "ETV6 fusion genes in hematological malignancies: a review," *Leukemia Research*, vol. 36, no. 8, pp. 945–961, 2012.

[29] M. Wall, K. C. Rayeroux, R. N. MacKinnon, A. Zordan, and L. J. Campbell, "ETV6 deletion is a common additional abnormality in patients with myelodysplastic syndromes or acute myeloid leukemia and monosomy 7," *Haematologica*, vol. 97, no. 12, pp. 1933–1936, 2012.

[30] R. Bejar, K. Stevenson, O. Abdel-Wahab et al., "Clinical effect of point mutations in myelodysplastic syndromes," *New England Journal of Medicine*, vol. 364, no. 26, pp. 2496–2506, 2011.

[31] R. Bejar, K. E. Stevenson, B. A. Caughey et al., "Validation of a prognostic model and the impact of mutations in patients with lower-risk myelodysplastic syndromes," *Journal of Clinical Oncology*, vol. 30, no. 27, pp. 3376–3382, 2012.

[32] M. J. Walter, D. Shen, J. Shao et al., "Clonal diversity of recurrently mutated genes in myelodysplastic syndromes," *Leukemia*, vol. 27, no. 6, pp. 1275–1282, 2013.

[33] S. Barjesteh van Waalwijk van Doorn-Kh, D. Spensberger, Y. de Knegt, M. Tang, B. Löwenberg, and R. Delwel, "Somatic heterozygous mutations in ETV6 (TEL) and frequent absence of ETV6 protein in acute myeloid leukemia," *Oncogene*, vol. 24, no. 25, pp. 4129–4137, 2005.

[34] Q. Wang, S. Dong, H. Yao et al., "ETV6 mutation in a cohort of 970 patients with hematologic malignancies," *Haematologica*, vol. 99, no. 10, pp. e176–e178, 2014.

[35] J. Di Paola and C. C. Porter, "ETV6-related thrombocytopenia and leukemia predisposition," *Blood*, vol. 134, no. 8, pp. 663–667, 2019.

[36] M. Wang, D. Gu, M. Du et al., "Common genetic variation in ETV6 is associated with colorectal cancer susceptibility," *Nature Communications*, vol. 7, no. 1, p. 11478, 2016.

[37] S. Topka, J. Vijai, M. F. Walsh et al., "Germline ETV6 mutations confer susceptibility to acute lymphoblastic leukemia and thrombocytopenia," *PLoS Genetics*, vol. 11, no. 6, Article ID e1005262, 2015.

[38] M. Y. Zhang, J. E. Churpek, S. B. Keel et al., "Germline ETV6 mutations in familial thrombocytopenia and hematologic malignancy," *Nature Genetics*, vol. 47, no. 2, pp. 180–185, 2015.

[39] L. Noetzli, R. W. Lo, A. B. Lee-Sherick et al., "Germline mutations in ETV6 are associated with thrombocytopenia, red cell macrocytosis and predisposition to lymphoblastic leukemia," *Nature Genetics*, vol. 47, no. 5, pp. 535–538, 2015.

[40] F. Melazzini, F. Palombo, A. Balduini et al., "Clinical and pathogenic features of ETV6-related thrombocytopenia with predisposition to acute lymphoblastic leukemia," *Haematologica*, vol. 101, no. 11, pp. 1333–1342, 2016.

[41] H. Hock and A. Shimamura, "ETV6 in hematopoiesis and leukemia predisposition," *Seminars in Hematology*, vol. 54, no. 2, pp. 98–104, 2017.

[42] International Council for Harmonisation of Technical Requirements for Pharmaceuticals for Human Use (ICH), *ICH Harmonised Guideline Integrated Addendum to ICH E6 (R1): Guideline for Good Clinical Practice E6 (R2)*, ICH, Geneva, Switzerland, 2016.

[43] G. L. McMichael, C. S. Gibson, M. E. O'Callaghan et al., "DNA from buccal swabs suitable for high-throughput 1 SNP multiplex analysis," *Journal of Biomolecular Techniques*, vol. 20, no. 5, pp. 232–235, 2009.

[44] J. E. Churpek and E. H. Bresnick, "Transcription factor mutations as a cause of familial myeloid neoplasms," *Journal of Clinical Investigation*, vol. 129, no. 2, pp. 476–488, 2019.

[45] P. Galera, A. Dulau-Florea, and K. R. Calvo, "Inherited thrombocytopenia and platelet disorders with germline predisposition to myeloid neoplasia," *International Journal of Laboratory Hematology*, vol. 41, no. S1, pp. 131–141, 2019.

[46] S. M. Amin, A. Beattie, X. Ling, L. J. Jennings, and J. Guitart, "Primary cutaneous mammary analog secretory carcinoma with ETV6-NTRK3 translocation," *The American Journal of Dermatopathology*, vol. 38, no. 11, pp. 842–845, 2016.

[47] M. L. Prasad, M. Vyas, M. J. Horne et al., "*NTRK* fusion oncogenes in pediatric papillary thyroid carcinoma in northeast United States," *Cancer*, vol. 122, no. 7, pp. 1097–1107, 2016.

[48] E. Sai, Y. Miwa, R. Takeyama et al., "Identification of candidates for driver oncogenes in scirrhous-type gastric cancer cell lines," *Cancer Science*, vol. 110, no. 8, pp. 2643–2651, 2019.

17

An Intriguing Case of Eosinophilia with FIP1L1/PDGFRA Rearrangement Who Presented as Thrombotic Thrombocytopenic Purpura

Hassan Alshehri,[1] Mohammad Alnomani,[1] Mubarak Alghamdi,[1] Ibrahim Motabi,[1] Imran Tailor,[1] Nawal Alshehry,[1] Mansour Alfayez,[1,2] Abdul Rehman Z. Zaidi,[1] Syed Altaf,[1] Azizah AlSwayyed,[3] Ammar AlSughayyer,[3] and Syed Z. A. Zaidi[1]

[1]*Department of Adult Hematology and BMT, King Fahad Medical City, Riyadh, Saudi Arabia*
[2]*Department of Leukemia, The University of Texas MD Anderson Cancer Center, Houston, TX, USA*
[3]*Department of Pathology and Clinical Laboratory Medicine, King Fahad Medical City, Riyadh, Saudi Arabia*

Correspondence should be addressed to Hassan Alshehri; hassan.shehri@gmail.com

Academic Editor: Eduardo Arellano-Rodrigo

Myeloid neoplasm with eosinophilia and FIP1-like-1-platelet-derived growth factor receptor-alpha (FIP1L1-PDGFRA) rearrangement is a multi-organ disease with diverse clinical presentation. Thrombotic thrombocytopenic purpura (TTP) is characterized by the concomitant occurrence of often severe thrombocytopenia, microangiopathic hemolytic anemia, and a variable degree of ischemic organ damage. To our knowledge, only one case of eosinophilia with FIP1L1-PDGFRA rearrangement presented as a case of thrombotic thrombocytopenic purpura reported in the literature. We herein report a case of a young male patient with hypereosinophilic syndrome and FIP1L1-PDGFRA rearrangement who presented with asthma, transient ischemic attacks (TIA), and confusion. He had an acquired TTP that was successfully treated with plasma exchanges (PLEX), corticosteroids, rituximab, and later with the addition of imatinib mesylate (Gleevec, Novartis). He remains in complete remission on imatinib 100 mg daily for more than 28 months of follow-up.

1. Introduction

Eosinophilia is commonly observed in diverse nonclonal and clonal disorders. In the majority of cases, it is reactive, associated with atopic conditions, autoimmune disorders, and infections or malignancies, while in other instances, it is a result of an underlying hematologic disorder [1].

Current evaluation of suspected hypereosinophilic syndrome (HES) includes a molecular/cytogenetic investigation with either reverse transcription polymerase chain reaction (RT-PCR) or fluorescent in situ hybridization (FISH) for the FIP1L1-PDGFRA rearrangement [2, 3]. It is categorized as a specific entity in the 2008 World Health Organization (WHO) classification of myeloid neoplasms (myeloid and lymphoid neoplasms with eosinophilia and abnormalities of PDGFRA, PDGFRB, and FGFR1) [4, 5]. In 2017 revision of WHO classification, myeloid and lymphoid neoplasms associated with *t* (8; 9) (p22; p24.1) and PCM1-JAK2 have been recognized as provisional entities to this group of eosinophilic disorders [6]. Tyrosine kinase inhibitors, such as imatinib, are effective in the treatment of FIP1L1-PDGFRA mutated disease. Given the striking sensitivity to imatinib, a dose of 100 mg daily is typically sufficient [7–10].

Thrombotic thrombocytopenic purpura (TTP) is characterized by the concomitant occurrence of often severe thrombocytopenia, microangiopathic hemolytic anemia, and a variable degree of ischemic organ damage, particularly affecting the brain, heart, and kidneys [11]. In acquired TTP, the underlying mechanism is deficiency of metalloprotease

ADAMTS13 (a disintegrin and metalloproteinase with a thrombospondin type 1 motif, member 13) due to the emergence of its inhibitor.

Simultaneous presentation of HES with FIP1L1-PDGFRA rearrangement and TTP is a unique phenomenon. To our knowledge, only one such a case has been reported in the literature [12].

2. Case Presentation

A 36-year-old man with past history of 36 pack-years of smoking and bronchial asthma presented to an outside facility on August 11, 2016 with one-hour duration of sudden onset right upper limb weakness that progressed to involve the lower limb along with slurring of speech and altered level of consciousness. CT scan of the brain and carotid ultrasound were reported as normal. His initial complete blood count (CBC) and biochemistry profile showed low hemoglobin and low platelets along with elevated bilirubin. Peripheral blood smear (PBS) showed fragmented red blood cells. TTP was suspected and fresh frozen plasma (FFP) infusion started (due to unavailability of PLEX) along with methylprednisolone intravenously (IV) 500 mg/day. He was then transferred to our facility on August 19, 2016 after 7 days of FFP infusions and methylprednisolone. Upon presentation at our emergency department, he was vitally stable; however, he was intermittently confused with a power of 3/5 in the right upper and lower limbs. His CBC with differential was remarkable for anemia, thrombocytopenia, and leukocytosis with eosinophilia (Table 1). The chest X-ray was normal (Figure 1). Peripheral blood film showed schistocytosis (4%) with eosinophilia in partly degranulated forms (Figures 2(a)–2(c). ADAMTS13 level and its inhibitor were sent to the reference laboratory; however, due to delay in processing, the sample was denatured and was not analyzable.

As he presented to our facility, PLEX with cryo-poor plasma 1.5 volumes daily was started along with methylprednisolone IV 500 mg/day for 3 days, followed by prednisolone 1 mg/kg/day. The patient's right sided weakness and confusion resolved after 2 sessions of PLEX.

As his eosinophilia persisted after giving pulse steroids, we called for a review of his old records. A blood analysis report of July 2012 had shown normal WBC (5.4×10^9) with normal absolute eosinophil count (0.378×10^9). Workup for eosinophilia including stool examination for ova and parasite, schistosoma serology, ANA, and ANCA was reported negative. Fluorescence in situ hybridization (FISH) screening on peripheral blood for FIP1L1-PDGFRA (4q12) rearrangement was positive in 20.5% of the 200 scored nuclei. T-cell receptor gene rearrangements study was negative.

Bone marrow aspirate and trephine core biopsies were performed. Bone marrow aspirate showed good spicules, and differential count revealed 2% blasts and 30% Eosinophils. Megakaryocytes were adequate and morphologically unremarkable. Erythroid and myeloid precursors showed progressive and orderly maturation (Figures 2(d) and 2(e)). Trephine core biopsy sections showed cellularity of 90% with trilineage hematopoiesis. Megakaryocytes and erythroid precursors were adequate and morphologically unremarkable. Myeloid precursors were adequate with prominently increased eosinophilic lineage cells (Figure 2(f)). Flow cytometry of the bone marrow (after steroid use) showed a T-cell population (about 78% of the lymphocytes analyzed) with no aberrant loss or aberrant expression of T-cell markers. Normal male karyotype (46, XY) without chromosomal aberrations was noted on the bone marrow specimen. FISH for *t* (9; 22) (q34; q11) and RT-qPCR for BCR : ABL1 p210 was negative. FISH study done on the bone marrow aspirate for FIP1L1/PDGFRA (4q12) rearrangement detected abnormal signals in 26% of the 200 scored nuclei (Figure 3).

After 18 sessions of PLEX, his LDH and platelet normalized. At this point, a trial to weaning off PLEX resulted in re-emergence of schistocytes with elevation in LDH accompanied by a drop-in platelet count, which did necessitate resuming PLEX. Rituximab 375 mg/m^2 weekly was started and was given for four doses (August 28, 2016, to September 18, 2016). Imatinib 100 mg daily was started on September 26, 2016 for steroid-refractory, FIPL1-PDGFRA rearrangement positive eosinophilia. Rapid resolution of his eosinophilia was noted, and absolute eosinophil count dropped from 3.57×10^9 to 0.14×10^9 after 3 days. In total, 30 PLEX sessions were needed to treat the TTP; the last session was 4 days after the initiation of Imatinib (September 30, 2016).

After more than 28 months of follow-up, the patient continues to be in remission, with normal eosinophil count and no TTP recurrence (Figure 4).

3. Discussion

Acquired TTP is relatively uncommon but a life-threatening disorder. ADAMTS13 deficiency is most frequently acquired via ADAMTS13 autoantibodies, but rarely, it is inherited via mutations of the ADAMTS13 gene. The first acute episode of TTP usually occurs during adulthood, with a predominant anti-ADAMTS13 autoimmune etiology. Rapid recognition of TTP is crucial to initiate appropriate treatment based on daily therapeutic plasma exchange supplying deficient ADAMTS13 (along with the removal of antibody), with or without steroids. Additional immune modulators targeting ADAMTS13 autoantibodies are mainly based on steroids and the anti-CD20 monoclonal antibody rituximab. In refractory or unresponsive TTP, more intensive therapies including twice-daily plasma exchange; pulses of cyclophosphamide, vincristine, or cyclosporine A; or salvage splenectomy may be considered [13]. Multiple reports from Oklahoma [14, 15] and other centers, including our facility, were published [13, 16–19]. There are many acquired associations of TTP; however, the co-occurrence of TTP with HES has rarely been reported, and it is even more unique when TTP-related symptoms are the primary presentation [12]. Chaudhary et al. reported unique association of

Table 1: Laboratory characteristics at baseline, after recovery from TTP post-PLEX and post-imatinib therapy.

Lab parameter	Baseline	After PLEX (pre-imatinib)	Post-imatinib 3 months	Reference range
WBC	13.62	5.78	10.57	$3.90–11.00 \times 10^9$/L
Abs. neutrophils	7.54	3.7	4.81	$1.35–7.50 \times 10^9$/L
Abs. lymphocytes	2.32	1.72	5.01	$1.50–4.30 \times 10^9$/L
Abs. monocytes	0.65	0.35	0.58	$0.25–1.00 \times 10^9$/L
Abs. eosinophils	3.06	1.01	0.02	$0.03–1.00 \times 10^9$/L
Abs. basophils	0.05	0.00	0.15	$0.25–1.00 \times 10^9$/L
Hemoglobin	7.5	11	15.1	13.50–18.00 g/dl
Platelet	30	319	416	$155.00–435.00 \times 10^9$/L
Coombs test	Negative	Negative	Negative	
Coagulation profile				
aPTT	34.6	31.2	35.2	28.0–41.0 sec
PT	16.5	14.6	13.6	11.5–15.0 sec
INR	1.3	1.1	1.0	0.9–1.2
Fibrinogen	2.6	2.2	4.8	1.4–4.4 g/L
D-dimer	2.4	0.5	0.3	0.0–0.5 μg/mL
Creatinine	110	83	81	62–106 μmol/L
Urea	11.6	7.2	4.4	2.5–6.4 mmol/L
Total bilirubin	94.9	5.2	10.9	0.0–21.0 μmol/L
Direct bilirubin	28.1	1.9	3.2	0.0–3.0 μmol/L
LDH	982	230	231	135–225 U/l
ALT	25	30	35	0–41 U/l
Alkaline phosphatase	90	86	101	40–129 U/l
Albumin	41	34	39	35–50 g/L
Haptoglobin	<0.07			0.3–1.8 g/L
FISH analysis for FIP1L1/PDGFRA (4q12) rearrangement (% of scored nuclei)	26% in bone marrow and 20.5% in peripheral blood	Not done	Negative	Negative

ADAMTS13 level and inhibitor sample were rejected by the reference lab.

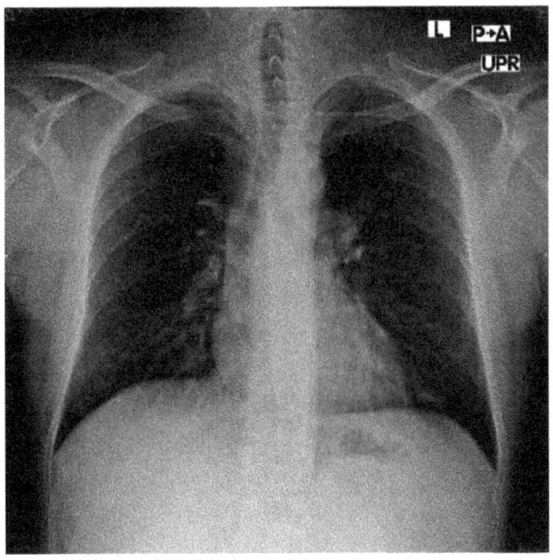

Figure 1: Baseline chest X-ray.

myeloid neoplasm with eosinophilia and abnormalities of PDGFRA with TTP [12]. Their patient was a female in whom TTP presented as one of the earlier manifestations of myeloproliferative HES with rearrangement of PDGFRA. Their patient was found to have a normal ADAMTS13 level which is not commonly seen with TTP [12]. Earlier than this report, two cases with FIP1L1-PDGFRA-negative hypereosinophilic syndrome and subsequent TTP have been reported [20, 21]. Ohguchi et al. reported a case of HES who subsequently developed TTP due to development of ADAMTS13 inhibitor and was successfully treated with corticosteroids and TPE [20]. Al Aly et al. reported a case who developed idiopathic HES [21]. She was treated with imatinib mesylate and subsequently developed TTP with renal failure. A kidney biopsy was performed and was diagnostic of thrombotic microangiopathy. The patient was treated with TPE and hemodialysis. Her eosinophilia resolved, but she remained dialysis-dependent. Our patient was unique as he had refractory TTP and HES. After 18 days of daily PLEX, an attempt of stopping of PLEX was made. Recurrence with increasing LDH and falling platelet count after 6 days was noted. PLEX was resumed on day 7 along with the addition of rituximab for refractory TTP. Meanwhile, we found evidence of FIP1L1-PDGFRA gene rearrangement by FISH analysis. Hence, we added imatinib on September 26, 2016 at a low dose of 100 mg/day. Absolute eosinophil count normalized within 3 days. This rapid response in eosinophil count can be related to concomitant use of steroids. The patient tolerated imatinib well without any adverse events. PLEX was successfully discontinued after a total of 30 PLEX. The patient was maintained on imatinib 100 mg daily and remains in remission for both TTP and HES after more than 28 months of follow-up.

Hypereosinophilic syndromes (HES) constitute a rare and heterogeneous group of disorders, defined as persistent and marked blood eosinophilia ($>1.5 \times 10^9$/L for more than

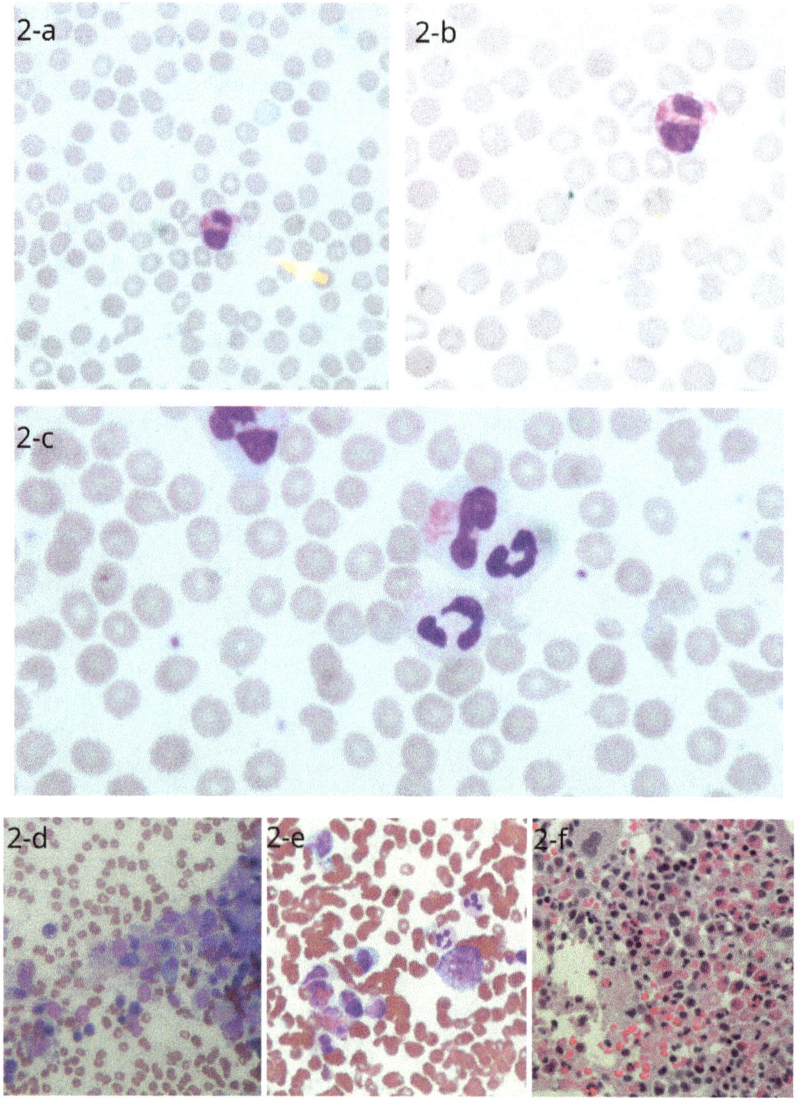

FIGURE 2: (a, b) Peripheral blood smear revealing schistocytes and eosinophil (May–Grüunwald stain). (c) Partially degranulated eosinophils and schistocytes (May–Grünwald stain). (d, e) Bone marrow aspirate (May–Grünwald stain, 400x magnification). (f) Bone marrow trephine biopsy (hematoxylin-eosin stain, 200x magnification).

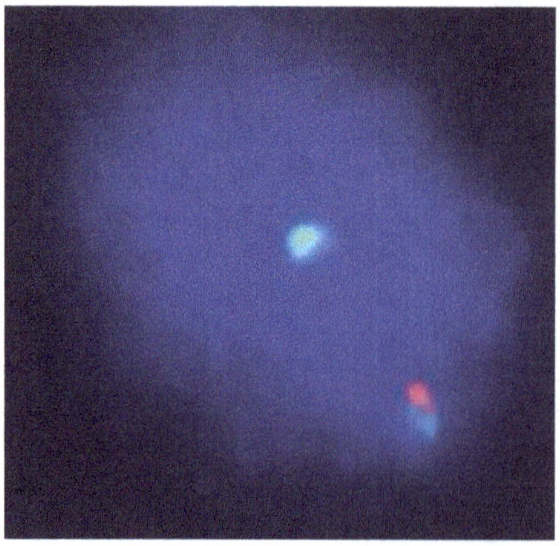

FIGURE 3: Fluorescence in situ hybridization (FISH) analysis for FIP1L1/CHIC/PDGFRA (using Vysis/Abbott FISH probes) revealed FIP1L1/PDGFRA (4q12) rearrangement in 20.5% of the scored nuclei. ISCN: nuc ish (FIP1L1x2, CHICx1, PDGFRAx2) (FIP1L1 con PDGFRA) (41/200).

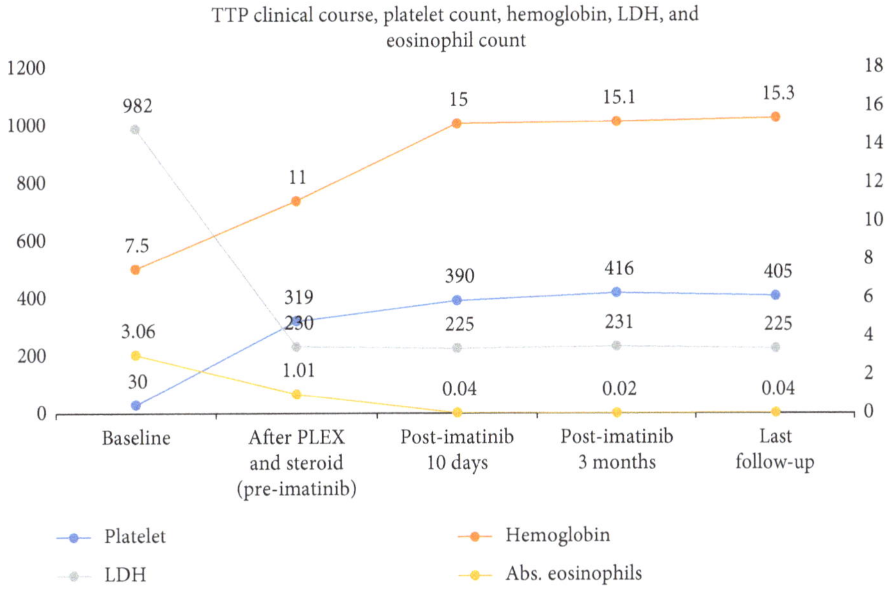

FIGURE 4: Clinical course, platelet count, hemoglobin, LDH, and eosinophil count of the patient. LDH, lactate dehydrogenase; PLEX, plasma exchange.

six consecutive months) associated with evidence of eosinophil-induced organ damage, where other causes of hypereosinophilia such as allergic, parasitic, and malignant disorders have been excluded [22]. Under normal physiologic conditions, eosinophil production is tightly controlled by the cytokine network. The normal eosinophil count in peripheral blood ranges between 0.05 and 0.5×10^9/L [23]. It can be reactive (secondary) or an integral phenotype of an underlying hematological neoplasm (primary). The diagnosis of clonal eosinophilia requires the demonstration of either a cytogenetic/molecular marker of clonality or bone marrow histological features that are not consistent with an otherwise classified myeloid malignancy [3]. FIP1L1 fusions with PDGFRA, PDGFRB, and FGFR1 were identified in 2002-2003 as recurrent rearrangements, with the FIP1L1-PDGFRA fusion being the most common fusion. Karyotype, although less sensitive, can show corresponding gene rearrangement (4q12 (PDGFRA), 5q31–33 (PDGFRB), or 8p11–12 (FGFR1) [24, 25].

Myeloproliferative neoplasms with FIP1L1-PDGFRA highlight the relevance of tyrosine kinases to both normal cellular physiology and disease states. PDGFRA is a member of type III-receptor tyrosine kinases. FIP1L1/PDGFRA protein fusion leads to deregulated PDGFRA kinase activity and abrogates normal growth factor-dependent stimulation of the receptor [26]. Imatinib at a dose of 100 mg is very effective in this disorder.

The plausible mechanism of the simultaneous presentation of TTP and HES is not clear to us. We ponder if neoantigen form FIP1L1-PDGFRA rearmament stimulated an immune response that cross-reacts with ADAMTS13 resulting in its subsequent depletion, or if this is related to eosinophilia/eosinophilic granules causing an independent platelets aggregation or devouring of ADAMTS13. However, the authors could not demonstrate the deficiency of ADAMTS13 or the presence of autoantibodies against ADAMTS13 due to logistic issues discussed. The eosinophilia in our case was clonal in nature; however, in lymphocyte-variant hypereosinophilia or with Th2/cytokines-mediated eosinophilia, TTP, in theory, can be a manifestation of this autoimmune dysregulation.

4. Conclusion

To our knowledge, this is the second case report on the simultaneous presentation of TTP with eosinophilia and FIP1L1-PDGFRA rearrangement. This presentation raises the possibility of a mechanistic association between the two disorders. Low dose imatinib resulted in an excellent and sustained response.

Abbreviations

Abs:	Absolute
ADAMTS13:	A disintegrin and metalloproteinase with a thrombospondin type 1 motif, member 13
FISH:	Fluorescence in situ hybridization
FIP1L1/ PDGFRA:	FIP1-like-1-platelet-derived growth factor receptor-alpha
LDH:	Lactate dehydrogenase
PLEX:	Plasma exchange
RDW:	Red cell distribution width
MCV:	Mean corpuscular volume
MCH:	Mean corpuscular hemoglobin.

References

[1] A. Reiter, D. Grimwade, and N. C. P. Cross, "Diagnostic and therapeutic management of eosinophilia-associated chronic

myeloproliferative disorders," *Haematologica*, vol. 92, no. 9, pp. 1153–1158, 2007.

[2] G. Loules, F. Kalala, N. Giannakoulas, E. Papadakis, P. Matsouka, and M. Speletas, "FIP1L1-PDGFRA molecular analysis in the differential diagnosis of eosinophilia," *BMC Hematology*, vol. 9, no. 1, p. 1, 2009.

[3] A. Tefferi, M. M. Patnaik, and A. Pardanani, "Eosinophilia: secondary, clonal and idiopathic," *British Journal of Haematology*, vol. 133, no. 5, pp. 468–492, 2006.

[4] S. H. C. E. Swerdlow, N. L. Harris, E. S. Jaffe et al., *WHO Classification of Tumours of Haematopoietic and Lymphoid Tissues*, International Agency for Research on Cancer, Lyon, France, 2008.

[5] A. Tefferi, J. Thiele, and J. W. Vardiman, "The 2008 World Health Organization classification system for myeloproliferative neoplasms," *Cancer*, vol. 115, no. 17, pp. 3842–3847, 2009.

[6] B. J. H. H.-P. Bain, D. A. Arber, A. Tefferi et al., *WHO Classification of Tumours of Haematopoietic and Lymphoid Tissues*, International Agency for Research on Cancer, Lyon, France, 4th edition, 2017.

[7] J. V. Jovanovic, J. Score, K. Waghorn et al., "Low-dose imatinib mesylate leads to rapid induction of major molecular responses and achievement of complete molecular remission in FIP1L1-PDGFRA positive chronic eosinophilic leukemia," *Blood*, vol. 109, no. 11, pp. 4635–4640, 2007.

[8] J. Cortes, P. Ault, C. Koller et al., "Efficacy of imatinib mesylate in the treatment of idiopathic hypereosinophilic syndrome," *Blood*, vol. 101, no. >12, pp. 4714–4716, 2003.

[9] M. Baccarani, D. Cilloni, M. Rondoni et al., "The efficacy of imatinib mesylate in patients with FIP1L1-PDGFR -positive hypereosinophilic syndrome. Results of a multicenter prospective study," *Haematologica*, vol. 92, no. 9, pp. 1173–1179, 2007.

[10] A. Pardanani, S. R. Brockman, S. F. Paternoster et al., "FIP1L1-PDGFRA fusion: prevalence and clinicopathologic correlates in 89 consecutive patients with moderate to severe eosinophilia," *Blood*, vol. 104, no. 10, pp. 3038–3045, 2004.

[11] J. A. Kremer Hovinga, P. Coppo, B. Lämmle, J. L. Moake, T. Miyata, and K. Vanhoorelbeke, "Thrombotic thrombocytopenic purpura," *Nature Reviews Disease Primers*, vol. 3, no. 1, p. 17020, 2017.

[12] L. N. Chaudhary, N. G. Bailey, J. A. Vos, and C. J. Stotler, "Unique association of myeloid neoplasm with eosinophilia and abnormalities of PDGFRA with TTP," *The West Virginia Medical Journal*, vol. 109, no. 2, pp. 6–9, 2013.

[13] B. S. Joly, P. Coppo, and A. Veyradier, "Thrombotic thrombocytopenic purpura," *Blood*, vol. 129, no. 21, pp. 2836–2846, 2017.

[14] J. N. George, S. K. Vesely, D. R. Terrell et al., "The Oklahoma thrombotic thrombocytopenic purpura-haemolytic uraemic syndrome registry. A model for clinical research, education and patient care," *Hämostaseologie*, vol. 33, no. 2, pp. 105–112, 2013.

[15] J. N. George, D. R. Terrell, K. K. Swisher, and S. K. Vesely, "Lessons learned from the Oklahoma thrombotic thrombocytopenic purpura-hemolytic uremic syndrome registry," *Journal of Clinical Apheresis*, vol. 23, no. 4, pp. 129–137, 2008.

[16] E. E. Page, J. A. Kremer Hovinga, D. R. Terrell, S. K. Vesely, and J. N. George, "Thrombotic thrombocytopenic purpura: diagnostic criteria, clinical features, and long-term outcomes from 1995 through 2015," *Blood Advances*, vol. 1, no. 10, pp. 590–600, 2017.

[17] J. N. George, "The remarkable diversity of thrombotic thrombocytopenic purpura: a perspective," *Blood Advances*, vol. 2, no. 12, pp. 1510–1516, 2018.

[18] J. N. George, "TTP: long-term outcomes following recovery," *Hematology*, Hematology American Society of Hematology Education Program, vol. 2018, no. 1, pp. 548–552, 2018.

[19] S. Iqbal, S. Z. Zaidi, I. H. Motabi, N. F. Alshehry, M. S. AlGhamdi, and I. K. Tailor, "Thrombotic thrombocytopenic purpura—analysis of clinical features, laboratory characteristics and therapeutic outcomeof 24 patients treated at a Tertiary Care Center in Saudi Arabia," *Pakistan Journal of Medical Sciences*, vol. 32, no. 6, pp. 1494–1499, 2016.

[20] H. Ohguchi, T. Sugawara, and H. Harigae, "Thrombotic thrombocytopenic purpura complicated with hypereosinophilic syndrome," *Internal Medicine*, vol. 48, no. 18, pp. 1687–1690, 2009.

[21] Z. Al Aly, J. M. Philoctête Ashley, M. E. Gellens, and E. A. González, "Thrombotic thrombocytopenic purpura in a patient treated with imatinib mesylate: true association or mere coincidence?," *American Journal of Kidney Diseases*, vol. 45, no. 4, pp. 762–768, 2005.

[22] F. E. Roufosse, M. Goldman, and E. Cogan, "Hypereosinophilic syndromes," *Orphanet Journal of Rare Diseases*, vol. 2, no. 1, p. 37, 2007.

[23] P. Valent, A. D. Klion, H.-P. Horny et al., "Contemporary consensus proposal on criteria and classification of eosinophilic disorders and related syndromes," *Journal of Allergy and Clinical Immunology*, vol. 130, no. 3, pp. 607–612, 2012.

[24] J. Gotlib and J. Cools, "Five years since the discovery of FIP1L1-PDGFRA: what we have learned about the fusion and other molecularly defined eosinophilias," *Leukemia*, vol. 22, no. 11, pp. 1999–2010, 2008.

[25] B. J. Bain, "Myeloid and lymphoid neoplasms with eosinophilia and abnormalities of PDGFRA, PDGFRB or FGFR1," *Haematologica*, vol. 95, no. 5, pp. 696–698, 2010.

[26] S. Coutré and J. Gotlib, "Targeted treatment of hypereosinophilic syndromes and chronic eosinophilic leukemias with imatinib mesylate," *Seminars in Cancer Biology*, vol. 14, no. 4, pp. 307–315, 2004.

18

Hereditary Hyperferritinemia-Cataract Syndrome in 3 Generations of a Family in East Tennessee

Heidi A. Worth, Zachary Marlette, David Aljadir, and Ronald Lands

Department of Medicine, Division of Hematology/Oncology, University of Tennessee Medical Center, Knoxville, TN, USA

Correspondence should be addressed to Heidi A. Worth; hworth@utmck.edu

Academic Editor: Sergio Storti

Hereditary hyperferritinemia and cataracts syndrome (HHCS) without iron overload is a syndrome first identified less than 3 decades ago. While investigators have dissected the gene where several responsible mutations reside, it remains a relatively unknown genetic disorder to clinicians. The result is often an expensive, invasive evaluation for iron overload, followed by a well-intended prescription for a series of phlebotomies that delivers morbidity instead of benefit. We present a father with an elevated ferritin and heterozygosity for H63D HFE mutation whose clinical course followed this path. His treatment rendered him symptomatic from iron deficiency with no reduction in his ferritin. On re-evaluation, a review of his past medical history clarified the cataract surgery noted in his record had occurred at a young age. Furthermore, one of his daughters required cataract surgery as a teenager. With this information, we strongly suspected HHCS. His phlebotomies were discontinued, and within weeks, his iatrogenic iron deficiency resolved and his health returned to normal.

1. Introduction

Ferritin is a protein that binds and sequesters intracellular iron. It is a hollow sphere where iron is oxidized and stored, composed of 24 heavy and light subunits in variable proportions in different tissues [1]. It is an indicator of iron stores. When low, it indicates iron deficiency. When elevated, it may indicate iron overload as in HFE hemochromatosis, thalassemia, and multiple blood transfusions. More commonly, it is elevated with very different implications due to a broad range of inflammatory states not associated with iron overloading including metabolic syndrome, autoimmune disease, chronic and acute infections, malignancy, and release of ferritin from hepatocytes in liver disease.

Hereditary hyperferritinemia-cataract syndrome (HHCS) was first described in 1995 in a family suspected of having a new genetic disease involving the contiguous L-ferritin gene (FTL) and the gene coding for the lens membrane protein thus accounting for the linkage of hereditary cataracts and elevations of L-ferritin [2]. Separate investigators soon reported another family with mutations in the iron-responsive element (IRE) of the L-ferritin gene that removed the inhibitory interaction with iron regulator protein (IRP) and deregulation of ferritin synthesis [3]. Since the initial discovery, other families in Western Europe, Australia, India, and the United States have been described. Over 32 different mutations were reported by 2013 [4]. The IRE, which is a noncoding stem loop, located in the 5′ untranslated region (5′ UTR) of L-ferritin mRNA plays an important role in the regulation of ferritin synthesis through its interaction with the IRP. Typically, the synthesis of ferritin is regulated by iron availability. When sufficient iron is present, a change in structure of the IRE occurs, preventing its binding to the IRP, leading to ferritin synthesis. In contrast, when levels of cellular iron are low, no change in structure of the IRE occurs, thus allowing the binding of IRP with IRE and inhibiting the translation of ferritin. The mutations of the IRE associated with HHCS lead to a structural change inhibiting the binding with the IRP, allowing for deregulated production of L-ferritin irrespective of cellular iron stores. The increased L-ferritin is due to increased synthesis and not due to elevated iron stores, so the serum iron and transferrin saturation remain normal. There are reports of associations of specific mutations in the IRE with the serum ferritin level, and the age of onset and severity of the cataracts. Other genetic and environmental modifiers are likely to play a role [5].

2. Case Presentation

A 61-year-old Caucasian male was referred to a hematologist for a presumed diagnosis of hemochromatosis after laboratory ordered in the course of evaluation of elevated transaminases demonstrated an elevated ferritin of 1,372 ug/L, and genetic testing demonstrated heterozygosity for H63D mutation. He was active and healthy, exercised regularly, and was a recreational runner and hiker. His past medical history was remarkable for bilateral cataract removal in separate procedures at the age of 12 years and at age 28. Family history was significant in that his father also had cataract surgery in separate procedures at age 40 and 60 years. One of the patient's daughters required surgery for congenital cataracts at the age of 15.

He was initially thought to have iron storage disease based on the presence of the heterozygous H63D mutation and the elevated ferritin. He was prescribed a series of monthly phlebotomies with no measurable reduction in his ferritin levels. A more aggressive treatment with weekly phlebotomies was abandoned when he developed a profound fatigue syndrome, exercise intolerance, and a microcytic anemia. Despite being symptomatic with iron deficiency, his serum ferritin remained elevated at levels consistently >1000 mcg/L. Prior to initiating chelation therapy, he was referred for a second opinion.

At the time of referral for another opinion, his lab studies demonstrated a ferritin of 1,963 ug/L, TIBC 489, iron 43, and transferrin saturation of 9%. An MRI of the liver demonstrated no evidence of iron overload. Because the H63D mutation may rarely be associated with iron overload when present with other risk factors, screening for porphyria, hemoglobinopathy, autoimmune disease, and viral hepatitis were confirmed to be normal. The association of early onset cataracts in three generations of this family, and the elevated ferritin in the absence of iron overload provided enough support to make the diagnosis of HHCS [6]. We discontinued the phlebotomies. While we considered treating him with oral iron to accelerate his recovery, he preferred to resume his normal diet and replete his iron stores without supplementation.

On his first follow-up visit after a month of freedom from the phlebotomies, he was near his previous level of work and recreational activities. His anemia resolved, and he was released to his primary internist for health maintenance. With his daughter's signed consent, we reviewed her medical record, but there were no ferritin levels documented. The patient's father was on hospice at the time of this diagnosis and we did not pursue lab work to determine his ferritin level. We considered submitting the patient's blood for analysis of the FTL gene, but availability and cost were barriers. Genetic testing is not necessary to make the diagnosis. An isolated elevated ferritin level in the absence of iron overload in 2 or more members of a family demonstrating an autosomal dominant pattern of early onset cataracts is usually sufficient [6].

3. Discussion

This case highlights the truth of the much-quoted aphorism that if we listen, the patient will tell us their diagnosis. In this case, the multicontributor past medical history in the electronic medical record noted only that the patient had "cataract surgery" and failed to describe the procedures, one performed in childhood and the other in young adulthood. The family history listed only a cursory list of the usual negatives. The history of cataract surgery in his daughter, which would have surely attracted some further inquiry, was not mentioned. A more detailed past medical history and a thorough family history made the diagnosis of HHCS likely before any images or lab studies were considered.

This presence of the heterozygous H63D mutation in our patient illustrates the importance of interpreting genetic tests with caution when considering hereditary hemochromatosis. Homozygous mutations of the HFE genotypes often do not predict the phenotype of iron overload. The C282Y mutation, a guanine to adenine substitution at nucleotide 845 of the HFE gene which leads to a cysteine to tyrosine substitution at amino acid 282 (C282Y), is variably reported to account for 60–90% of hereditary hemochromatosis when homozygous. Heterozygotes rarely develop iron overload without other risk factors. The H63D mutation, a guanine to cytosine substitution at HFE nucleotide 187 which leads to a histidine to aspartic acid substitution at amino acid 63 (H63D), is much more common than the C282Y mutation and rarely causes iron overload even in homozygotes. Combinations of doubly heterozygous hemochromatosis mutations and heterozygous mutations occurring with other illnesses may result in ferritin elevation with or without iron overload [7]. Pertinent to our patient, an interaction between the H63D mutation and the L-ferritin mutation has not been shown [8].

This case also highlights the lack of awareness of a potential connection between early onset cataracts with elevated ferritin. The prevalence of this disease is considered to be rare, but what was once thought to be a disease located in one or two European countries has now been diagnosed in several areas of the United States and other parts of the world. It is probably better characterized as unrecognized. Many cases are only diagnosed after misdiagnosis of hemochromatosis because of the elevated ferritin and after a significant investment in expensive, painful tests followed by iatrogenic iron deficiency. Ophthalmologists who remove early onset cataracts are often unaware of the HHCS syndrome and do not order iron studies or refer the patient for evaluation. There were missed opportunities in this case. Our patient had two separate cataract surgeries while very young. His elevated ferritin was discovered many years later during an evaluation of abnormal liver functions. His referral to a hematologist was based on the erroneous presumption of iron overload due to the H63D mutation and an elevated ferritin. The patient's daughter, also with two cataract surgeries as a teenager, did not have further evaluation.

4. Conclusion

HHCS is an autosomal dominant genetic disorder that causes hyperferritinemia without iron overload and early onset cataracts. Clues to the diagnosis require a detailed medical and surgical history and a thorough family history. It should be considered in any patient with cataracts at a young age, even in the absence of a family history. Anyone found to have an elevated ferritin in the absence of iron overload without another explanation should have an ophthalmology evaluation. Patients should be counseled regarding the autosomal dominant pattern of heredity, the absence of any organ pathology other than eyes, and that the only treatment necessary is cataract surgery.

References

[1] C. Camaschella and E. Poggiali, "Towards explaining "unexplained hyperferritinemia"" *Haematologica*, vol. 94, no. 3, pp. 307–309, 2009.

[2] D. Bonneau, I. Winter-Fuseau, M.-N. Loiseau et al., "Bilateral cataract and high serum ferritin: a new dominant genetic disorder?" *Journal of Medical Genetics*, vol. 32, no. 10, pp. 778-779, 1995.

[3] D. Girelli, R. Corrocher, L. Bisceglia et al., "Hereditary hyperferritinemia-cataract syndrome caused by a 29-base pair deletion in the iron responsive element of ferritin L-subunit gene," *Blood*, vol. 90, no. 5, pp. 2084–2088, 1997.

[4] J. Muñoz-Muñoz, N. Cuadrado-Grande, M.-I. Moreno-Carralero et al., "Hereditary hyperferritinemia cataract syndrome in four patients with mutations in the IRE of theFTLgene," *Clinical Genetics*, vol. 83, no. 5, pp. 491–493, 2013.

[5] J. Shekunov, P. C. de Groen, N. M. Lindor et al., "Hereditary hyperferritinemia-cataract syndrome in two large multigenerational American families," *Journal of American Association for Pediatric Ophthalmology and Strabismus*, vol. 15, no. 4, pp. 356–361, 2011.

[6] P. C. Adams and J. C. Barton, "A diagnostic approach to hyperferritinemia with a non-elevated transferrin saturation," *Journal of Hepatology*, vol. 55, no. 2, pp. 453–458, 2011.

[7] H. A. Leitch and E. Nemeth, "Iron physiology, iron overload, and the porphyrias," in *American Society of Hematology -Self Assessment Program*, A. Cuker, J. K. Altman, A. T. Gerds, and T. Wun, Eds., pp. 120–122, American Society of Hematology, Washington, DC, USA, 2019, http://ash-sap.org/, 7th edition.

[8] J. C. Barton, E. Beutler, and T. Gelbart, "Coinheritance of alleles associated with hemochromatosis and hereditary hyperferritinemia-cataract syndrome," *Blood*, vol. 92, no. 11, pp. 4480-4481, 1998.

19

Addressing the Challenges to Diagnose Neonatal Hemolytic Anemia's Aetiologies in Low Ressources Countries: A Case Report

Lydie Ocini Ngolet[1] **Josue Simo Louokdom,**[1] **Nelly Guembo,**[2] **and Ocko Ngokaba Thibault**[3]

[1]*Department of Medical Hematology, Brazzaville Teaching Hospital, 13 Avenue Auxence Ikonga, BP 32, Brazzaville, Congo*
[2]*Department of Pediatry, Brazzaville Blanche Gomes Hospital, Sassou Nguesso Boulevard, Brazzaville, Congo*
[3]*Department of laboratory, Brazzaville Teaching Hospital, 13 Avenue Auxence Ikonga, BP 32, Brazzaville, Congo*

Correspondence should be addressed to Lydie Ocini Ngolet; lngolet@yahoo.fr

Academic Editor: Håkon Reikvam

Background. The diagnosis of neonatal hemolysis is an easy exercise. However, the diagnosis of its etiology can be very challenging especially in low ressources countries where laboratory capacities are limited. We report the case of hemolytic anemia episodes that started in the neonatal period, for which the trigger factor, infectious of paracetamol, is debatable.

1. Case Presentation

A 3-month-old and 2-day-old male infant was referred to the hematology department of the University Hospital for anemia.

The patient was the product on an uncomplicated full-term pregnancy. His medical history revealed neonatal jaundice at 5 days of life and 2 episodes of acute anemia following febrile runny nose, respectively, at 1 and 2 months. They required blood transfusion (80 mL each) and antipyretic (paracetamol 10 mg/Kg every 6 hours when needed) and empiric antibiotics for the second episode (amoxicillin 50 mg/kg every 12 hours during 5 days). The malaria smear was negative. The hemoglobin electrophoresis was also negative for the hemoglobin S. The rate of the hemoglobin F was 12%, which for the age of 1 monthwas normal.

Since the hemolytic anemia reoccurred 32 days after the last episode, the infant was referred to the hematology clinic at the University Hospital (June 12, 2019).

On physical examination, the patient was in good health, dynamic, and reactive. His rectal temperature was 36.6°C. There was pallor but no jaundice. The blood pressure was 129/88 mmHg and pulse rate was 120 beats per min, with enlarged spleen but no hepatomegaly. The rest of the physical was unremarkable.

After examination, we performed several blood tests (Table 1). The initial thin smear revealed at the microscopic inclusions in the red cells. Eleven percent of the patient's red cells were infected by parasites identified as *Plasmodium falciparum*. The malaria rapide test was positive for *Plasmodium falciparum*. We made the diagnosis of severe malaria based on the parasitemia and anemia. The mother tested also positive for *Plasmodium falciparum*. An antimalarial treatment with artesunate IV (3 mg/kg/j) was initiated for the mother and the baby for 3 days. The infant's smear was repeated after three days of antimalarial treatment. The results were still positive for *Plasmodium falciparum* (1% of the red cell infected). We decided to extend the antimalarial treatment for a total of 7 days. We requested additional laboratory studies to investigate the cause of the hemolytic anemia. The second hemoglobin electrophoresis was again negative for the hemoglobin S. The direct antiglobulin test was negative. The Glucose 6 Phosphate dehydrogenase level was low at 3.1 U/GHb (6.6 to 17.2). Table 1. We concluded that the patient was Glucose 6 Phosphate Dehydrogenase deficient (G6PD). The trigger factor of the hemolytic anemia was malaria.

TABLE 1: Results of blood work.

Age Date	5 days 15-03-2019	1 month ½ 15-04-2019	2 months 14-05-2019	3 months 12-06-2019	4 months 17-07-2019	5 months 20-08-2019
Laboratory studies						
White cell count (G/L)	6.4	3.8	8.5	6.9	8.58	7.30
Differential count						
Neutrophils (%)	38	20	27.4	16.0	15.3	12.9
Lymphocytes (%)	54	70.8	60.9	73.5	76.9	61.6
Hemoglobin (g/dL)	9.6	5.0	8.6	7.9	6.9	12.5
Hematocrit (%)	28.9	15.0	28	25.9	27.5	30.7
Platelets (10^9 g/L)	172	157	207	243	381	281
Reticulocyte count (G/L)	156.3	214	175.9	186.2	192.3	98.8
Serum bilirubin total (mg/L)	183.4			21.2	22	6.2
Serum bilirubin indirect (mg/L)	172.9			12.13	12.7	3.2
ALT (UI/L)					17	
AST (UI/L)					13	
Ferritin (μg/L)				1518.4		390.4
Direct Coombs test		Negative		Negative		
Hemoglobin electrophoresis		A1 : 88% F.12%				A1 : 97.9% A2 : 2.1%
G6PD level (U/GHb)				3.1		

At the follow-up visit (July 17, 2019), no improvement was noticed. The hemoglobin level was at 6.9 g/d, and the hemolysis was persistent (Table 1). The family denied any febrile episodes or drug intake. We reviewed carefully the environmental agents (as naphthalene ball) to which the infant was exposed and also the diet of the infant's mother and medication intake, since she was breastfeeding. The interview revealed that the mother had been self-medicating with paracetamol for a migraine condition since she was pregnant and she had presented two malaria episodes. We stopped the paracetamol and scheduled the infant for a follow-up.

The patient consulted 4 weeks and 3 days later. The hemoglobin rate was normal and, there were no biological signs of hemolysis.

2. Discussion

This case demonstrates the difficulty in diagnosing neonatal hemolytic anemia's etiology in Sub-Saharian Africa. The difficulties were related to not only the limit of diagnosis capacities but also the complexity of the case.

(1) It was unclear to deduce if the patient developed congenital malaria or was infected in the postnatal period. Congenital malaria is defined as the presence of plasmodium asexual stages in newborn's cord or peripheral blood during the first week of life as a result of maternofetal transfer of parasites [1]. In areas endemic for malaria, symptomatic malaria infection is rare because of the effectiveness of the placenta as a barrier and the high level of maternal's antibodies and hemoglobin F [2, 3]. It is reported that it might take 3 to 4 weeks before congenitally-infected infants present symptoms [4]. Neonatal jaundice when related to malaria is usually associated with fever, irritability, and hepatosplenomegaly. Congenital malaria is characterized by low parasitemia, and the diagnosis is often missed because malaria smears, used in low ressources countries as a tool diagnosis, are often negative. The presence of *Plasmodium falciparum* in the blood of the mother and malaria history during the pregnancy concurred to the hypothesis of congenital malaria. The Polymerase Chain Reaction technique which is very sensitive in the detection of low parasite density, if available in the Congo, would have been helpful in the revision of our primary care but also our initial management. Repeated malaria smears turned out to be positive at the age of 3 months. The high density in *Plasmodium falciparum* may be the result of the progression of the disease or new contamination. Severe malaria is rare in the infant population and the population with G6PD deficiency [5]. An article from Mali examined the relationship between G6PD deficiency and severe malaria and reported that the G6PD deficiency confers highly significant protection against severe malaria in hemizygous males but not in heterozygous females [6].

(2) The diagnosis of acquired hemolytic anemia triggered only by malaria was revised because the anemia was persistent despite the antimalarial treatment. The usual presentation of the X-linked disease is, in the Sub-Saharian African region, acute hemolytic anemia triggered by a factor. Between the crisis, the hemoglobin rate is usually back to normal [6]. The persistence of the anemia between crisis and absence of acute hemolytic anemia in the infant's male sibling contributed to delay in the diagnosis of G6PD deficiency. Since he got a femoral fracture during the delivery, the pediatrician assessed neonatal nonimmune hemolytic anemia due to trauma. The jaundice was related to the hematoma resorption. The repetition of the hemolysis episodes led to the diagnosis. A blood specimen sent to France helped in diagnosis of G6PD deficiency.

(3) The nature of the triggered factor of the acute hemolysis anemia remains unclear. Despite the malaria treatment, the patient kept hemolyzing. Potential triggering factors were reviewed. There was no exposure to environmental factors as naphtalene balls or diet-related cause. The mother was exclusively breastfeeding. She reported paracetamol intake during her pregnancy. Paracetamol or acetaminophen is not an oxidant medication. It is not considered as a drug that can cause acute the hemolytic reaction. However, we found 2 case reports of hemolytic crisis following paracetamol ingestion through the database from Pubmed [7, 8]. Per the authors, the interindividual reaction to the drug intake in patients with G6PD deficient may explain that fact. The same agent may cause hemolysis to one patient and not to another one. Differences result not only from multiple factors such as genetics but also from maturation of liver enzymes [9]. It is not clear in our case to determine if the acute and prolonged anemia were associated with the mother's consumption of paracetamol. However, the hemolysis resolved since the mother stopped taking paracetamol.

At that stage, we can state the following:

(a) The anemia was hemolytic and regenerative, which excluded aplastic anemia.

(b) The hemolytic anemia was prolonged which is not common in G6PD deficiency. A G6PD genotype investigation, if available, would have been helpful.

(c) The hyperbilirubinemia initially hemolytic turned out to be progressively mixt without liver enzymes elevation which eliminated liver disease and conforted a chronic hemolytic anemia.

(d) The repeated hemoglobin electrophoresis was normal.

This observation highlights three points:

(1) There is a need to build our diagnosis capacity but also to develop and implement a neonatal G6PD screening program in the Congo where the disease rate is theoretically high.

(2) The need to establish guidelines for the diagnosis and management of neonatal jaundice and acute hemolytic anemia.

(3) Congenital malaria should be suspected in all neonates in the Congo, endemic for malaria, who present with fever. Malaria smears and the rapid malaria test in the absence of the PCR technique should be repeated. Early diagnosis could prevent unnecessary antibiotic usage and avert the progression of malaria.

3. Conclusion

G6PD deficiency is a condition frequently underdiagnosed among infants in the Congo when symptoms are atypical. G6PD deficiency should be considered as a differential diagnosis in male infants with neonatal jaundice or hemolytic anemia.

Consent

Written informed consent was obtained from the parents of the patient for publication of this case report.

Authors' Contributions

Lydie Ocini Ngolet drafted the paper. Josue Simo Luokdom, Nelly Guembo, and Thibault Oko helped in the diagnosis. All authors read and approved the final paper.

Acknowledgments

The authors wish to thank Ms. Ngenyi Ousman for her help in translating and editing the manuscript.

References

[1] U. D'Allessandro, D. Ubber, K. Homeed et al., "Malaria in infants aged less than six months-is-it an area of unmet medical need?" *Malaria Journal*, vol. 11, p. 4400, 2012.

[2] C. Menendez and A. Mayor, "Congenital malaria: the least known consequence of malaria in pregnancy," *Seminars in Fetal and Neonatal Medicine*, vol. 12, no. 3, pp. 207–213, 2007.

[3] S. Uyoga, C. M. Ndila, A. W. Macharia et al., "Glucose-6-phosphate dehydrogenase deficiency and the risk of malaria and other diseases in children in Kenya: a case-control and a cohort study," *The Lancet Haematology*, vol. 2, no. 10, pp. e437–e444, 2015.

[4] J. Stassijns, W. Van Den Boogaard, P. Pannus et al., "Prevalence and diagnosis of congenital malaria in rural Burundi: a cross-sectionnal study," *Malaria Journal*, vol. 15, no. 443, pp. 1–6, 2016.

[5] A. K. Ouattara, P. Yameogo, B. Diarra et al., *BMC Medical Genetics*, vol. 18, pp. 2–8, 2017.

[6] A. Guindo, R. M. Fairhust, O. K. Doumbo et al., "X-linked G6PD deficiency protects hemizigous males but not heterozygous females against severe malaria," *PLoS Medecine March*, vol. 4, no. 3, 2007.

[7] K. R. Dobbs and A. E. Dent, "Plasmodium malaria and antimalarial antibodies in the first year of life," *Parasitology*, vol. 143, no. 2, pp. 129–138, 2016.

[8] C. S. Bartsocas, J. D. Schulman, and L. Corash, "Can acetaminophen cause hemolysis in G6PD deficiency?" *Acta Haematologica*, vol. 67, no. 3, p. 228, 1982.

[9] M. Olivier, T. Coton, C. Badens et al., "Homozygous G6PD deficiency and propacetamol induced hemolysis," *Haematologica*, vol. 86, pp. 987-988, 2001.

The Implications of Liver Biopsy Results in Patients with Myeloproliferative Neoplasms Being Treated with Ruxolitinib

Douglas Tremblay,[1] Juan Putra,[2] Alexander Vogel,[3] Adam Winters,[3] Ronald Hoffman,[1] Thomas D. Schiano,[4] Maria Isabel Fiel,[2] and John O. Mascarenhas[1]

[1]*Tisch Cancer Institute, Icahn School of Medicine at Mount Sinai, New York, NY, USA*
[2]*Department of Pathology, Icahn School of Medicine at Mount Sinai, New York, NY, USA*
[3]*Department of Medicine, Icahn School of Medicine at Mount Sinai, New York, NY, USA*
[4]*Department of Medicine, Division of Liver Diseases, Recanati/Miller Transplantation Institute, Icahn School of Medicine at Mount Sinai, New York, NY, USA*

Correspondence should be addressed to John O. Mascarenhas; john.mascarenhas@mssm.edu

Academic Editor: Akimichi Ohsaka

Ruxolitinib is increasingly being utilized for the treatment of myelofibrosis and polycythemia vera, but the potential for hepatic toxicity is poorly understood. We performed a retrospective review of hepatic damage occurring in patients with myeloproliferative neoplasms receiving ruxolitinib. Relevant histologic images of liver biopsies were reviewed by an experienced liver pathologist and reported to a multidisciplinary team including hepatology and hematology. A variety of liver pathology was observed including extramedullary hematopoiesis, obliterative portal venopathy, and drug-induced liver injury. In all cases reviewed, the liver biopsy had significant treatment implications. We conclude that hepatology referral and liver biopsy in patients receiving ruxolitinib therapy with biochemical evidence of liver injury reveals a variety of etiologies which have significant treatment impact. Clinicians should be aware of the potential causes of liver damage in this population and initiate prompt referral and liver biopsy.

1. Introduction

Ruxolitinib is a JAK1/2 inhibitor and is the sole FDA-approved therapy for patients with intermediate-/high-risk myelofibrosis (MF), and it is also approved to treat patients with polycythemia vera (PV) that have previously failed therapy with hydroxyurea. Ruxolitinib treatment has been associated with transient mild aminotransferase elevations during preapproval clinical trials, with grade 1, by Common Terminology Criteria for Adverse Event (CTCAEs), alanine aminotransferase (ALT), and aspartate aminotransferase (AST) elevations seen in 25.2% and 17.4% of patients, respectively [1]. Another estimate based on preapproval regulatory reviews cites the incidence of aminotransferase elevations as 18% in those receiving ruxolitinib [2]. No cases of acute hepatic failure have been reported to date.

MF itself is also associated with hepatic dysfunction. Examples include invasion of hepatic tissue with hematopoietic cells in the setting of extramedullary hematopoiesis (EMH), portal vein thrombosis, and obliterative portal venopathy (OPV) [3]. EMH in particular is important to identify as it is a disease manifestation that may respond favorably to ruxolitinib therapy [4]. With the increasingly widespread use of ruxolitinib in the treatment of MF and PV patients, clinicians may be faced with the dilemma as to whether ruxolitinib is the cause of hepatic enzyme elevations or is in fact beneficial for the treatment of hepatic dysfunction arising from EMH. Herein, we describe a series of patients without known liver disease or pathology receiving ruxolitinib who experienced hepatocellular damage and had a liver biopsy performed that assisted in their subsequent management.

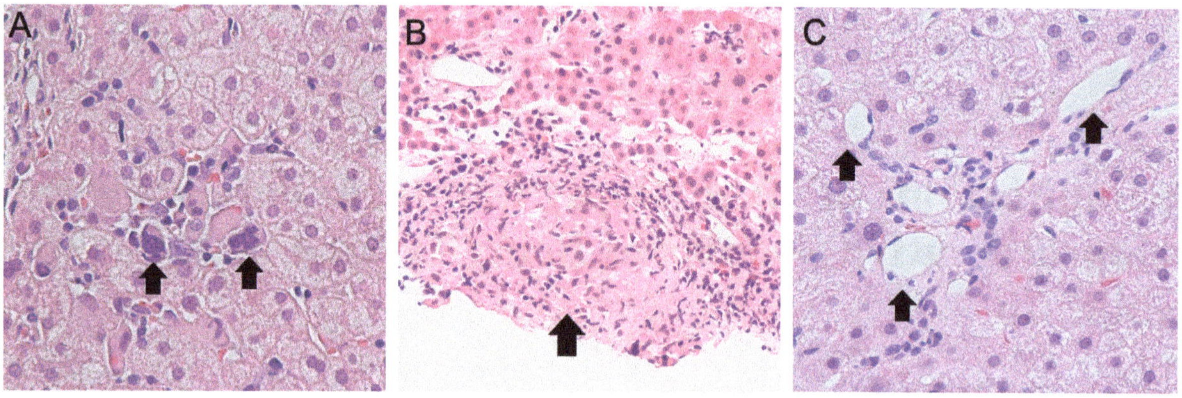

FIGURE 1: (A) The liver biopsy specimen shows prominent extramedullary hematopoiesis in the sinusoids. Megakaryocytes are marked by the arrows. (B) An epithelioid granuloma (arrow) is noted in the portal tract. An adjacent area shows sinusoidal dilatation. (C) A portal tract with herniated portal veins(arrows). The findings are compatible with obliterative portal venopathy.

2. Cases

2.1. Case 1. A 55-year-old male with a history of *CALR*-positive, low-risk MF by the Dynamic International Prognostic Scoring System (DIPSS) was initiated on 5 mg twice daily ruxolitinib treatment given progressive splenomegaly and worsening night sweats. He experienced an outstanding symptomatic response without significant improvement in splenomegaly. His aminotransferases, which were normal prior to ruxolitinib initiation, became mildly elevated, with ALT rising from 64 U/L at initiation to 232 U/L after 5 months of therapy. The patient was not on other hepatotoxic medications. A transjugular liver biopsy was obtained, which demonstrated significant EMH and diffuse sinusoidal infiltration with atypical appearing megakaryocytes, without evidence of steatohepatitis or drug-induced liver injury (DILI) (Figure 1(A)). Given the finding of EMH, the ruxolitinib dose was increased to 10 mg twice daily with immediate and sustained improvement in ALT to 85 U/L. He is currently being evaluated for an allogeneic hematopoietic stem cell transplantation.

2.2. Case 2. A 66-year-old male with a history of PV was initiated on ruxolitinib 10 mg twice daily for worsening leukocytosis and massive splenomegaly. He experienced an excellent initial response with significant reduction in palpable splenomegaly by 50%. However, serum levels of alkaline phosphatase (ALP) began to rise from a baseline of 113 U/L to 311 U/L after 2 weeks of exposure to drug. The ALP peaked at 1286 U/L after approximately 8 months of ruxolitinib exposure. He did not start any other medications or supplements during this time. He was continued on a higher dose of ruxolitinib at 15 mg twice daily for presumed EMH. The ALP remained elevated at 334 U/L, so a liver biopsy was performed at that time, demonstrating granulomatous hepatitis with ductopenia (Figure 1(B)), which was attributed to DILI. Shortly afterwards, he expired from hypoxemic respiratory failure in the setting of a lobar pneumonia. This represents a potential case of DILI due to ruxolitinib given the temporal relationship between ruxolitinib initiation and a grade 3 ALP rise, and further supported by the liver biopsy findings.

2.3. Case 3. A 74-year-old male with high-risk JAK2V617F-positive post-PV MF was initiated on ruxolitinib 10 mg twice daily to address worsening splenomegaly and debilitating fatigue. The patient experienced improvement in symptom burden and a decrease in palpable spleen size by 20%. However, he began to experience worsening ascites requiring large-volume paracentesis. Additionally, the ALP rose to 335 U/L from a baseline of around 180 U/L. Given the unknown cause of his liver dysfunction, he underwent a transjugular liver biopsy, demonstrating the presence of both EMH and OPV (Figure 1(C)). Because of these findings, the ruxolitinib dose was increased to 20 mg twice daily with improvement in symptoms and ascites and decrease in ALP to 151 U/L within 5 months.

2.4. Case 4. A 49-year-old male with DIPSS intermediate-2 risk, JAK2V617F-positive post-PV MF, and a history of portal vein thrombosis was started on ruxolitinib at 10 mg twice daily for splenomegaly. He attained an excellent symptomatic response but was noted to have an increase in total bilirubin to 2.6 mg/dL (44.5 μmol/L) from a normal baseline. During this time, no new medications were started. Although some hyperbilirubinemia can be attributed to hemolysis, he underwent a liver biopsy which demonstrated OPV with extensive EMH. He was continued on ruxolitinib 15 mg with improvement in total bilirubin to 1.3 mg/dL (22.23 μmol/L).

3. Discussion

There is a significant but incompletely understood relationship between MPNs and liver disease. Noncirrhotic portal hypertension (NCPH), a broad category of diseases including OPV, has been described in the setting of MPNs with the sequela including ascites, esophageal and gastric varices, and subsequent variceal bleeding. The development of NCPH is at least in part a consequence of thrombotic disease; however, inappropriate endothelial cell activation associated with *JAK2V617F* expression has been implicated [5]. OPV involves variable obliteration of the portal vein, particularly in the terminal branches of the intrahepatic portal vein, and has been observed in patients with MPNs [3]. Finally, EMH can manifest as a focal hepatic nodule [6], diffuse hepatomegaly and portal hypertension [7], or laboratory manifestations as in the first, second, and fourth cases described in the current series [8].

As demonstrated in a retrospective study of 398 PMF patients, the most common hepatic laboratory derangement was an elevated ALP, which was CTCAE grade 1 in 40% of patients, grade 2 in 7%, and grade 3 or above in 1%. When grade 2 or above, an elevated ALP was associated with a higher leukocyte count and worse prognosis. AST elevations were also present in this population, with 9% having elevations which were mostly grade 1. No findings were reported for other liver chemistry tests such as ALT or bilirubin levels [9]. The pathological basis of these laboratory findings was not reported, nor were concomitant medications including ruxolitinib noted.

The cases described in the current series illustrate the variety of liver pathology seen in PV/MF patients with liver dysfunction. However, it is unclear the prevalence of liver pathology in MPN patients without liver dysfunction. We also report a possible case of ruxolitinib-associated DILI. There are no known mechanisms to explain possible hepatotoxicity with this agent. Ruxolitinib is metabolized by the liver through the CYP3A4 system, with metabolites mainly excreted in the urine. It is plausible that liver injury may be related to the production of a toxic intermediate [10]. If DILI is suspected with ruxolitinib exposure, discontinuation may be warranted. However, abrupt discontinuation of ruxolitinib in any context can lead to a serious and potentially life-threatening withdrawal syndrome characterized by worsening cytopenias and progressive splenomegaly, the most severe form of which can mimic septic shock with hemodynamic instability [11]. Therefore, when ruxolitinib is discontinued, it should be done as a taper under close supervision and in certain cases overlapped with prednisone to blunt the potential cytokine rebound phenomenon. Thus, utilizing a liver biopsy to diagnose DILI is of paramount importance before considering withdrawal of ruxolitinib.

Although some liver abnormalities can be attributed to ruxolitinib itself, the majority of patients in our series had abnormalities as a consequence of EMH. This series emphasizes that obtaining a liver biopsy is a crucial and necessary step for adaptive management in patients with evidence of hepatocellular damage receiving ruxolitinib treatment. The liver biopsy may be instrumental in determining if ruxolitinib therapy should be discontinued or continued.

References

[1] United States Food and Drug Administration, *JAKAFI (Ruxolitinib) Label*, USFDA, Silver Spring, MD, USA, 2011.

[2] R. R. Shah, J. Morganroth, and D. R. Shah, "Hepatotoxicity of tyrosine kinase inhibitors: clinical and regulatory perspectives," *Drug Safety*, vol. 36, no. 7, pp. 491–503, 2013.

[3] J. E. Mayer, T. D. Schiano, M. I. Fiel, R. Hoffman, and J. O. Mascarenhas, "An association of myeloproliferative neoplasms and obliterative portal venopathy," *Digestive Diseases and Sciences*, vol. 59, no. 7, pp. 1638–1641, 2014.

[4] M. Maccaferri, G. Leonardi, R. Marasca et al., "Ruxolitinib for pulmonary extramedullary hematopoiesis in myelofibrosis," *Leukemia & Lymphoma*, vol. 55, no. 9, pp. 2207-2208, 2014.

[5] S. Sozer, M. I. Fiel, T. Schiano, M. Xu, J. Mascarenhas, and R. Hoffman, "The presence of JAK2V617F mutation in the liver endothelial cells of patients with Budd-Chiari syndrome," *Blood*, vol. 113, no. 21, pp. 5246–5249, 2009.

[6] F. S. Cardoso, J. V. Pires, J. S. Miranda, and J. M. Araujo, "Hepatic nodule: a case of primary myelofibrosis," *BMJ Case Reports*, vol. 2011, article bcr0520114220, 2011.

[7] P. Amarapurkar, S. Parekh, A. Amarapurkar, and D. Amarapurkar, "Portal hypertension and ascites in extramedullary hematopoiesis," *Journal of Clinical and Experimental Hepatology*, vol. 2, no. 2, pp. 188–190, 2012.

[8] M. Yotsumoto, F. Ishida, T. Ito, M. Ueno, K. Kitano, and K. Kiyosawa, "Idiopathic myelofibrosis with refractory massive ascites," *Internal Medicine*, vol. 42, no. 6, pp. 525–528, 2003.

[9] D. Barraco, M. Mudireddy, S. Shah et al., "Liver function test abnormalities and their clinical relevance in primary myelofibrosis," *Blood Cancer Journal*, vol. 7, no. 4, p. e557, 2017.

[10] S. Galli, D. McLornan, and C. Harrison, "Safety evaluation of ruxolitinib for treating myelofibrosis," *Expert Opinion on Drug Safety*, vol. 13, no. 7, pp. 967–976, 2014.

[11] A. Tefferi and A. Pardanani, "Serious adverse events during ruxolitinib treatment discontinuation in patients with myelofibrosis," *Mayo Clinic Proceedings*, vol. 86, no. 12, pp. 1188–1191, 2011.

21

Relapse of *NPM1*-Mutated AML with Extramedullary Manifestation 17 Years after Allogeneic Hematopoietic Stem Cell Transplantation

Jan Braune,[1] **Kathrin Rieger**,[1] **Olga Blau**,[1] **Ulrich Keller**,[1,2,3] **Lars Bullinger**,[1,2,3] **and Jan Krönke**[1,2,3]

[1]*Department of Hematology, Oncology and Cancer Immunology, Charité-Universitätsmedizin Berlin, Freie Universität Berlin and Humboldt-Universität zu Berlin, Berlin, Germany*
[2]*German Cancer Consortium (DKTK) Partner Site Berlin and German Cancer Research Center (DKFZ), Heidelberg, Germany*
[3]*Berlin Institute of Health (BIH), Berlin, Germany*

Correspondence should be addressed to Jan Braune; jan.braune@charite.de

Academic Editor: Håkon Reikvam

The majority of patients with acute myeloid leukemia (AML) with the *NPM1* mutation achieve remission with intensive chemotherapy. However, many patients subsequently relapse, which occurs frequently within the first 2–3 years after therapy, while late relapse after more than 10 years is rare and can also represent secondary/therapy-associated AML without the NPM1 mutation. Here, we present a case of *NPM1*-mutated AML that developed medullary and extramedullary relapse 17 years after allogeneic stem cell transplantation, maintaining the *NPM1* mutation and all other genetic alterations detected at first diagnosis. This exceptionally long latency between diagnosis and relapse of a genetically highly related leukemic clone implies the existence of therapy-resistant, persisting dormant leukemic stem cells in *NPM1* mutant AML.

1. Introduction

NPM1 mutations are among the most frequent genetic alterations in acute myeloid leukemia (AML) and are associated with distinct morphological, genetic, and clinical features. Intensive chemotherapy with or without allogeneic stem cell transplantation (allo-HSCT) leads to remission in 70–90% of patients with *NPM1*^{mut} AML, but about 30–50% of patients relapse due to persistent leukemic stem cells [1]. Most AML relapses occur early, usually within 12–18 months after the first complete remission (CR1), while late (LR) and very late relapses (VLR), defined as >3 years and >5 years after CR1, respectively, are rare and occur in 1–3% of the patients [2, 3], with only a few case studies describing relapses after more than 10 years [2, 4–7]. Recent studies revealed that many very late relapses are secondary, therapy-related AMLs with a distinct genetic profile as compared to the first AML at diagnosis [8, 9]. Extramedullary (EM) AML is a rare manifestation of AML and occurs in only 2–9% of newly diagnosed patients [10]. Nevertheless, it occurs more frequently in relapsed patients, and EM relapses have been reported more frequently in transplant recipients than in patients treated with chemotherapy alone.

Here, we report the case of a patient with *NPM1*-mutated AML who developed a bone marrow (BM) and EM relapse 17 years after the first diagnosis (Figure 1).

2. Case Presentation

A 23-year-old male patient was diagnosed with AML (initial white blood cell count: 50/nL; hemoglobin: 3.6 g/dL; platelet count: $67 \times 10^3/\mu L$) in 2003. A BM biopsy showed 80% blasts with monocytic features without evidence of extramedullary disease. Conventional cytogenetics revealed a 46, XY, del(9q) karyotype. Flow cytometry revealed the expression of CD33 and HLA-DR, without CD34 or CD117 expression. Molecular genetics and MRD assessment were initially not

(a)

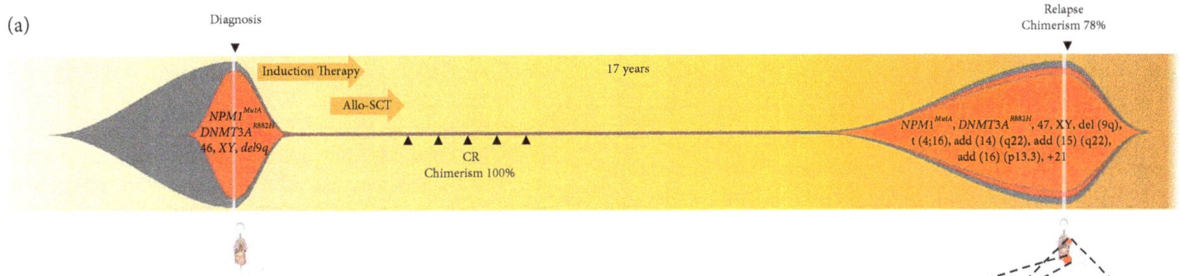

(b)

	Diagnosis	Relapse
Blasts	80%	30%
FACS	CD33+, HLA-DR+, CD34-, CD117-	CD33+, CD13+, CD34+, CD117+
Karyotype	46, XY, del9q	47, XY, del (9q), t (4;16), add (14) (q22), add (15) (q22), add (16) (p13.3), +21
NPM1	Mut A	Mut A
DNMT3A	R882H	R882H
FLT3	wt	wt
IDH1	wt	wt
IDH2	wt	wt
RUNX1	wt	wt
ASXL1	wt	wt
TP53	wt	wt

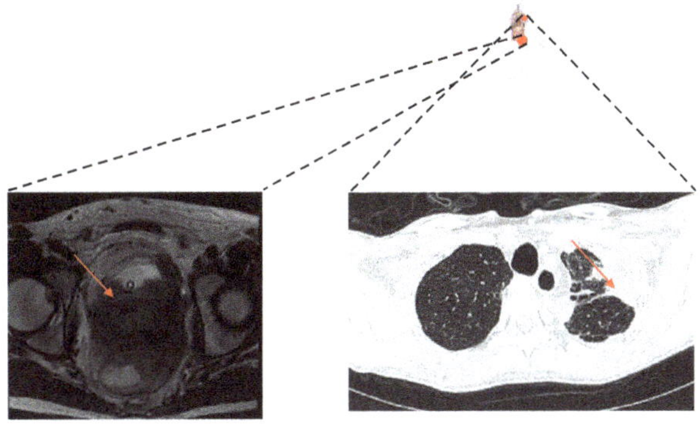

FIGURE 1: (a) Schematic presentation of treatment and genetic evolution in a patient with *NPM1*-mutated AML. The patient had no evidence of extramedullary disease at diagnosis and presented with a chloroma in the lesser pelvis and pulmonary lesions at relapse, as shown in the MRI and CT scan, respectively. (b) AML characteristics of leukemia at diagnosis and relapse.

performed as they were not available at that time. No relevant comorbidities, no family history of malignancies, and no known environmental exposures to substances that damage DNA were reported. The patient received intensive induction therapy with cytarabine, daunorubicin, and thioguanine and achieved a complete remission. He then underwent allogeneic HSCT from an HLA-identical sibling, which was well tolerated without the development of GvHD. Bone marrow assessment revealed a CR with complete donor chimerism one month after transplantation until the end of follow-up seven years after transplantation.

In 2020, 17 years after transplantation, the patient was admitted to the hospital suffering from severe renal impairment, urine retention, and a mechanical ileus. MRI of the abdomen revealed a 12 × 9 cm large mass infiltrating the lesser pelvis. Furthermore, a computed tomography (CT) scan of the chest revealed lesions in both lungs suspicious of metastases. However, histologic analysis of the tumor that infiltrated the colon mucous membrane showed myeloid leukemic cells that were strongly positive for CD33 and CD117 and negative for CD34.

Next, a BM biopsy was taken, which revealed a 30% infiltration of the BM by myeloid leukemia blasts with monocytic differentiation positive for CD13, CD33, CD34, and CD117. By molecular diagnostics, we detected an *NPM1*-Type A mutation and a *DNMT3A* R882H mutation, while no mutations were found in *FLT3*, *IDH1/IDH2*, *RUNX1*, *TP53*, or *ASXL1*. Cytogenetics revealed the same del(9) (q22q34) as 17 years before, in addition to further chromosomal aberrations in the same metaphases 47, XY, t(4; 6) (p16; p21), del(9) (q22q34)x2, add(14) (q22), add(15) (q22), add(16) (p13.3),and +21.

Retrospective analyses of the diagnostic AML sample obtained 17 years before revealed that the *DNMT3A* R882H and *NPM1* Type A mutations were already present at initial diagnosis, while no other mutations were found in *FLT3*, *IDH1/IDH2*, *RUNX1*, *TP53*, or *ASXL1*. A drop in donor chimerism revealed that leukemia originated from the host and not the donor. The persistence of two identical gene mutations and one chromosomal aberration highly implies that relapse evolved directly from persisting cells of the initial leukemic clone rather than an independent clone with newly acquired aberrations.

After induction therapy with cytarabine and daunorubicin, followed by consolidation therapy with intermediate-dose cytarabine and radiation of the pelvic chloroma, a second complete hematologic remission was achieved with complete regression of the pelvic tumor. Radiotherapy of the lung and pelvis was performed. A second HSCT from an HLA haploid donor was planned, but unfortunately, the patient died due to neutropenic sepsis during consolidation therapy.

3. Discussion

This case represents one of the latest relapses described in AML with a confirmed *NPM1* mutation at both diagnosis and relapse. The presence of the same gene mutations, $NPM1^{\text{mutA}}$ and $DNMT3A^{\text{R882H}}$, as well as a del(9q), strongly argues that the second AML directly evolved from the initial AML clone [8]. While a complex karyotype that was detected in the relapsed AML in addition to the initial alterations is frequently observed in patients exposed to DNA damaging agents, typical therapy-associated aberrations such as deletions 5 or 7 or mutations in *TP53* [11] were absent. This is in contrast to our previous findings that very late reoccurrence of leukemia in $NPM1^{\text{mut}}$ AML often represents a genetically distinct, therapy-associated AML without *NPM1* mutation [8, 9].

Bertoli et al. showed that "true," genetically stable, very late relapses after 5 years are more common in patients with the *NPM1* mutation than in AML without the *NPM1* mutation [3]. Watts et al. recently described four cases with very late relapse [12] that were similar to our patient: they had a monocytic phenotype, underwent allo-HSCT, and relapsed with the extramedullary disease. While molecular diagnostic data was not available for any of these cases, monocytic differentiation and extramedullary disease are indicative that these cases harbored an *NPM1* mutation. Bolli et al. described a case of a myeloid sarcoma with an *NPM1* mutation occurring 20 years after the first diagnosis of AML but no genetic information was available at the initial diagnosis [5]. EM disease, although a rare manifestation of AML, is more frequently seen at relapse and after allo-HSCT compared to standard chemotherapy, suggesting a differing underlying pathogenic mechanism [10, 12]. Characteristics that seem to correlate with EM relapse are VLR, monocytic differentiation, favorable cytogenetics, younger age, and *NPM1* mutations [3, 10, 12], all of which were present in our case.

The underlying pathophysiologic mechanisms of such long quiescence of a leukemic stem cell are unclear. The microenvironment has a strong influence on normal and leukemic stem cells, and the transition of such a cell outside the bone marrow may have induced an awakening from dormancy. Decreased immunosurveillance may be a possible factor. Graft versus leukemia might not be that effective outside the BM, explaining the higher rates of EM relapse after allo-HSCT [13–15].

Very late relapse AML with clear proof of a genetic relationship, as in our case, has several implications. From a clinical perspective, the occurrence of very late hematologic and extramedullary relapse in $NPM1^{mut}$ AML has to be considered and warrants awareness of the possibility of EM relapse. AML cases with VLR further demonstrate that leukemia stem cells (LSCs) may persist for many years, most likely in a dormant state that is invisible to the immune system, even after allo-HSCT. It is conceivable that many patients in long-term remission also have persisting, dormant LSCs, as also suggested by the detection of low MRD levels in patients in long-term remission [16]. The reasons for the "awakening" of persisting LSCs are not clear and warrant the further molecular and functional characterization of dormant LSCs. Furthermore, understanding how AML cells persist in therapy over many years may help find ways to eradicate them and cure patients.

References

[1] H. Döhner, D. J. Weisdorf, and C. D. Bloomfield, "Acute myeloid leukemia," in *New England Journal of Medicine*, D. L. Longo, Ed., vol. 373, no. 12, pp. 1136–1152, 2015.

[2] J. M. Watts, X. V. Wang, M. R. Litzow et al., "Younger adults with acute myeloid leukemia in remission for ≥3 years have a high likelihood of cure: the ECOG experience in over 1200 patients," *Leukemia Research*, vol. 38, no. 8, pp. 901–906, 2014.

[3] S. Bertoli, S. Tavitian, E. Bérard et al., "More than ten percent of relapses occur after five years in AML patients with *NPM1* mutation," *Leukemia and Lymphoma*, vol. 61, no. 5, pp. 1226–1229, 2020.

[4] C. Rautenberg, J. Kaivers, U. Germing, R. Haas, T. Schroeder, and G. Kobbe, "Spontaneous remission in a patient with very late relapse of acute myeloid leukemia 17 years after allogeneic blood stem cell transplantation," *European Journal of Haematology*, vol. 103, no. 2, pp. 131–133, 2019.

[5] N. Bolli, S. Galimberti, M. P. Martelli et al., "Cytoplasmic nucleophosmin in myeloid sarcoma occurring 20 years after diagnosis of acute myeloid leukaemia," *The Lancet Oncology*, vol. 7, no. 4, pp. 350–352, 2006.

[6] K. Takahashi, W. Roh, J. Zhang et al., "Clonal evolution of acute myeloid leukemia relapsed after 19 years of remission: late relapse of AML," *American Journal of Hematology*, vol. 90, no. 7, pp. E134–E135, 2015.

[7] G. D. Unis, N. VanderVeen, M. Fletcher, and R. J. Vasquez, "Very late relapse in pediatric acute myeloid leukemia: a case report and brief literature review," *Journal of Pediatric Hematology*, vol. 43, no. 6, pp. 236–239, 2021.

[8] S. Cocciardi, A. Dolnik, S. Kapp-Schwoerer et al., "Clonal evolution patterns in acute myeloid leukemia with NPM1 mutation," *Nature Communications*, vol. 10, no. 1, p. 2031, 2019.

[9] J. Krönke, L. Bullinger, V. Teleanu et al., "Clonal evolution in relapsed NPM1-mutated acute myeloid leukemia," *Blood*, vol. 122, no. 1, pp. 100–108, 2013.

[10] M. Solh, S. Solomon, L. Morris, K. Holland, and A. Bashey, "Extramedullary acute myelogenous leukemia," *Blood Reviews*, vol. 30, no. 5, pp. 333–339, 2016.

[11] T. N. Wong, G. Ramsingh, A. L. Young et al., "Role of TP53 mutations in the origin and evolution of therapy-related acute myeloid leukaemia," *Nature*, vol. 518, no. 7540, pp. 552–555, 2015.

[12] J. M. Watts, X. V. Wang, R. T. Swords et al., "Very late relapse of AML after allogeneic hematopoietic cell transplantation is often extramedullary," *Bone Marrow Transplantation*, vol. 51, no. 7, pp. 1013–1015, 2016.

[13] E. Risson, A. R. Nobre, V. Maguer-Satta, and J. A. Aguirre-Ghiso, "The current paradigm and challenges ahead for the dormancy of disseminated tumor cells," *Naturaliste Canadien*, vol. 1, no. 7, pp. 672–680, 2020.

[14] S. Lee and C. A. Schmitt, "The dynamic nature of senescence in cancer," *Nature Cell Biology*, vol. 21, no. 1, pp. 94–101, 2019.

[15] A. Trumpp and S. Haas, "Cancer stem cells: the adventurous journey from hematopoietic to leukemic stem cells," *Cell*, vol. 185, no. 8, pp. 1266–1270, 2022.

[16] A. L. Boyd, L. Aslostovar, J. Reid et al., "Identification of chemotherapy-induced leukemic-regenerating cells reveals a transient vulnerability of human AML recurrence," *Cancer Cell*, vol. 34, no. 3, pp. 483–498, 2018.

22

Relapse after Prolonged Remission in Philadelphia-Like Acute Lymphoblastic Leukemia

Gaurav Shah,[1] Fady M. Mikhail,[2] Andrew J. Carroll III,[2] Matthew Kutny,[3] and Nikolaos Papadantonakis[4]

[1]*Internal Medicine, University of Alabama at Birmingham, Birmingham, AL, USA*
[2]*Department of Genetics, University of Alabama at Birmingham, Birmingham, AL, USA*
[3]*Division of Hematology/Oncology, Department of Pediatrics, University of Alabama at Birmingham, Birmingham, AL, USA*
[4]*Division of Hematology/Oncology, Department of Medicine, University of Alabama at Birmingham, Birmingham, AL, USA*

Correspondence should be addressed to Nikolaos Papadantonakis; papadan@uab.edu

Academic Editor: Pier P. Piccaluga

We describe a case of late relapse of Philadelphia-like acute lymphoblastic leukemia. The patient relapsed several years from diagnosis and responded to second salvage treatment. The case highlights the open questions regarding management of Philadelphia-like acute lymphoblastic leukemia.

1. Introduction

Recent advances identified a subgroup of Philadelphia (Ph) negative acute lymphoblastic leukemia (ALL) patients with dismal outcomes [1]. This group of patients has an expression profile similar to that of Ph positive ALL patients but lacks the characteristic *BCR-ABL1* gene fusion due to the translocation 9;22. This group encompasses a variety of kinase-activating lesions and is referred to as Ph-like ALL [2].

2. Case Description

We report the case of a 25-year-old young adult patient with relapsed Ph-like ALL at over 15 years from his initial ALL diagnosis at age 9. Patient's initial treatment included a multiagent chemotherapy regimen for standard risk (SR) pre-B ALL in accordance with the Pediatric Oncology Group (POG) 9905 regimen D [3]. Cytogenetics at initial diagnosis showed a balanced translocation t(3;12)(q21;q24), and *BCR-ABL1* gene fusion was negative. Flow cytometry revealed immature B-lineage phenotype. This initial diagnosis was during an era prior to the recognition of Ph-like ALL. The patient achieved first complete remission (CR) at end of induction therapy, and he completed the full regimen of chemotherapy for SR pre-B ALL. He remained in remission until 13 years off therapy (over 15 years from initial diagnosis) when he presented with a one-month history of night sweats, generalized weakness, petechiae, weight loss, lymphadenopathy, and splenomegaly.

Initial laboratory evaluation showed white blood count (WBC) of $44 \times 10^3/\text{mm}^3$ with a differential of 54% blast, hemoglobin of 8.3 g/dL, and platelet count of $24.6 \times 10^3/\text{mm}^3$. CT scans revealed scattered lymphadenopathy throughout chest, abdomen, and pelvis. The patient underwent a BM biopsy with an aspirate revealing 85% blasts. The bone marrow (BM) core biopsy had cellularity of 95% mostly composed by lymphoblasts. Flow cytometry on BM revealed atypical precursor B-cells with the following phenotype: CD19+, CD10hi, CD34 heterogenous, CD20+, CD9+, CD5−, and CD33− (see Table 1 for details). This phenotype was similar to his original diagnosis over 15 years prior. BM karyotype was 46,XY,t(3;12)(q21;q24) [20]. The same karyotype was present in previous samples, and later remission testing revealed that this translocation was constitutional. FISH analysis revealed that 86% of the cells had a rearrangement involving the *CRLF2* gene at Xp22.33/Yp11.32. BM metaphase FISH analysis demonstrated the

Table 1: Summary of hematological and flow cytometry findings, molecular aberrations, and cytogenetics at various stages of clinical course.

	Relapse	Postcycle 1 blinatumomab	Blinatumomab treatment failure	Postcycle 1 inotuzumab ozogamicin	Prior to AlloHSCT
WBC in $10^3/mm^3$ (blast percentage)	44 (54%)	7.51 (5%)	108 (79%)	7.45 (0%)	6.45 (0%)
Platelet count ($10^3/mm^3$)	24.6	158	112	194	167
Flow cytometry	Precursor B-ALL (76% blast)	Precursor B-ALL (32% blast)	Precursor B-ALL (79% blast)	No evidence of ALL	No evidence of ALL
Bone marrow diagnosis	Aspirate: 85% blasts	Aspirate: 41% blasts	Not performed	Aspirate/core: no morphologic or phenotypic evidence of B-ALL	Aspirate/core: no morphologic or phenotypic evidence of B-ALL
Pertinent CD markers on bone marrow (peripheral blood at blinatumomab treatment failure)	CD19+, CD10 high, CD45 low, CD34±, CD20+, zCD9+, CD38+, CD58+, sIg−, CD5−, CD22+, CD13−/low, and CD33−	CD19+, CD10 high, CD45 low, CD34±, CD20+, CD22+, CD38+, CD58+, sIg−, CD13−, and CD33−	CD19+, CD20+, CD10hi, CD45lo, CD34 heterogeneous, CD117−, CD22+, CD38+, CD58lo, CD9+, surface Ig−, CD13−, and CD33−		
CRLF2 rearrangement at Xp22.33/Yp11.32	86% of cells positive	40% of cell positive	76% of cell positive	Negative	Negative
Karyotype	46,XY,t(3;12)(q21; q24) [20]	46,XY,t(3; 12)(q21; q24.1) [20]	46,XY,t(3; 12)(q21; q24.1) [20]	46,XY,t(3; 12)(q21; q24.1)c [20]	46,XY,t(3; 12)(q21; q24.1)c [20]
Pertinent molecular genetics	1 copy of the pathogenic variant in the kinase region of the *JAK2* gene		Fusion of PAX5-ZCCHC7. Mutation in JAK2, CHD2, FIP1L1, and KDM6A		

presence of the t(X; 14)(p22.33;q32.3), which results in *IGH/CRLF2* fusion. BM FISH analysis was negative for the *BCR/ABL1* gene fusion, *MLL* gene rearrangement, and the *ETV6/RUNX1* gene fusion. Initial analysis revealed one copy of pathogenic variant in the kinase region of the *JAK2* gene (Nationwide Children's Hospital). Notably, subsequent molecular analysis (Neogenomics) at a later point on his treatment was positive for a fusion (*PAX5/ZCCHC7*) transcript involving *PAX5* and *ZCCHC7* genes resulting from t(9;9)(p13.2;p13.2) translocation. In addition, significantly high levels of *CRLF2* expression were detected. Moreover, mutations in *JAK2, CHD2, FIP1L1,* and *KDM6A* were detected. Of note, *JAK2* mutations are common among *CRLF2* rearranged cases [4]. The findings of *CRLF2* rearrangement with *JAK2* mutation are diagnostic of Ph-like ALL. Importantly, CSF assessment did not reveal presence of lymphoblasts.

The patient was treated with blinatumomab without significant complications. The BM biopsy after cycle 1 of blinatumomab revealed a reduction to the aspirate blasts to 41% while cellularity was decreased to 50–60% composed mostly by lymphoblasts. The peripheral WBC reduced to $7.51 \times 10^3/mm^3$ with 3% blasts. The hemoglobin improved to 11.4 g/dl and platelets to $158 \times 10^3/mm^3$. The patient then proceeded to the second cycle of blinatumomab, but within a few days, the WBC had increased from 5.84 to $108.6 \times 10^3/mm^3$ with 70% blasts.

Blinatumomab was discontinued, and after cytoreduction, the patient received inotuzumab ozogamicin (InO) at the recommended dose and schedule. Repeat BM biopsy after cycle 1 of InO showed no morphologic evidence of leukemia. Flow cytometry as well as FISH analysis for *CRLF2* rearrangement were negative (see table); karyotype was 46,XY,t(3;12)(q21;q24) [20]. The repeat CT scan showed improvement in diffuse lymphadenopathy and splenomegaly. The patient completed 2nd cycle without any complication, and another BM biopsy was performed again without morphological or flow cytometry evidence of ALL. Karyotype was again 46,XY,t(3;12)(q21;q24) [20], and therefore, it was considered to be most consistent with constitutional translocation.

Following further imaging studies, allogeneic bone marrow transplant (AlloHSCT) was pursued. Conditioning regimen was based on total body irradiation and cyclophosphamide while the donor was matched unrelated. The patient developed infectious complications, electrolyte abnormalities, and arrhythmias during his AlloHSCT course and expired. There was no evidence of veno-occlusive disease at the time of death.

3. Discussion

Children, adolescents, and adults with Ph-like ALL have a dismal prognosis [2, 5]. The use of dasatinib or ruxolitinib with chemotherapy in this subgroup of patients is underway (ClinicalTrials.gov Identifier: NCT02420717) in an attempt to improve outcomes [6].

Patients in CR remain at risk of relapse; the median EFS was 17.2 months for adult patients treated on the study of

Jain et al. [7]. In a recent report of pediatric patients, the median relapse free survival was less than 3 years with a patient relapsing 10.86 years after diagnosis [8].

The Ph-like ALL patient described in this case report relapsed 15 years after initial diagnosis. Our case is one of the very late relapses in ALL reported in the literature and further highlights that such late relapses can occur in Ph-like ALL patients. The mechanisms that can lead to such a late relapse are not well defined (discussed in Norkin et al.) [9]. One hypothesis is that a leukemic clone persists in a semidormant state kept in check by the immune system but then escapes immune system surveillance many years later. Alternatively, a quiescent leukemic stem cell can survive the course of initial treatments and later through further mutational events attain a proliferative state that becomes clinically apparent.

The optimal management of Ph-like ALL patients that relapse remains uncertain. Although the sensitivity of Ph-like ALL to therapy with kinase inhibitors (including the JAK2 inhibitor ruxolitinib and the ABL1 kinase inhibitor dasatinib) has been reported, many aspects of the optimal use of these agents remain unclear. Moreover, the safety of the combination of dasatinib or ruxolitinib with immunotherapies (including the immunoconjugate InO and the bispecific T-cell engaging antibody Blinatumomab) that are FDA approved for relapsed ALL has not been extensively studied [10].

We utilized blinatumomab as salvage regimen as it has been associated with favorable outcomes in relapsed/refractory ALL compared with conventional chemotherapy [11]. Our patient did not respond to blinatumomab. We next attempted treatment with InO as it is also approved for relapsed/refractory ALL [12]. Moreover, in a case series after treatment failure with blinatumomab, the InO was able to achieve 75% response [13]. In this single institution experience, 7 of 12 patients who achieved response received InO in combination with chemotherapy. Our patient responded to InO and was able to proceed to AlloHSCT.

Notably, we were not able to find guidance in the literature regarding the optimal management of relapsed Ph-like ALL patients. Studies focusing on the outcomes of salvage treatments in the Ph-like ALL would be very helpful to inform a preferred approach. For example, the association of specific molecular aberrations in Ph-like ALL patients with FDA approved and NCCN category 1 recommended treatments such as blinatumomab or InO would be of particular interest.

4. Conclusion

Our case of very late relapse of a Ph-like ALL patient highlights that although uncommon, late occurrence can happen. Moreover, optimal salvage regimen for Ph-like ALL is not defined, and further studies are eagerly awaited.

Consent

Patient consent was not obtained as deidentified information was used.

References

[1] C. G. Mullighan, X. Su, J. Zhang et al., "Deletion of IKZF1 and prognosis in acute lymphoblastic leukemia," *New England Journal of Medicine*, vol. 360, no. 5, pp. 470–480, 2009.

[2] K. G. Roberts, Y. Li, D. Payne-Turner et al., "Targetable kinase-activating lesions in Ph-like acute lymphoblastic leukemia," *New England Journal of Medicine*, vol. 371, no. 11, pp. 1005–1015, 2014.

[3] N. Winick, P. L. Martin, M. Devidas et al., "Delayed intensification (DI) enhances event-free survival (EFS) of children with B-precursor acute lymphoblastic leukemia (ALL) who received intensification therapy with six courses of intravenous methotrexate (MTX): POG 9904/9905: a childrens Oncology group study (COG)," *Blood*, vol. 110, no. 11, p. 583, 2007.

[4] S. K. Tasian, M. L. Loh, and S. P. Hunger, "Philadelphia chromosome-like acute lymphoblastic leukemia," *Blood*, vol. 130, no. 19, pp. 2064–2072, 2017.

[5] K. G. Roberts, Z. Gu, D. Payne-Turner et al., "High frequency and poor outcome of Philadelphia chromosome-like acute lymphoblastic leukemia in adults," *Journal of Clinical Oncology*, vol. 35, no. 4, pp. 394–401, 2017.

[6] National Library of Medicine (US), *Identifier NCT02420717, Ruxolitinib or Dasatinib with Chemotherapy in Patients with Philadelphia Chromosome (Ph)-Like Acute Lymphoblastic Leukemia (ALL)*, National Library of Medicine (US), Bethesda, MD, USA, 2000, https://clinicaltrials.gov/ct2/show/NCT02420717.

[7] N. Jain, K. G. Roberts, E. Jabbour et al., "Ph-like acute lymphoblastic leukemia: a high-risk subtype in adults," *Blood*, vol. 129, no. 5, pp. 572–581, 2017.

[8] S. L. Heatley, T. Sadras, C. H. Kok et al., "High prevalence of relapse in children with Philadelphia-like acute lymphoblastic leukemia despite risk-adapted treatment," *Haematologica*, vol. 102, no. 12, pp. e490–e493, 2017.

[9] M. Norkin, J. P. Uberti, and C. A. Schiffer, "Very late recurrences of leukemia: why does leukemia awake after many years of dormancy?," *Leukemia Research*, vol. 35, no. 2, pp. 139–144, 2011.

[10] R. Assi, H. Kantarjian, N. J. Short et al., "Safety and efficacy of Blinatumomab in combination with a tyrosine kinase inhibitor for the treatment of relapsed Philadelphia chromosome-positive leukemia," *Clinical Lymphoma Myeloma and Leukemia*, vol. 17, no. 12, pp. 897–901, 2017.

[11] H. Kantarjian, A. Stein, N. Gökbuget et al., "Blinatumomab versus chemotherapy for advanced acute lymphoblastic leukemia," *New England Journal of Medicine*, vol. 376, no. 9, pp. 836–847, 2017.

[12] H. M. Kantarjian, D. J. DeAngelo, M. Stelljes et al., "Inotuzumab ozogamicin versus standard therapy for acute lymphoblastic leukemia," *New England Journal of Medicine*, vol. 375, no. 8, pp. 740–753, 2016.

[13] M. Yilmaz, H. Kantarjian, D. Thomas et al., "Outcomes after Blinatumomab failure in patients with relapsed/refractory (R/R) B-cell ALL (ALL)," *Clinical Lymphoma, Myeloma and Leukemia*, vol. 16, pp. S12–S13, 2016.

23

Efficacy of Omalizumab in Indolent Systemic Mastocytosis

Calum Slapnicar,[1] **Martina Trinkaus**,[2] **Lisa Hicks**,[2] **and Peter Vadas**[1]

[1]*Division of Allergy and Clinical Immunology, St. Michael's Hospital, University of Toronto, Toronto, Ontario, Canada*
[2]*Division of Hematology, St. Michael's Hospital, University of Toronto, Toronto, Ontario, Canada*

Correspondence should be addressed to Peter Vadas; vadasp@smh.ca

Academic Editor: Stephen E. Langabeer

Background. Systemic mastocytosis (SM) comprises a heterogeneous group of disorders characterized by the proliferation of clonal mast cells in skin and various internal organs. Omalizumab is an established, labelled therapy for allergic asthma and chronic urticaria, but its experience in the efficacy of SM is limited. *Methods.* A retrospective analysis of 6 patients diagnosed with indolent SM treated with omalizumab at St. Michael's Hospital between 2009 and 2018 is described. Reported frequency of anaphylaxis, baseline and follow-up tryptase levels, and SM-related symptoms were captured to measure the control of the disease. *Results.* Of the 5 patients who had experienced unprovoked anaphylaxis prior to treatment with omalizumab, 3 had no further episodes of anaphylaxis following initiation of omalizumab, while the remaining 2 patients had milder multisystem reactions. Significant improvement in cutaneous symptoms was also observed. *Conclusion.* These data suggest that omalizumab provides benefit to patients with SM who remain highly symptomatic in spite of treatment with conventional therapies.

1. Background

Systemic mastocytosis (SM) comprises a heterogeneous group of disorders characterized by accumulation of clonal mast cells (MCs) in various internal organs, including the bone marrow (BM), spleen, liver, and gastrointestinal tract (GI) as well as the skin [1–3]. In 2016, the World Health Organization revised the major and minor diagnostic criteria for SM [1]. Binding of the kit ligand, stem cell factor (SCF), to the kit receptor is important for the normal development and function of MCs from their hematopoietic progenitors [4]. Most individuals with SM carry a mutation at codon 816, wherein aspartic acid is replaced by valine (D816V), resulting in ligand-independent autophosphorylation of the kit receptor [4, 5]. Constitutive activation of MCs results in secretion of multiple MC-derived mediators, including histamine and prostaglandin D2. Alpha tryptase is released constitutively from MC and reflects the total body MC burden, whereas beta tryptase is a marker of MC activation [6, 7]. In Canadian laboratories, reports of tryptase levels reflects the total of both alpha and beta tryptase. Circulating IgE or cytokines as well as extrinsic factors such as physical stimuli, heat, alcohol, insect stings, or infection can all induce MC activation and, potentially, anaphylaxis [8, 9].

Classification of SM can fall into one of the five major subvariants: (i) indolent SM (ISM, the most common and carrying the most favourable prognosis); (ii) smoldering SM (SSM); (iii) SM with an associated nonmast cell clonal hematological disease (SM-AHN); (iv) aggressive SM (ASM); and (v) MC leukemia (MCL) [1, 10, 11]. SM is a rare disease with an annual incidence of 5–10 new cases per million population [12, 13].

SM has no cure apart from hematopoietic stem cell transplant [14], and treatment algorithms focus for the most part on symptom control. Treatment ladders are used in highly symptomatic patients to capture control [15]. These include use of H1 and H2 antagonists, leukotriene modifiers, and mast cell stabilizers, such as ketotifen and sodium cromoglycate [15]. In patients with a suboptimal response, omalizumab, a monoclonal anti-IgE antibody, may be considered [16, 17]. This therapy was licensed for use in patients with severe asthma and chronic spontaneous urticaria. However, a number of studies [16, 17] suggest that omalizumab may provide additional benefit for patients with SM with recurrent anaphylaxis despite maximal mast cell blockade.

Herein, we describe the efficacy of omalizumab in 6 patients with indolent SM, who experienced recurrent anaphylaxis refractory to maximal medical therapy.

2. Methods

Data were collected retrospectively on patients diagnosed with ISM and treated with omalizumab at our institution between January 2009 and May 2018. This study was approved by the St. Michael's Hospital Research Ethics Board. Only those patients who fulfilled the World Health Organization (WHO) diagnostic criteria for ISM were included. All patients underwent bone marrow biopsies for diagnosis. Those diagnosed with a different SM subvariant were excluded. Tryptase levels, frequency of anaphylaxis, and other mastocytosis-related symptoms were collated to assess control of symptoms. Severity of anaphylaxis was graded according to Brown [18].

3. Results

3.1. Patient 1. A 28-year-old male developed urticaria pigmentosa confirmed by skin biopsy in 2008. The number of skin lesions had been gradually increasing over the course of 6 years. A bone marrow biopsy confirmed the presence of ISM with c-kit D816V mutation and serum tryptase of 134 ng/ml. He complained of nausea, palpitations, and presyncope, which recurred every 2–4 weeks [19]. More severe multisystem reactions occurred approximately twice per year, usually triggered by respiratory tract infections, resulting in itchy skin, flushing, nausea, lightheadedness, severe joint pain, and mild throat constriction with no loss of consciousness. Symptoms were poorly controlled in spite of sodium cromoglycate, ketotifen, and cetirizine. In late 2014, treatment with omalizumab 150 mg at 4-week intervals was started (Table 1). In early 2015, due to a suboptimal response to therapy, his omalizumab dosage was increased to 300 mg every four weeks. Four months later, tryptase levels had fallen from 134 ng/ml to 84 ng/ml (Table 1), with complete control of all symptoms by seven months. A trial of dose reduction of omalizumab back to 150 mg every 4 weeks resulted in a return of episodic flushing, nausea, bone pain, palpitations, and diarrhea as well as 2 anaphylactic reactions, both requiring hospitalization within a span of 6 weeks. Basal tryptase levels had increased to 100 ng/ml. Omalizumab dosage was increased to 300 mg at 2-week intervals and later maintained at 4-weeks intervals. By early 2017, he had experienced only one reported flare of symptoms with facial flushing, dizziness, and diarrhea. In April 2018, the patient reported his first anaphylactic reaction in nearly two years, 3 months after omalizumab injections had been discontinued. The number of skin lesions of urticaria pigmentosa was not controlled by omalizumab, and later, he required ultraviolet therapy with a good clinical response.

3.2. Patient 2. A 49-year-old woman was diagnosed with c-kit-positive ISM with tryptase 11.4 ng/ml (Table 1). Symptoms of SM included daily headaches, sporadic flushing, itchy throat, mild coughing, loose stools, lightheadedness, and palpitations. No cutaneous manifestations of mastocytosis were observed. She was markedly intolerant to exercise, heat, and strong emotion, all of which triggered the symptoms in spite of medications, which included ranitidine, loratadine, cetirizine, ketotifen, and montelukast. In early 2017, she experienced 5 anaphylactic reactions, requiring emergency department visits and treatment with epinephrine as well as 5 milder reactions managed at home (Table 1). Omalizumab was started at 300 mg at 4-week intervals (Table 1). On omalizumab, multisystem reactions were entirely suppressed, with only breakthrough flushing once per week, loose stools roughly twice per month, and occasional lightheadedness. A follow-up one year later revealed complete resolution of symptoms with no adverse reactions to her medications and reduced tryptase to 8.3 ng/ml (Table 1).

3.3. Patient 3. A 51-year-old female with c-kit-positive ISM and tryptase 31.8 ng/ml (Table 1) reported intermittent episodes of shortness of breath, chest tightness, abdominal pain, and diarrhea. She had generalized lesions of urticaria pigmentosa involving her entire body, although numerous on her lower extremities. Ketotifen and ranitidine failed to control the symptoms. Omalizumab injections were started at 300 mg every two weeks (Table 1). At follow-up, her shortness of breath and chest tightness were controlled and GI symptoms had improved. Furthermore, her urticaria pigmentosa had improved and was now only observed on the lower abdomen and upper thighs. After the fourth cycle of omalizumab, she experienced an immediate multisystem reaction with respiratory distress and tongue swelling. A fifth cycle was attempted but again resulted in a similar reaction, leading to discontinuation of omalizumab therapy. At follow-up, she reported a worsening respiratory and functional status as well as 3-4 loose bowel movements per day. Basal tryptase levels had increased up to 41.2 ng/ml (Table 1).

3.4. Patient 4. A 40-year-old female with c-kit-positive ISM had daily flushing, nausea, abdominal discomfort, and loose stools 3-4 times per day. She had cutaneous lesions of telangiectasia macularis eruptiva perstans and tryptase 55.2 ng/ml (Table 1). She complained of debilitating bone pain, episodic presyncope, shortness of breath, and frequent palpitations. Ongoing medications included cetirizine, ranitidine, ketotifen, and cromolyn. Treatment with omalizumab 300 mg every 4 weeks was started (Table 1). After 3 injections, bone pain and GI symptoms had subsided. After 6 cycles of omalizumab, cutaneous lesions had decreased in number, daily palpitations and syncopal episodes had subsided, and tryptase had increased to 61.7 ng/ml (Table 1). She was subsequently able to discontinue both ketotifen and cromolyn with ongoing treatment with omalizumab.

Table 1: Clinical characteristics and response to therapy of patients diagnosed with indolent systemic mastocytosis.

Patient #	Age	Gender	Disease duration	Optimal omalizumab dosage	Tryptase preomalizumab therapy	Tryptase during omalizumab therapy	Annualized frequency of anaphylaxis before treatment with omalizumab	Annualized frequency of anaphylaxis on optimal dose of omalizumab
1	38	M	10 years	150 mg·q. 4 weeks	134 ng/ml	84.1 ng/ml	2	2
2	51	F	3 years	300 mg·q. 4 weeks	11.4 ng/ml	8.3 ng/ml	60	0
3[1]	55	F	4 years	300 mg·q. 2 weeks	31.8 ng/ml	N/A	—	—
4	42	F	2 years	300 mg·q. 4 weeks	55.2 ng/ml	61.7 ng/ml	1	0
5	42	M	10 years	300 mg·q. 4 weeks	42.2 ng/ml	34 ng/ml	1	0
6	75	F	3 years	300 mg·q. 4 weeks	40.5 ng/ml	36.8 ng/ml	1	0

[1]This patient had poorly controlled manifestations of ISM but no history of anaphylaxis.

3.5. Patient 5. A 32-year-old male with lesions of urticaria pigmentosa was diagnosed with c-kit-positive ISM. During the summer of 2015, while working outside, he experienced 3 Hymenoptera stings resulting in immediate onset of flushing and presyncope (Table 1). In spite of administration of epinephrine, he developed nausea and vomiting, generalized hives, and worsening presyncope. He was resuscitated in an emergency department but continued to experience daily diarrhea, numbness, and tingling sensation in his extremities, night sweats, severe headaches, and flushing upon strenuous physical activity. Because the symptoms were refractory to a combination of cetirizine, ranitidine, montelukast, and cromolyn, he was started on omalizumab 300 mg at 4-week intervals (Table 1). A follow-up 8 months later revealed improved symptomatic control and a fall in tryptase from 42.2 to 34 ng/ml (Table 1). However, he has continued to experience intermittent itching, flushing, and diarrhea. A follow-up in late 2018 revealed that he had chosen to discontinue omalizumab, with continued control of disease.

3.6. Patient 6. A 72-year-old female was diagnosed with c-kit-positive ISM. She had no cutaneous manifestations of mastocytosis. Her initial presentation was that of Hymenoptera anaphylaxis, with flushing, palpitations, and loss of consciousness (Table 1). She was treated with cetirizine and ranitidine but continued to experience occasional facial flushing, vomiting, lightheadedness, drenching night sweats, and bone pain. Given her history of venom anaphylaxis, omalizumab was started at 300 mg every 4 weeks (Table 1) for 14 months followed by rush venom desensitization [20, 21]. Symptoms of her underlying ISM resolved completely on ongoing omalizumab therapy. Tryptase had also fallen from 40.5 to 36.8 ng/ml.

4. Discussion

The current treatment of indolent systemic mastocytosis focuses on symptom control and suppression of mast cell mediator release [1]. Newer targeted agents such as avapritinib and midostaurin are only available for treatment of symptomatic ISM via clinical trials or through limited compassionate access programs. Neither drug was available for the patients described in this report. In accordance with other reports [22–26], treatment with omalizumab was effective in suppressing symptoms in patients with ISM, including recurrent anaphylaxis and other mast-cell-related symptoms refractory to maximal pharmacotherapy.

A number of studies [16, 17] describe omalizumab as being the most effective in controlling frequency and severity of recurrent anaphylaxis in ISM. In one cohort, ten of twelve patients treated with omalizumab 300 mg at 4-week intervals had a good therapeutic response [16], whereas two of twelve patients were maintained on 150 mg at 2- and 4-week intervals. In keeping with these reports, our patients had optimal control of disease manifestations on a maintenance dose of 300 mg at 4-week intervals. One patient achieved complete control on this regimen and was subsequently tapered down to 150 mg every 4 weeks, leading to the return of unprovoked anaphylaxis, and daily symptoms attributed to uncontrolled disease.

Not only did patients experience a reduction in frequency and severity of anaphylaxis but also four of six patients had a decline in tryptase levels (134 ng/ml to 84.1 ng/ml; 11.4 ng/ml to 8.3 ng/ml; 42.2 ng/ml to 34 ng/ml; 40.5 ng/ml to 36.8 ng/ml). One patient had an increase (55.2 ng/ml to 61.7 ng/ml), and the patient who discontinued omalizumab due to an adverse reaction had an increase from baseline (31.8 ng/ml to 41.2 ng/ml). Chang et al. [27] present evidence that IgE binding to FcεRI, but without cross linking, will modulate the mast cell function. Specific effects include increased mast cell proliferation and survival and a reduction in the threshold of degranulation of mast cells with a corresponding increase in sensitivity to various allergens. Conversely, depletion of IgE by omalizumab will result in reduction of the ability of mast cells to degranulate, with a concomitant fall in mediator release.

Although the results of this study are encouraging, this study is a retrospective, single-center study with a small cohort of patients. Nonetheless, the results in this small group of patients with symptoms refractory to routine pharmacotherapy are promising and suggest that omalizumab should be considered in highly symptomatic patients with ISM. Future prospective studies of omalizumab or other potential therapies would benefit by use of methodologies such as ISM-specific quality-of-life questionnaire developed by van Anrooij et al. [28].

This case series describes the response to therapy in 6 patients with ISM treated with omalizumab. These data lend further support to the use of omalizumab in treatment of patients with clonal mast cell disorders, including mastocytosis and monoclonal mast cell activation syndrome [29], adding to the existing evidence in the literature, supporting the efficacy of omalizumab in highly symptomatic patients.

References

[1] P. Valent, C. Akin, and D. D. Metcalfe, "Mastocytosis: 2016 updated WHO classification and novel emerging treatment concepts," *Blood*, vol. 129, no. 11, pp. 1420–1427, 2017.

[2] A. Pardanani, "Systemic mastocytosis in adults: 2019 update on diagnosis, risk stratification and management," *American Journal of Hematology*, vol. 94, no. 3, pp. 363–377, 2019.

[3] M. Castells and J. Butterfield, "Mast cell activation syndrome and mastocytosis: initial treatment options and long-term management," *The Journal of Allergy and Clinical Immunology: In Practice*, vol. 7, no. 4, pp. 1097–1106, 2019.

[4] C. Akin, "Molecular diagnosis of mast cell disorders," *The Journal of Molecular Diagnostics*, vol. 8, no. 4, pp. 412–419, 2006.

[5] H. Nagata, A. S. Worobec, C. K. Oh et al., "Identification of a point mutation in the catalytic domain of the protooncogene c-kit in peripheral blood mononuclear cells of patients who have mastocytosis with an associated hematologic disorder," *Proceedings of the National Academy of Sciences*, vol. 92, no. 23, pp. 10560–10564, 1995.

[6] L. B. Schwartz and A.-M. A. Irani, "Serum tryptase and the laboratory diagnosis of systemic mastocytosis," *Hematology/Oncology Clinics of North America*, vol. 14, no. 3, pp. 641–657, 2000.

[7] P. Valent, W. R. Sperr, K. Sotlar et al., "The serum tryptase test: an emerging robust biomarker in clinical hematology," *Expert Review of Hematology*, vol. 7, no. 5, pp. 683–690, 2014.

[8] A. Matito, J. M. Morgado, P. Sánchez-López et al., "Management of anesthesia in adult and pediatric mastocytosis: a study of the Spanish network on mastocytosis (REMA) based on 726 anesthetic procedures," *International Archives of Allergy and Immunology*, vol. 167, no. 1, pp. 47–56, 2015.

[9] T. Gülen, C. Ljung, G. Nilsson, and C. Akin, "Risk factor analysis of anaphylactic reactions in patients with systemic mastocytosis," *The Journal of Allergy and Clinical Immunology: In Practice*, vol. 5, no. 5, pp. 1248–1255, 2017.

[10] H.-P. Horny, K. Sotlar, and P. Valent, "Mastocytosis: state of the art," *Pathobiology*, vol. 74, no. 2, pp. 121–132, 2007.

[11] P. Valent, C. Akin, L. Escribano et al., "Standards and standardization in mastocytosis: consensus statements on diagnostics, treatment recommendations and response criteria," *European Journal of Clinical Investigation*, vol. 37, no. 6, pp. 435–453, 2007.

[12] S. S. Cohen, S. Skovbo, H. Vestergaard et al., "Epidemiology of systemic mastocytosis in Denmark," *British Journal of Haematology*, vol. 166, no. 4, pp. 521–528, 2014.

[13] J. J. van Doormal, S. Arends, K. L. Brunekreeft et al., "Prevalence of indolent systemic mastocytosis in a Dutch region," *The Journal of Allergy and Clinical Immunology*, vol. 131, pp. 1429–1431, 2013.

[14] P. Valent, W. R. Sperr, and C. Akin, "How I treat patients with advanced systemic mastocytosis," *Blood*, vol. 116, no. 26, pp. 5812–5817, 2010.

[15] F. Siebenhaar, C. Akin, C. Bindslev-Jensen, M. Maurer, and S. Broesby-Olsen, "Treatment strategies in mastocytosis," *Immunology and Allergy Clinics of North America*, vol. 34, no. 2, pp. 433–447, 2014.

[16] S. Broesby-Olsen, H. Vestergaard, C. G. Mortz et al., "Omalizumab prevents anaphylaxis and improves symptoms in systemic mastocytosis: efficacy and safety observations," *Allergy*, vol. 73, no. 1, pp. 230–238, 2018.

[17] R. Lemal, G. Fouquet, L. Terriou et al., "Omalizumab therapy for mast cell-mediator symptoms in patients with ISM, CM, MMAS, and MCAS," *The Journal of Allergy and Clinical Immunology: In Practice*, vol. 7, no. 7, pp. 2387–2395.e3, 2019.

[18] S. G. A. Brown, "Clinical features and severity grading of anaphylaxis," *Journal of Allergy and Clinical Immunology*, vol. 114, no. 2, pp. 371–376, 2004.

[19] C. A. Slapnicar, C. S. Smeenk, L. Hicks, M. Trinkaus, and P. Vadas, "Omalizumab and systemic mastocytosis: a single centre case series," *Journal of Allergy and Clinical Immunology*, vol. 143, no. 2, Article ID AB182, 2019.

[20] İ. Yılmaz, S. N. Bahçecioğlu, and M. Türk, "Combination of omalizumab and bee venom immunotherapy: does it work?," *Asia Pacific Allergy*, vol. 8, no. 1, 2018.

[21] C. Galera, N. Soohun, N. Zankar, S. Caimmi, C. Gallen, and P. Demoly, "Severe anaphylaxis to bee venom immunotherapy: efficacy of pretreatment and concurrent treatment with omalizumab," *Journal of Investigational Allergology & Clinical Immunology*, vol. 19, no. 3, pp. 225–229, 2009.

[22] G. J. Molderings, M. Raithel, F. Kratz et al., "Omalizumab treatment of systemic mast cell activation disease: experiences from four cases," *Internal Medicine*, vol. 50, no. 6, pp. 611–615, 2011.

[23] T. J. Pitt, N. Cisneros, C. Kalicinsky, and A. B. Becker, "Successful treatment of idiopathic anaphylaxis in an adolescent," *Journal of Allergy and Clinical Immunology*, vol. 126, no. 2, pp. 415-416, 2010.

[24] M. C. Carter, J. A. Robyn, P. B. Bressler, J. C. Walker, G. G. Shapiro, and D. D. Metcalfe, "Omalizumab for the treatment of unprovoked anaphylaxis in patients with systemic mastocytosis," *Journal of Allergy and Clinical Immunology*, vol. 119, no. 6, pp. 1550-1551, 2007.

[25] L. Kibsgaard, T. Skjold, M. Deleuran, and C. Vestergaard, "Omalizumab induced remission of idiopathic anaphylaxis in a patient suffering from indolent systemic mastocytosis," *Acta Dermato Venereologica*, vol. 94, no. 3, pp. 363-364, 2014.

[26] P. Jandus, O. Hausmann, G. Haeberli, T. Gentinetta, U. Mueller, and A. Helbling, "Unpredicted adverse reaction to omalizumab," *Journal of Investigational Allergology & Clinical Immunology*, vol. 21, no. 7, pp. 563–566, 2011.

[27] T. W. Chang, C. Chen, C.-J. Lin, M. Metz, M. K. Church, and M. Maurer, "The potential pharmacologic mechanisms of omalizumab in patients with chronic spontaneous urticaria," *Journal of Allergy and Clinical Immunology*, vol. 135, no. 2, pp. 337–342, 2015.

[28] B. van Anrooij, J. C. Kluin-Nelemans, M. Safy, B. M. J. Flokstra-de Blok, and J. N. G. Oude Elberink, "Patient-reported disease-specific quality-of-life and symptom severity in systemic mastocytosis," *Allergy*, vol. 71, no. 11, pp. 1585–1593, 2016.

[29] A. Jagdis and P. Vadas, "Omalizumab effectively prevents recurrent refractory anaphylaxis in a patient with monoclonal mast cell activation syndrome," *Annals of Allergy, Asthma & Immunology*, vol. 113, no. 1, pp. 115-116, 2014.

24

Reactivation of *Coccidioides immitis* in a Prosthetic Knee after Initiation of Chemotherapy

Zachary Ciochetto,[1,2] Maria Georgen,[1,2] Adam Hadro,[1,2] Lauren Jurkowski,[1,2] Kimberly Ridolfi,[2] Adam Wooldridge,[1,2] Nathan Gundacker,[1,2] and Javeria Haque[1,2]

[1]*Medical College of Wisconsin Affiliated Hospitals, Milwaukee, WI, USA*
[2]*Zablocki VA Medical Center, Milwaukee, WI, USA*

Correspondence should be addressed to Zachary Ciochetto; zciochetto@mcw.edu and Javeria Haque; jhaque@mcw.edu

Academic Editor: Kostas Konstantopoulos

Coccidioides is an endemic fungus in the Southwestern United States and Central and South America. Coccidioidomycosis primary infections are typically of the lung with an asymptomatic or self-limiting course. Some infections disseminate to other parts of the body and a few can remain latent for many years. Reactivation of latent fungal disease can occur following an insult to the host immune system. Here, we describe a case of a 76-year-old Caucasian male patient who moved from California to Wisconsin with a history of coccidioidomycosis infection of the left knee that reactivated decades later in his prosthetic knee shortly after being initiated on ibrutinib (Imbruvica), a Bruton tyrosine kinase (BTK) inhibitor, for chronic lymphocytic leukemia (CLL)/small lymphocytic lymphoma (SLL). There have been some case reports regarding coccidioidomycosis infections after initiating ibrutinib therapy but none with a 50 year latency period before reactivation. Readers will learn the immunological effects of ibrutinib on the hosts' innate and adaptive immunity and its role in putting the host at risk for invasive fungal infections. We also review the literature and data on treatment regimens and recommendations based on current guidelines.

1. Introduction

Coccidioidomycosis, also known as Valley Fever, is an uncommon infection in the upper Midwest as it is endemic to the southwestern United States and Central and South America. Infections are generally acquired from inhalation of arthroconidia, the spores of the dimorphic organism *Coccidioides immitis,* whereas those acquired elsewhere are from *Coccidioides posadasii.* This fungus causes asymptomatic or mild infections in most patients with some developing acute or subacute pulmonary infections 1–3 weeks after inoculation. An estimated 5–10% of patients develop residual pulmonary disease consisting of nodules or cavitary lesions and about 1% develop disseminated disease. Extrapulmonary sites typically involve the skin and skeletal system [1].

Disruption in the innate immunity with reduced activation of neutrophils by cytokines and INF-γ, as well as poor T-cell response and function, can lead to disseminated fungal infections [2]. Patients with CLL/SLL develop a secondary immunodeficiency through lymphocyte dysfunction that is further compounded by immunomodulating treatment therapies, such as ibrutinib, a BTK inhibitor. BTK is important in B-cell receptor signaling maturation and activation. It also has been observed in the pathways activating innate and adaptive immunities with key targets being neutrophils, macrophages, and monocytes. Through BTK inhibition, ibrutinib dysregulates downstream T-cell signaling and maturation, thus leading to ineffective Th2 effector cells, predisposing hosts to invasive fungal infections (IFIs) such as invasive aspergillosis, cryptococcus, and Pneumocystis jiroveci pneumonia (PJP) [3], and as in our case, coccidioidomycosis.

Herein, we present a report of a patient with reactivation of *Coccidioides immitis* knee prosthetic joint infection (PJI)

three months after initiation of ibrutinib for CLL/SLL after a 50-year latency period. There are only a few case reports [4, 5] regarding reactivation of articular infection; however, none are described with such a prolonged latency period. We further present relevant literature available thus far on the topic and discuss immunologic mechanisms that may be involved in the fungal pathogenesis in such patients.

2. Case Presentation

A 75-year-old male with history of CLL/SLL presented to the emergency department (ED) with complaints of left knee pain and swelling for one week. Patient had undergone left total knee arthroplasty (TKA) for osteoarthritis twelve years prior without post-operative complications. Three months prior to presentation, he was started on ibrutinib for his CLL/SLL due to worsening anemia, leukocytosis, and lymphadenopathy. In the ED, his physical exam was notable for a left knee effusion with tenderness and limited range of motion. His effusion was aspirated, and synovial fluid analysis revealed a total WBC count of 6,404 cells/mm^3 with 53% monocytes, 29% neutrophils, and 19% lymphocytes. On presentation, his WBC was 7.4×10^9/L (normal 4–12$\times10^9$/L), with 57% lymphocytes and 30% neutrophils, with a hemoglobin of 9.6 g/dl (normal male 13.5–17.5 g/dL) and platelet count of 131×10^9/L (normal 150–450$\times10^9$/L). His erythrocyte sedimentation rate (ESR) and c-reactive protein (CRP) were both elevated at 74 mm/h (normal male 0–20 mm/hr) and 76.9 mg/L (normal male <10 mg/L), respectively. He was started on intravenous (IV) vancomycin and cefepime and his ibrutinib was held.

The next day he underwent left knee incision and drainage with synovectomy and exchange of his tibial polyethylene component with orthopedic surgery with intraoperative specimens sent off for Gram stain and cultures. Forty-eight hours post-operative fungal stains turned positive for mold, and he was started on IV liposomal amphotericin B 5 mg/kg daily and antibiotics were discontinued.

Patient reported he was originally born in Southern California and lived there for 25 years. In his early 20's, he had acute onset of left knee pain and swelling, underwent left knee aspiration, and was told he had "Valley Fever" in his knee. Records from 1970s were not available; however, as per the patient, he was given 2 intra-articular injections followed by one year of antifungal treatment with complete resolution of his symptoms. He reported no problems with his knee until 2008 when he underwent left TKA for osteoarthritis. A CT scan of his chest four months prior to presentation for his CLL workup was noted to have a calcified granuloma in his left lower lobe suggestive of possible previous coccidioidomycosis inoculation.

After 12 days of incubation, the cultures were visualized in the lab (Figures 1 and 2) and confirmed to be *Coccidioides immitis*. He underwent explantation of his left total knee arthroplasty with extensive synovectomy and conversion to a rigid spacer. He was switched to oral fluconazole 400 mg daily on post-operative day one after receiving 12 days of IV liposomal amphotericin B. Coccidioides complement fixation came back positive at 1:16 (normal <1:2) and patient was discharged on hospital day 15 with his ibrutinib on hold.

Six months later his left knee was re-aspirated which demonstrated no fungal growth and his ESR and CRP had also normalized. He then underwent second-stage revision of his left knee with reimplantation of hardware without complications. He is currently following the expected post-operative course and will be continued on lifelong suppressive fluconazole therapy.

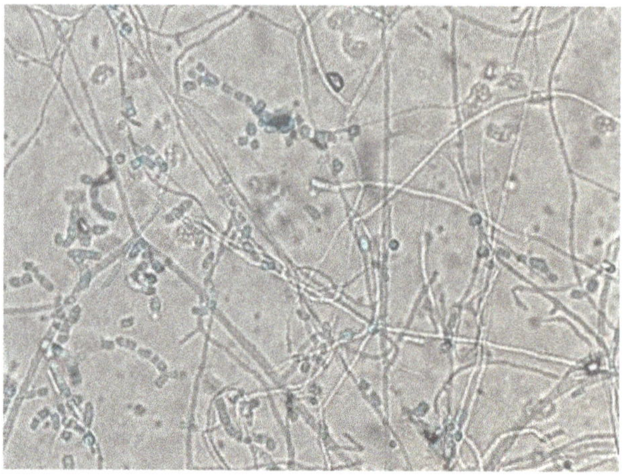

FIGURE 1: *Coccidioides immitis* under 10x magnification.

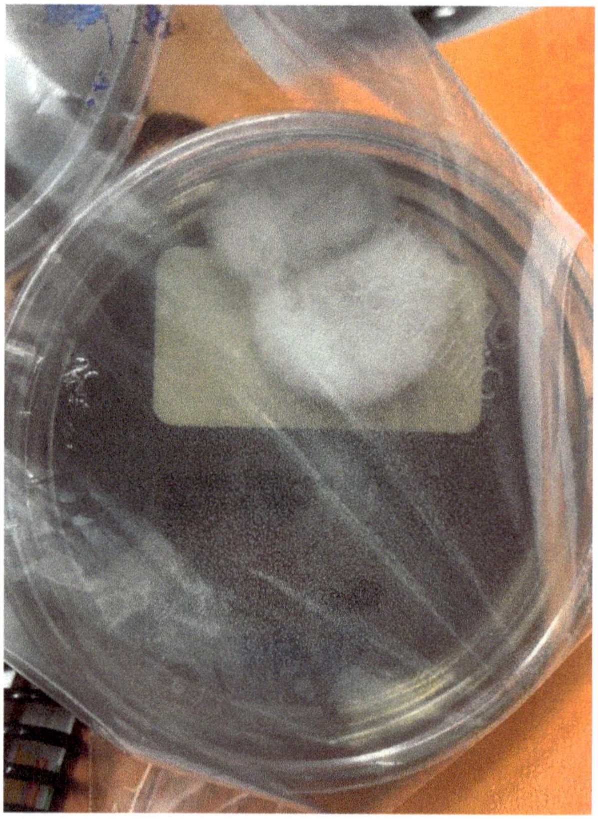

FIGURE 2: *Coccidioides immitis* gross visualization on culture media plates.

Table 1: Reported coccidioidomycosis native and prosthetic joint infections and their treatments.

Source	Case	Site of infection	Native vs. prosthetic	Type of surgery	Treatment course	Treatment response
Taxy et al. [6]		Ankle	Native	None	Oral fluconazole × 14 months	Successful
Ellerbrook et al. [7]		Knee	Native	Debridement	Oral fluconazole 600 mg/d indefinitely	Successful
Weisenberg [8]		Knee	Native	Debridement, extensive synovectomy, and meniscectomy	Oral flucaonazole 800 mg/d × 5 months and then itraconazole 200 mg/d indefinitely	Successful
Arbeloa-Gutierrez et al. [4]		Knee	Prosthetic	Prosthesis removal with amphotericin spacer and knee fusion	Oral itraconazole indefinitely	Successful
Austen et al. [9]		Knee	Prosthetic	None	Oral fluconazole 800 mg/d × 4 months and then 400 mg/d indefinitely	Successful
Kuberski et al. [5]	1	Knee	Prosthetic	Debridement, prosthesis removal, and knee fusion	Oral fluconazole 200 mg BID indefinitely	Successful
	2	Knee	Native	Synovectomy and total knee replacement	IV amphotericin (total 1000 mg) and then oral fluconazole 200 mg BID indefinitely	Successful
	3	Knee	Native	None	IV amphotericin (total 1000 mg) and then oral fluconazole 400 mg/d indefinitely	Unsuccessful
	4	Bilateral knees and ankles	Native	Right knee debridement	IV amphotericin (total 920 mg) and then oral itraconazole indefinitely	Unsuccessful
	5	Hip	Prosthetic	None	Oral fluconazole 800 mg/d indefinitely	Successful
	6	Knee	Native	Synovectomy and total knee replacement	Oral fluconazole 400 mg/d indefinitely	Unknown
Nasrawi et al. [10]		Wrist, knee, and ankle	Native	None	IV amphotericin × 12 weeks and then isavuconazonium indefinitely	Unknown

3. Discussion

We present this case of reactivation of a latent *Coccidioides immitis* infection in a prosthetic knee 3 months after starting ibrutinib therapy for CLL/SLL in a patient who was previously treated for native knee infection 50 years ago. Host cell-mediated and adaptive immunity are required to prevent disseminated infections with *Coccidioides immitis.* Our patient experienced a two-fold disruption in these pathways with his underlying CLL/SLL, as well as with treatment with ibrutinib, predisposing him to reactivation of latent coccidioidomycosis infection in his prosthetic joint.

There have been few reports of coccidioidomycosis reactivation in the literature (Table 1), but none with a prolonged indolence of 50 years as seen in this patient. A similar scenario was described when a patient from an endemic coccidioidomycosis region moved to Spain and 30 years later underwent TKA. Then, seven years after her surgery, she had coccidioidomycosis reactivation which was treated with fluconazole suppression alone [4]. Another case series reviewed 6 cases of coccidioidomycosis infections in prosthetic joints and described their treatment regimens which included delayed two-stage arthroplasty followed by azole therapy or azole suppression alone. Two of the patients' azole therapy was stopped after 1 year and relapsed shortly after discontinuation [4]. Another unique factor in our patient's case was quick reactivation of his PJI after starting ibrutinib therapy for his CLL/SLL. Ibrutinib is a BTK inhibitor which affects neutrophil maturation and activation through inhibiting key signal cascades which directly interferes with the innate defense against fungal infections [11]. One study looked at 378 patients in which ibrutinib was used to treat leukemia where they observed 37% of patients developed an invasive fungal infection (IFI). None of these patients had the classic risk factors for IFIs which include neutropenia, lymphopenia, or high-dose corticosteroid use. Patients were at highest risk of reactivation in the first 6 months with a mean of 4.5 months. Infection rates were higher in those receiving combined corticosteroids and chemotherapy. The first infections described were invasive aspergillosis and cryptococcal meningoencephalitis followed by mucormycosis, primary central nervous system lymphoma, PJP, and even disseminated coccidioidomycosis infection [12]. It was observed that disrupting the TH2 pathway and INF-y production led to poor host fungal defense predisposing patients to IFIs.

Maintenance therapy for coccidioidomycosis infections primarily consists of the azole class of drugs that inhibits the CYP3A4 enzyme which can cause ibrutinib toxicity [11]. Under-dosing of these medications can lead to poorly controlled malignancy and high risk of infection relapse while overdosing can lead to systemic toxicities. The Infectious Disease Society of America (IDSA) recommends azole therapy for bone and joint coccidioidomycosis infections unless there is severe osseous disease or life-threatening infection, in which case amphotericin B should be utilized. Patients on biological modifiers with active coccidioidomycosis infections should be treated with azole therapy unless severe pneumonia, meningitis, or soft tissue and osseous dissemination is present, in which case liposomal amphotericin B again is recommended [12]. There are no current recommendations on which azole to use, but itraconazole is favored over fluconazole for skeletal infections, with some studies evaluating voriconazole and posaconazole use. One clinical trial involving 198 patients with various coccidioidomycosis infections involving skin, lung, and bone disease compared fluconazole versus itraconazole and found that, after 12 months, 57% responded to fluconazole at 400 mg per day and 72% of those on itraconazole 200 mg twice a day. There was no statistical superior efficacy of either treatment, but itraconazole was favored by those involved in the study [13].

Current literature suggests lifelong azole therapy, if possible, given the high risk of relapse seen in patients who stopped their azole treatment, especially in patients with a periprosthetic joint infection [5, 14]. Serial coccidioides complement fixation is a useful tool for monitoring therapeutic response [1]. Timing and utility of one versus two-stage revision surgeries is unknown, especially in the context of lifelong suppression. It is also unclear when resumption of chemotherapeutics is safe, especially given the interaction with azoles. Our patient underwent second stage of his revision 6 months after initial explant and his ibrutinib is still on hold as his CLL/SLL is stable.

In summary, this case highlights the importance of clinical history taking especially regarding infections prior to initiation of chemotherapeutics. *Coccidioides immitis* can have an extraordinary long latency period requiring clinicians to be cognizant of a patient's historical geography and raises the question for secondary prophylaxis in high-risk patients. An urgency exists for further data related to infections, specifically fungal, seen with ibrutinib.

Consent

Written informed consent was obtained from the patients for publication of this case report and any accompanying images. A copy of the written consent is available for review by the Editor of this journal.

Authors' Contributions

ZC put together the manuscript with the help of MG. ZC took the real time pictures of Figures 1–4. LJ put together Table 1 with some additions to the discussion. AH and JW added details regarding orthopedic interventions and hospital course. NG, JH, and KR were key contributors in overseeing, editing, and adding to the manuscript.

References

[1] J. N. Galgiani, N. M. Ampel, J. E. Blair et al., "Coccidioidomycosis," *Clinical Infectious Diseases*, vol. 41, no. 9, pp. 1217–1223, 2005.

[2] T. N. Kirkland and J. Fierer, "Coccidioides immitis and posadasii; a review of their biology, genomics, pathogenesis, and host immunity," *Virulence*, vol. 9, no. 1, pp. 1426–1435, 2018.

[3] L. Pagano, D. Facchinelli, G. Nadali, and L. Pagano, "Invasive fungal infections in patients with chronic lymphoproliferative disorders in the era of target drugs," *Mediterranean Journal of Hematology and Infectious Diseases*, vol. 10, no. 1, Article ID e2018063, 2018.

[4] L. Arbeloa-Gutierrez, T. Kuberski, S. M. Johnson, I. Sagastibelza, J. I. Alaez, and D. Pappagianis, "Reactivation of coccidioidomycosis: a prosthetic joint infection in Spain," *European Journal of Clinical Microbiology & Infectious Diseases*, vol. 35, no. 2, pp. 183–186, 2016.

[5] T. Kuberski, V. Ianas, T. Ferguson, J. Nomura, and R. Johnson, "Treatment of prosthetic joint infections associated with coccidioidomycosis," *Infectious Diseases in Clinical Practice*, vol. 19, no. 4, pp. 252–255, 2011.

[6] J. B. Taxy and S. Kodros, "Musculoskeletal coccidioidomycosis," *American Journal of Clinical Pathology*, vol. 124, no. 5, pp. 693–696, 2005.

[7] L. Ellerbrook and S. Laks, "Coccidioidomycosis osteomyelitis of the knee in a 23-year-old diabetic patient," *Radiology Case Reports*, vol. 10, no. 1, Article ID 1034, 2015.

[8] S. A. Weisenberg, "Coccidioides immitis septic knee arthritis," *BMJ Case Reports*, vol. 2018, Article ID bcr2017222585, 2018.

[9] S. Austen, W. van der Weegen, C. M. Verduin, M. van der Valk, and H. J. Hoekstra, "Coccidioidomycosis infection of a total knee arthroplasty in a nonendemic region," *The Journal of Arthroplasty*, vol. 28, no. 2, pp. 375.e13–375.e15, 2013.

[10] F. Nasrawi, A. Heidari, T. Aljashamy et al., "Disseminated coccidioidomycosis presenting as polyarticular septic arthritis: a case report," *Journal of investigative medicine high impact case reports*, vol. 8, pp. 2324709620974894–2324709620974898, 2020.

[11] R. Maffei, M. Maccaferri, L. Arletti et al., "Immunomodulatory effect of ibrutinib: reducing the barrier against fungal infections," *Blood Reviews*, vol. 40, Article ID 100635, 2020.

[12] J. N. Galgiani, N. M. Ampel, J. E. Blair et al., "2016 infectious diseases society of America (IDSA) clinical practice guideline for the treatment of coccidioidomycosis," *Clinical Infectious Diseases*, vol. 63, no. 6, pp. e112–e146, 2016.

[13] J. N. Galgiani, A. Catanzaro, G. A. Cloud et al., "Comparison of oral fluconazole and itraconazole for progressive, non-meningeal coccidioidomycosis," *Annals of Internal Medicine*, vol. 133, no. 9, pp. 676–686, 2000.

[14] A. Catanzaro, J. N. Galgiani, B. E. Levine et al., "Fluconazole in the treatment of chronic pulmonary and nonmeningeal disseminated coccidioidomycosis," *The American Journal of Medicine*, vol. 98, no. 3, pp. 249–256, 1995.

25

Acute Myeloid Leukemia in an Infant with t(8;19 (p11.2;q13) Translocation: Case Report and a Review of the Literature

Ashley C. Eason,[1] Silvia T. Bunting,[2] Jess F. Peterson,[3] Debra Saxe,[4] and Himalee S. Sabnis[1]

[1]*Department of Pediatrics, Aflac Cancer and Blood Disorders Center, Children's Healthcare of Atlanta and Emory University, Atlanta, GA, USA*
[2]*Department of Pathology, Children's Healthcare of Atlanta, Atlanta, GA, USA*
[3]*Department of Laboratory Medicine and Pathology, Mayo Clinic, Rochester, MN, USA*
[4]*Department of Pathology and Laboratory Medicine, Emory University, Atlanta, GA, USA*

Correspondence should be addressed to Himalee S. Sabnis; hsabnis@emory.edu

Academic Editor: Håkon Reikvam

Acute myeloid leukemia (AML) patients with t(8;16)(p11.2;p13) constitute a small subgroup with a distinct genetic and clinical profile. We present a unique case of a female infant with monocytic AML associated with t(8;19)(p11.2;q13.3), a rarely reported variation of t(8;16)(p11.2;p13). The patient presented with leukemia cutis and demonstrated erythrophagocytosis in the diagnostic bone marrow. She responded well to standard AML chemotherapy and is currently in remission. Here, we highlight her case as the youngest AML patient with t(8;19) described in the literature, discuss the significance and prognostic implications of this genetic variant, and review 8p11.2 fusion proteins in AML.

1. Introduction

In acute myeloid leukemia (AML), genetic mutations are often associated with specific disease subtypes which have biologic and prognostic implications [1]. While AML continues to be a predominantly adult disease, it is the second most common acute leukemia in children and is associated with high morbidity and mortality. Among the cytogenetic abnormalities seen in AML, translocation between 8p11.2 and 16p13 is a rare gene rearrangement seen in <1% of adult and pediatric patients [2–4]. It results in fusion of *KAT6A* (lysine acetyltransferase 6A) with *CREBBP* (CREB-binding protein), and the gene expression profile of these leukemias resembles that of AML with MLL (mixed lineage leukemia) gene rearrangement [5]. Additionally, it is characterized by a monocytic phenotype, leukemia cutis at presentation, histologic evidence of erythro/hemophagocytosis and spontaneous remission, specifically in congenital cases [3, 4, 6, 7]. Aside from transient myelopoiesis associated with Down's syndrome, this is the only described self-limited neonatal leukemia [3]. However, in adults, t(8;16)(p11.2;p13) AML has been shown to have a poor prognosis, which may be related to the increased frequency of this translocation with therapy-related AML [4].

AML associated with t(8;19)(p11.2;q13) is an extremely rare variant of 8p11.2-rearranged acute leukemias. Although infrequently reported in the literature, it is believed to behave similarly to t(8;16)(p11.2;p13) AML [7–10]. We report a case of a 3-month-old female infant presenting with skin nodules, who upon further evaluation was confirmed to have leukemia cutis and a diagnosis of AML with myelomonocytic differentiation. Cytogenetic evaluation demonstrated t(8;19)(p11.2;q13). This rare translocation has been previously described in only four patients in the literature. Here, we highlight the youngest reported case of t(8;19)(p11.2;q13) AML and review the disease characteristics and clinical outcomes associated with 8p11.2-rearranged leukemias.

2. Case Description

A 3-month-old Caucasian female presented to her pediatrician with a spreading erythematous maculopapular rash with bluish raised lesions, most prominent over her back and scalp. Her first skin lesion was noted shortly after she received vaccinations at 2 months of age. A skin biopsy was notable for a monocytic infiltrative process consistent with leukemia cutis (Figures 1(a)–1(c)). She was subsequently referred to pediatric oncology for further evaluation and treatment. Her initial complete blood count showed a normal leukocyte count ($14.63 \times 10^3/\mu L$) with a normal differential, hemoglobin (11.1 g/dL) and platelet count ($281 \times 10^3/\mu L$). Flow cytometry of the bone marrow aspirate revealed a distinct population of cells totaling 26% of the sample, expressing bright CD4, CD11c, dim CD13, CD15, CD16, and CD33, CD36, CD38, CD58, CD123, HLA-DR, myeloperoxidase (MPO), dim terminal deoxynucleotidyl transferase (TdT), and moderate CD45. These findings confirmed the diagnosis of AML with monocytic differentiation (French-American-British (FAB) M4). Striking erythrophagocytosis was noted in the bone marrow biopsy (Figure 1(d)). Chromosome analysis showed translocation between the short arm of chromosome 8 and the long arm of chromosome 19 with resulting karyotype t(8;19)(p11.2;q13) (Figure 1(e)). Fluorescence *in situ* hybridization (FISH) was performed on a bone marrow aspirate smear using a *KAT6A* break-apart probe set (CytoTest Inc., Rockville, MD), confirming a *KAT6A* rearrangement in metaphases (seen in 50% of 200 interphase nuclei analyzed) (Figure 1(f)).

The patient was treated per our institutional standard of care for AML patients. She received induction therapy with ADE which included cytarabine 3.3 mg/kg every 12 hours for days 1–10, daunorubicin 1.7 mg/kg for three doses on days 1, 3, and 5, and etoposide 3.3 mg/kg daily for days 1–5. She had no evidence of minimal residual disease (MRD), defined as <0.1% disease in bone marrow by flow cytometry, at the end of induction. Her subsequent chemotherapy included three more cycles of chemotherapy: Induction II with cytarabine 33 mg/kg every 12 hours on days 1–4 and mitoxantrone 0.4 mg/kg daily on days 3–6, Intensification I with cytarabine 33 mg/kg every 12 hours on days 1–5 and etoposide 85 mg/kg daily on days 1–5, and Intensification II with cytarabine 100 mg/kg every 12 hours on days 1-2 and 8-9 and Erwinia asparaginase 830 units/kg on days 2 and 9. Per institutional standard, she remained hospitalized following chemotherapy through count recovery. She tolerated each course of chemotherapy well with minimal toxicity and continues to remain in remission now two years from initial diagnosis.

3. Discussion

Cytogenetic abnormalities play a prominent role in risk stratification of AML, with t(8;16)(p11.2;p13)-associated AML demonstrating a unique phenotype [4]. This translocation creates a fusion of *KAT6A* (previously *MOZ* or *MYST3*) gene on chromosome 8 with the *CREBBP* gene on chromosome 16 [4]. Both *KAT6A* and *CREBBP* modulate gene transcription and induce hematopoietic cell transformation [11]. In adults, this rare translocation has been noted with increased frequency in patients with therapy-related AML compared to patients with *de novo* AML [4, 12]. Most patients with t(8;16) AML demonstrated M4/M5 FAB subtype, erythrophagocytosis, and a gene signature similar to *MLL* (*KMT2A*)-rearranged leukemias. Median overall survival in two large cohorts was poor (4.7–8.5 months), which may be related to the high number of therapy-related AML cases most often seen following treatment for solid tumors in these groups [4, 12]. In addition, the majority of patients in these cohorts were adults with only two pediatric cases reported [4, 12]. Interestingly, both were infants less than 6 months of age [12].

Similar to adults, pediatric AML with t(8;16)(p11.2;p13) has been characterized as a distinct subgroup commonly associated with leukemia cutis and hemophagocytosis at diagnosis. In the largest pediatric evaluation of this translocation to date, the International Berlin-Frankfurt-Munster (I-BFM) AML study group reviewed 62 patients with t(8;16)(p11.2;p13) and compared them with a pediatric AML reference cohort [3]. Nearly all patients had *de novo* disease (60/62) and presented with M4/M5 FAB AML (97% compared to only 41% in the reference group). Leukemia cutis occurred more commonly in infants and with higher frequency (58% versus 8%) as compared to other AML patients. Selective activation of HOXA (homeobox A cluster) genes without activation of HOXB (homeobox B cluster) genes was noted in gene expression profiling, similar to *KMT2A*-rearranged AML. Disseminated intravascular coagulation (DIC) at presentation was noted in 15/38 of the t(8;16)(p11.2;p13) patients at diagnosis. A substantial subgroup of patients (17/62) was diagnosed in the first month of life which was significantly higher than the reference cohort. Seven of these seventeen infants were initially untreated and noted to have a spontaneous remission. Four patients subsequently developed recurrence requiring treatment; however, 5/7 patients were alive at last follow-up. Five-year overall survival rate for the entire cohort was 59% (±9%) similar to the rate for the reference group (62% ± 2%).

While t(8;16)(p11.2;p13)-associated AML is described in several studies, AML involving t(8;19)(p11.2;q13) has been rarely reported and is considered a subgroup of the t(8;16) subtype. In 1988, Brizard et al. first noted the t(8;19)(p11.2;q13) variant in an 8-month-old infant with M5 AML and marked erythrophagocytosis [8]. The infant achieved remission following standard chemotherapy, but later died due to veno-occlusive disease following hematopoietic stem cell transplantation. Since then, three other patients have been reported (Table 1) [7, 9, 10]. To the best of our knowledge, this is the youngest patient to be described in the literature harboring this translocation. Most of these patients (3/5) were males and had *de novo* AML (4/5). Other coexisting cytogenetic mutations were rare (1/5), suggesting this is likely an initiating event in leukemogenesis. All patients with *de novo* disease had a favorable response to standard chemotherapy alone, and only one patient underwent stem cell transplantation. The one patient with therapy-related AML did not respond to initial chemotherapy and died shortly after.

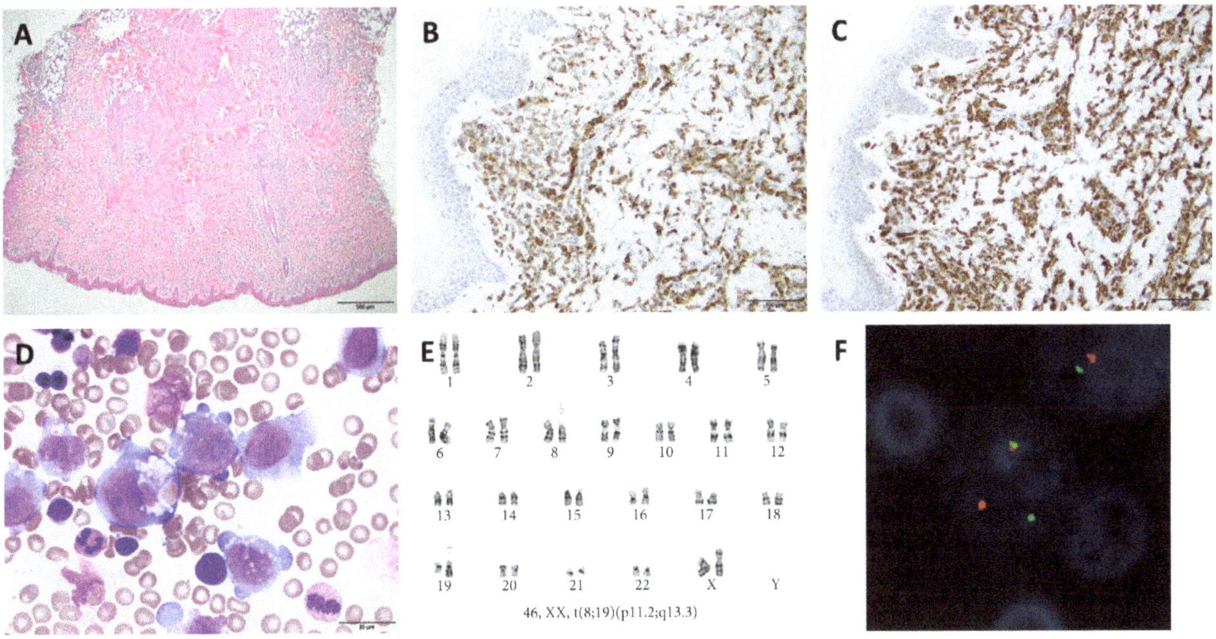

FIGURE 1: Histopathology and cytogenetic features of the case. (a) Skin biopsy shows diffuse infiltrates in the dermis and subcutis, concentrated around the vessels and appendages. (b and c) Cells are positive for CD68 and myeloperoxidase, respectively. (d) Blasts show evidence of erythrophagocytosis. (e) Patient karyotype demonstrating t(8;19) (p11.2;q13.3). (f) Representative interphase cell demonstrating a *KAT6A* rearrangement by fluorescence *in situ* hybridization.

TABLE 1: Summary of t(8;19)(p11.2;q13) cases in the literature.

Age/sex	Disease	FAB	Karyotype	AML treatment	Outcome	Reference (year)
8 months/M	*De novo*	M5	46,XY,t(8;19)(p11.2;q13.2)[8]/46,XY,t(8;19),−1,+1q+[22]/46,XY,t(8;19),−16,+16q+[6]	Chemotherapy ⟶ BMT	Remission ⟶ death due to VOD	Brizard et al. [8] (1988)
15 years/F	*De novo*	M4	46,XX,t(8;19)(p11;q13) [6]/46,XX [15]	Chemotherapy alone	Remission (14 months)	Stark et al. [9] (1995)
76 years/M	*De novo*	M5a	46,XY,t(8;19)(p11;q13.3)[18]/46,XY [2]	Chemotherapy alone	Remission (8 months)	Gervais et al. [7] (2008)
71 years/M	Secondary AML	M4	46,XY,t(8;19)(p11;q13)[20]	Chemotherapy alone	No response to therapy—death due to disease progression	Chinen et al. [10] (2014)
3 months/F	*De novo*	M4	46,XX,t(8;19)(p11.2;q13.3)[16]/46,XX [4]	Chemotherapy alone	Remission (24 months)	Current case

FAB, French-American-British classification; AML, acute myeloid leukemia; BMT, bone marrow transplantation; VOD, veno-occlusive disease.

The fusion partner of the *KAT6A* gene in t(8;19)(p11.2;q13) was recently identified in a patient with therapy-related AML to be the leucine twenty homeobox (*LEUTX*) gene located on chromosome 19q13 [10]. It plays an important role in preimplantation embryo development and is known to be primarily expressed in human embryos; however, the exact mechanism of leukemogenesis in t(8;19)(p11.2;q13) AML remains unclear [13]. In addition to *CREBBP* and *LEUTX*, four other *KAT6A* fusion partners have been identified, namely, *EP300*, *NCOA2*, *NCOA3*, and *ASXL2* [14]. Similar to *CREBBP*, all except *ASXL2* and *LEUTX* contain a histone acetyltransferase domain. Cases involving *KAT6A-CREBBP* fusions have demonstrated gain of *MYB* and overexpression of *HOXA9*, *HOXA10*, *HOXA11*, *CEBPA*, *LMO2*, and *PTPN6* genes [14]. *C-MYB* gene is a downstream target of *HOXA9* and upregulation of *HOXA9*, and other *HOX* genes have been implicated in leukemic transformation via increased self-renewal of leukemic stem cells [15]. *KAT6A* leukemias are classified with M4/M5 AML with the exception of those having *ASXL2* as a partner [10].

AML associated with t(8;19)(p11.2;q13) remains a rarely described entity in both pediatric and adult patients. Similar to other infant cases of AML with t(8;16)(p11.2;p13), our patient presented with leukemia cutis, demonstrated erythrophagocytosis in the bone marrow, and was able to achieve remission with standard AML therapy supporting the biologic similarities between the two disease subtypes. While there likely are similar underlying pathways for leukemogenesis between the two 8p11.2-translocated subgroups, our case suggests that the t(8;19) variant is associated with a favorable prognosis in pediatric patients, similar to previously reported cases of t(8;19)(p11.2;q13) AML.

References

[1] M. Moarii and E. Papaemmanuil, "Classification and risk assessment in AML: integrating cytogenetics and molecular profiling," *Hematology*, vol. 2017, no. 1, pp. 37–44, 2017.

[2] L. Bullinger, K. Döhner, and H. Döhner, "Genomics of acute myeloid leukemia diagnosis and pathways," *Journal of Clinical Oncology*, vol. 35, no. 9, pp. 934–946, 2017.

[3] E. A. Coenen, C. M. Zwaan, D. Reinhardt et al., "Pediatric acute myeloid leukemia with t(8; 16)(p11; p13), a distinct clinical and biological entity: a collaborative study by the international-Berlin-Frankfurt-Munster AML-study group," *Blood*, vol. 122, no. 15, pp. 2704–2713, 2013.

[4] T. Haferlach, A. Kohlmann, H.-U. Klein et al., "AML with translocation t(8; 16)(p11; p13) demonstrates unique cytomorphological, cytogenetic, molecular and prognostic features," *Leukemia*, vol. 23, no. 5, pp. 934–943, 2009.

[5] M. Camós, J. Esteve, P. Jares et al., "Gene expression profiling of acute myeloid leukemia with translocation t(8; 16)(p11; p13) and *MYST3-CREBBP* rearrangement reveals a distinctive signature with a specific pattern of *HOX* gene expression," *Cancer Research*, vol. 66, no. 14, pp. 6947–6954, 2006.

[6] R. Barrett, M. Barbara, R. David et al., "FISH identifies a *KAT6A/CREBBP* fusion caused by a cryptic insertional t(8; 16) in a case of spontaneously remitting congenital acute myeloid leukemia with a normal karyotype," *Pediatric Blood & Cancer*, vol. 64, no. 8, 2017.

[7] C. Gervais, A. Murati, C. Helias et al., "Acute myeloid leukaemia with 8p11 (MYST3) rearrangement: an integrated cytologic, cytogenetic and molecular study by the groupe francophone de cytogénétique hématologique," *Leukemia*, vol. 22, no. 8, pp. 1567–1575, 2008.

[8] A. Brizard, F. Guilhot, J. L. Huret, E. Benz-Lemoine, and J. Tanzer, "The 8p11 anomaly in "monoblastic" leukaemia," *Leukemia Research*, vol. 12, no. 8, pp. 693–697, 1988.

[9] B. Stark, P. Resnitzky, M. Jeison et al., "A distinct subtype of M4/M5 acute myeloblastic leukemia (AML) associated with t(8 : 16)(p11 : p13), in a patient with the variant t(8 : 19)(p11 : q13)-Case report and review of the literature," *Leukemia Research*, vol. 19, no. 6, pp. 367–379, 1995.

[10] Y. Chinen, T. Taki, Y. Tsutsumi et al., "The leucine twenty homeobox (*LEUTX*) gene, which lacks a histone acetyltransferase domain, is fused to *KAT6A* in therapy-related acute myeloid leukemia with t(8; 19)(p11; q13)," *Genes, Chromosomes and Cancer*, vol. 53, no. 4, pp. 299–308, 2014.

[11] P. J. F. Troke, K. B. Kindle, H. M. Collins, and D. M. Heery, "MOZ fusion proteins in acute myeloid leukaemia," *Biochemical Society Symposium*, vol. 73, pp. 23–39, 2006.

[12] A. Diab, L. Zickl, O. Abdel-Wahab et al., "Acute myeloid leukemia with translocation t(8; 16) presents with features which mimic acute promyelocytic leukemia and is associated with poor prognosis," *Leukemia Research*, vol. 37, no. 1, pp. 32–36, 2013.

[13] E.-M. Jouhilahti, E. Madissoon, L. Vesterlund et al., "The human PRD-like homeobox gene *LEUTX* has a central role in embryo genome activation," *Development*, vol. 143, no. 19, pp. 3459–3469, 2016.

[14] A. Murati, C. Gervais, N. Carbuccia et al., "Genome profiling of acute myelomonocytic leukemia: alteration of the MYB locus in MYST3-linked cases," *Leukemia*, vol. 23, no. 1, pp. 85–94, 2009.

[15] B. Argiropoulos and R. K. Humphries, "Hox genes in hematopoiesis and leukemogenesis," *Oncogene*, vol. 26, no. 47, pp. 6766–6776, 2007.

26

Tibial Plasmablastic Lymphoma in a HIV-Negative Child: A Novel Extraoral Localisation

Ali Mala, Yameena Noman Khan, Akbar Ahmed, Naema Khayyam, and Kanwal Aftab

Indus Hospital and Health Network, Plot C-76, Sector 31/5, Opposite Darussalam Society Korangi Crossing, Karachi 75190, Pakistan

Correspondence should be addressed to Ali Mala; ali9173@zu.edu.pk

Academic Editor: Kostas Konstantopoulos

Plasmablastic lymphoma is an aggressive, high-grade non-Hodgkin lymphoma predominantly seen in HIV-infected individuals. Alongside a strong correlation with HIV, PBL can manifest in immunocompromised HIV-negative patients. A rare case of PBL in an immunocompetent and otherwise healthy child presented to Indus Hospital & Health Network (IHHN), Karachi, Pakistan. The patient had complaints of swelling and pain in the right leg and was referred from a city in Interior Sindh. Histopathological analysis revealed sheets and aggregates of neoplasm replacing bone marrow interspersed with sclerotic bony fragments. Large, monomorphic, multinucleated neoplastic cells containing abundant cytoplasm and scattered pleomorphic cells were also noted, leading to the diagnosis of tibial plasmablastic lymphoma. A FAB/LMB96 group C chemotherapy regimen for aggressive and high-risk cancer was administered with a marked improvement in clinical symptoms.

1. Introduction

Plasmablastic lymphoma (PBL) is an aggressive, high-grade non-Hodgkin's lymphoma (NHL). Initially considered a variation of diffuse large B-cell lymphoma (DLBCL), PBL was later classified as a distinctive mature B-cell lymphoma and separated from the class of DLBCL by WHO [1]. PBL is predominantly seen in HIV-infected individuals with a preponderance of adults with children accounting for only a handful of cases [2].

Plasmablastic lymphoma was first reported in 1997, when a series of sixteen diffuse large B-cell lymphomas with unique immunohistochemistry were presented in HIV-positive patients with predominant involvement of the oral cavity [3]. Along with the oral cavity, it may also occur in sites including but not exclusive to skin, bone, genitourinary tract, nasal cavity and paranasal sinuses, CNS, liver, lungs, and orbits [4].

Herein, we report a rare case of HIV-negative plasmablastic lymphoma in a 9-year-old male child who presented with swelling and pain in the right leg.

2. Case Presentation

A 9-year-old male, resident of Larkana, presented to the ER of Indus Hospital with complaints of swelling and pain in his right leg. The patient reported trauma to the right leg 16 months prior after which he developed a swelling that gradually increased over time. It was associated with moderate pain, exacerbated on walking. An examination revealed a vitally stable child with a limping gait. A hard and nontender swelling was palpable in the middle of the right lower limb measuring 4-5 cm. The patient had received treatment for osteomyelitis after a presumptive diagnosis made by a primary care physician in Larkana a year back. Biopsy was conducted from the right tibia at a primary care hospital in Larkana four months prior to presenting at Indus Hospital, and histopathological analysis confirmed a diagnosis of plasmablastic lymphoma.

On admission at IHHN, staging workup and routine baseline investigations were conducted. Magnetic resonance imaging (MRI) of the primary site demonstrated lobulated abnormal signal intensity enhancing soft tissue mass arising from the medullary cavity of the right tibia. These soft tissue lesions had an exophytic component along the anterior and posterior aspect of the right tibia. The anterior lesion had an axial dimension of 3.7 cm × 2.5 cm with a craniocaudal diameter of 5.3 cm. The lesion arising from the posterior aspect had an axial dimension of 5.1 cm × 4.1 cm with a craniocaudal dimension of 5.7 cm. The posterior lesion showed gastrocnemius infiltration. The peroneal neurovascular bundle was encased and the popliteal fossa remained intact. Anteriorly, the lesion extended subcutaneously, showing postcontrast enhancement within the cutaneous and subcutaneous soft tissues. The anterior tibial neurovascular bundle was intact along with the absence of intraarticular extension of the lesion. No synchronous lesion was identified in fibula. Medullary bone involvement of the tibia was 10.7 cm in length.

Computed tomography (CT) neck, chest, and abdomen were negative for metastasis. A lumbar puncture was done and the CSF findings were unremarkable. Bilateral bone marrow biopsy exhibited trilineage hematopoiesis with absence of neoplastic cellular infiltration leading to categorization as stage 1, limited to the right tibia. Histopathology of the right tibial lesion was reviewed at IHHN, revealing sheets and aggregates of neoplastic cells replacing bone marrow interspersed with sclerotic bony fragments. Large, monomorphic multinucleated neoplastic cells containing abundant cytoplasm and scattered pleomorphic cells were also noted. Cells with plasmacytoid features were imparted from visible plasma cells. Immunohistochemical stains CD138, CD 38, VS38c, and MUM1 plasma cell markers were positive in neoplastic cells. Ki-67 was positive and expressed an increased proliferative index, approximately 98%. Pax 5 was negative in neoplastic cells. The B-cell markers CD20 and CD79a were negative. Leukocyte common antigen CD45, NK cell marker CD56, CD30, and Alk-1 and T-cell markers CD3 and CD5 were negative. Monoclonal pattern of distribution with kappa strong positive in neoplastic cells was noted on immunohistochemistry. The patient was found to be HIV and Hepatitis B and C negative on screening. Epstein–Barr encoding region (EBER) test was not conducted due to high cost of testing.

The patient received chemotherapeutic protocol FAB/LMB96 group C for aggressive and high-risk non-Hodgkin's lymphoma. Chemotherapeutic regimen involved first cycle of prephase COP (cyclophosphamide, vincristine, and prednisolone) followed by 2 cycles of induction chemotherapy COPADM (cyclophosphamide, vincristine, prednisone, adriamycin, and high-dose methotrexate) along with intrathecal chemotherapy administered over 3-week intervals. The patient proceeded with consolidation courses of chemotherapy and received 2 cycles of CYVE (cytarabine, etoposide) followed by maintenance cycles. A marked reduction in the size of the externally visible swelling in the right lower limb along with improvement in gait and pain was noted via clinical assessment conducted over the course of 4 months. MRI scan posttreatment demonstrated soft tissue anterior compartment lesion measuring 0.8 cm anterior posterior ×0.5 cm transverse ×3.7 cm craniocaudal. These findings hence showed a marked reduction in the size of the lesion posttreatment. Medullary bone involvement was 10.4 cm in length. The posterior compartment lesion was not visible. These findings hence showed a marked reduction in the size of the lesion posttreatment. Following maintenance chemotherapy, positron emission tomography computed tomography (PET-CT) of skeletal system revealed nonfluorodeoxyglucose (FDG) avid irregular cortical sclerosis with multiple small breaks present in the mid two thirds of the shaft of the right tibia rated at 1 on a Deauville 5-point PET-CT scale. The size of sclerotic areas in the tibia was not available. No evidence of hypermetabolic lesions was seen in the skeletal system. Subcentimeter level II lymph nodes were noted with SUV max ranging up to 1.62, appearing infective. Hence, it is concluded that the patient is currently in remission and is being monitored clinically for any signs of recurrence. The patient experienced chemotherapy-related toxicities including mucositis, nausea, vomiting, and febrile neutropenia which were treated with antibiotics, filgrastim, and supportive care. Chemotherapy-induced myelosuppression causes anemia and thrombocytopenia leading to perirectal bleeding requiring blood transfusions in the form of packed red blood cells and platelets.

3. Discussion

Plasmablastic lymphoma is an aggressive B-cell malignancy that is recognized as a subtype of non-Hodgkin's lymphoma. It is highly associated with human immunodeficiency virus (HIV) and its estimated incidence accounts for approximately 5% of all HIV-positive NHL cases. Regardless of its strong relationship with HIV, PBL can also manifest in HIV-negative patients; however, such patients are presumed to have history of autoimmune or lymphoproliferative disorders [5]. This entity not only occurs in the clinical setting of HIV/AIDS but has also been reported in cases of latent Epstein–Barr virus (EBV) infections [6]. Even though features of PBL in an HIV-negative individual have previously been reported, the etiology of HIV-negative PBL is still uncertain. According to a comprehensive analysis, HIV-negative PBL occurs in a wide spectrum of patients with average age at the time of diagnosis found to be 58.9 years with a range of (2–86) years old. Moreover, the statistical data shows male predominance with male: female (2.29 : 1) occurring more in elderly patients (greater than 60 years old, 56.14%) [7]. Another report of 8 cases showed the mean age to be 53.0 years with a range of (27.0–69.0) years [8].

PBL almost as a rule presents as a mass in extranodal regions of the head and neck, in particular the oral cavity and only >1% of cases of extranodal localisations are reported [4]. However, recently, PBL has been discovered to invade extraoral regions which is supported by a number of cases, including a case of vulvar plasmablastic lymphoma in a HIV-positive child [9] and a cutaneous presentation of plasmablastic lymphoma in an EBV positive child [10]. Furthermore, there have been PBL reports on immunocompetent

TABLE 1: Panel of immunohistochemical markers performed and results are as follows.

CD138	Diffuse strong positive in neoplastic cells
CD38	Positive in few neoplastic cells
CD56	Negative in neoplastic cells
Ki-67	Increased proliferative index approximately 98%
Kappa and lambda	Monoclonal pattern of distribution with kappa strong positive in neoplastic cells
CD20	Negative in neoplastic cells. Highlight mature B-lymphocytes in background
CD79a	Negative in neoplastic cells
PAX-5	Negative in neoplastic cells
CD30	Negative in neoplastic cells
Alk-1	Negative in neoplastic cells
CD3	Negative in neoplastic cells. Highlight mature T-lymphocytes in background.
CD45	Negative in neoplastic cells
CD5	Negative in neoplastic cells

and HIV-negative individuals with lesions of the stomach and anorectal junction, respectively [11, 12].

In this case, the patient tested negative for HIV but was not tested for EBV due to its high cost and unavailability at IHHN.

The cell from which the tumour originates is itself an active, postgerminal centre B-lymphocyte which could be a likely reason for its plasma cell traits and plasmacytic differentiation markers. Such a distinct set of characteristics of PBL poses a diagnostic challenge and requires a strong observation for its recognition [13].

Since PBL is described by an immunoblastic or plasmablastic morphology and a plasma cell immunophenotype, its separation from other large B-cell lymphoma or plasmablastic plasma cell neoplasm is often difficult [14]. Hence, the articulation of immunohistochemical markers is an imperative component of the diagnostic protocol [15]. Plasmablastic lymphoma is diagnosed on the basis of specific histopathological features consisting of cohesive cellular proliferation of large atypical cells resembling immunoblasts with plasmacytic differentiation [4]. The immunohistochemical panel of these neoplastic cells expresses a plasma cell phenotype along with positivity for CD138, CD38, VS38c, IRF4/MUM1, PRDM1 (also called BLIMP1), and XBP1. However, CD45, CD20, and PAX5 appear to be either negative or sometimes weakly positive in a minority of cells. Moreover, cytoplasmic immunoglobulin is commonly expressed with the Ki-67 proliferation index being very high (>90%) [4]. It was demonstrated in this case an immunohistochemical profile that mirrored plasmablastic lymphoma containing CD138 (+) plasma cells and scattered linear recticulin with no intersections. The Ki-67 antigen exhibited an increased proliferative index of approximately 98%. CD20 and CD3 were found to be negative in neoplastic cells, indicating the presence of mature B and T lymphocytes. Kappa and lambda were positive and exhibited a monoclonal pattern along with negative CD79a.

The recent parameters for the treatment of lymphoma in initial stages include CHOP or similar chemotherapy regimens [11]. However, the treatment is not fixed and varies according to the case presentation. Chemotherapy using prednisolone, cyclophosphamide, adriamycin, and/or vincristine with or without field radiation therapy can be considered. However, the implementation of chemotherapy,

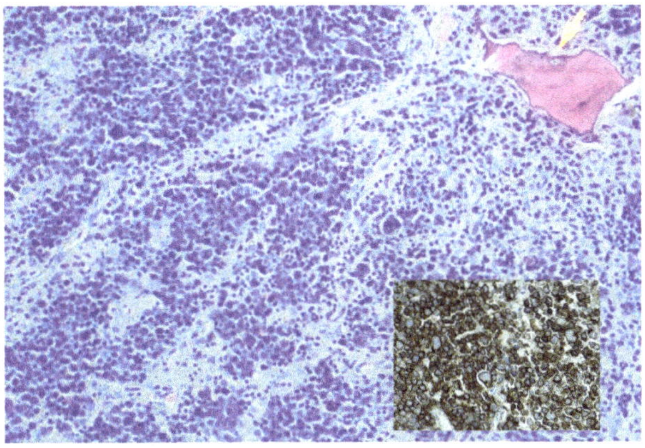

FIGURE 1: Photomicrograph showing sheets of tumor cells in the intertrabecular areas (hematoxylin and eosin stain, 400x). Inset shows strong positivity with CD138 (immunohistochemical stain, 400x).

radiotherapy, or a merger of both is observed in 38%, 27%, and 22% of cases, respectively. Some researchers have utilised highly active antiretroviral drugs in HIV-related PBL with a response rate of 14% [15]. Prognosis is generally poor in cases of PBL with patients surviving less than 12 months. Nonetheless, there are case reports documenting longer survival rates of more than 5–6 years in adults [16] (see Table 1).

The reported patient was treated with cyclophosphamide, vincristine, daunorubicin, and high-dose methotrexate. He received five cycles of chemotherapy, which showed a substantial decrease in lesion size on CT scans and of the externally visible swelling along with improvement in gait. Our patient belonged to a low socioeconomic background with decreased access to quality healthcare, a likely reason for the initial misdiagnosis of osteomyelitis and delay in diagnosis and treatment. Delay in seeking medical care, disorganised referral systems, and lack of specialists are other major factors in the lack of cases reported overall. Due to the unique histological nature and clinical presentation of plasmablastic lymphoma, there is a need for further research on diagnostic protocols and treatment trials along with the identification of predisposing factors such as causative genetic mutations and alterations.

An article in the American Journal of Hematology recorded a satisfactory initial response to therapy in 113

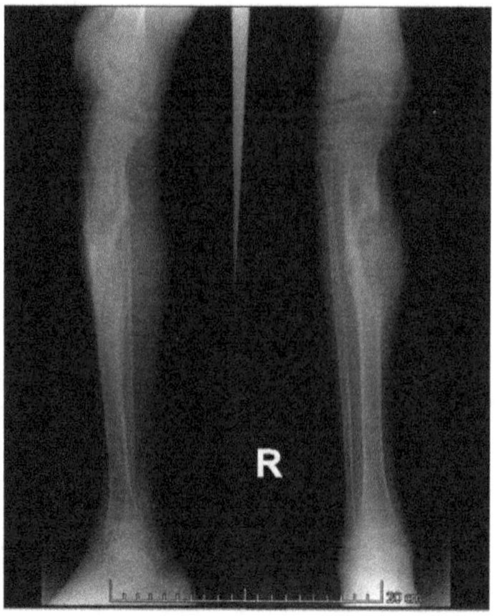

(a)

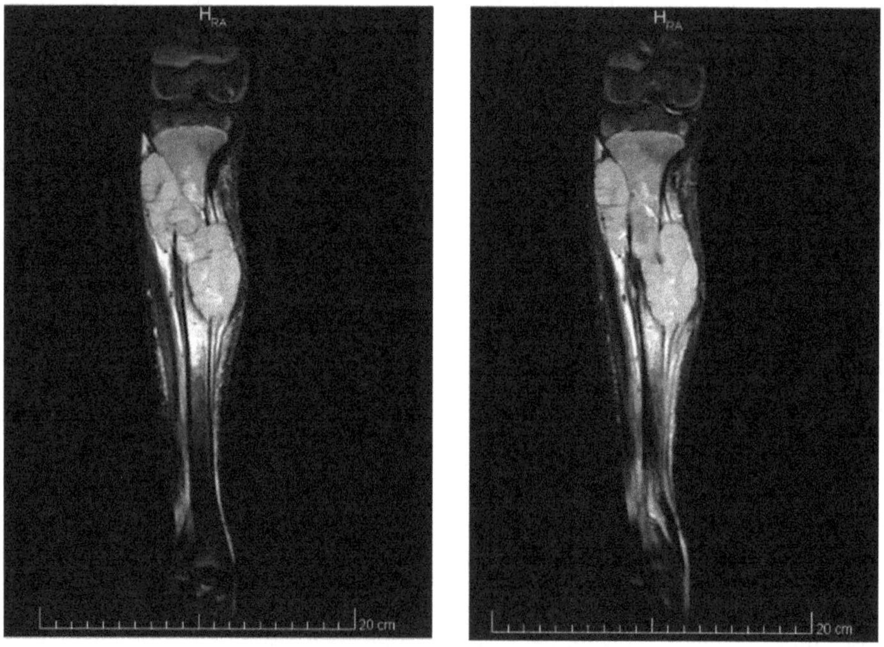

(b)

FIGURE 2: Continued.

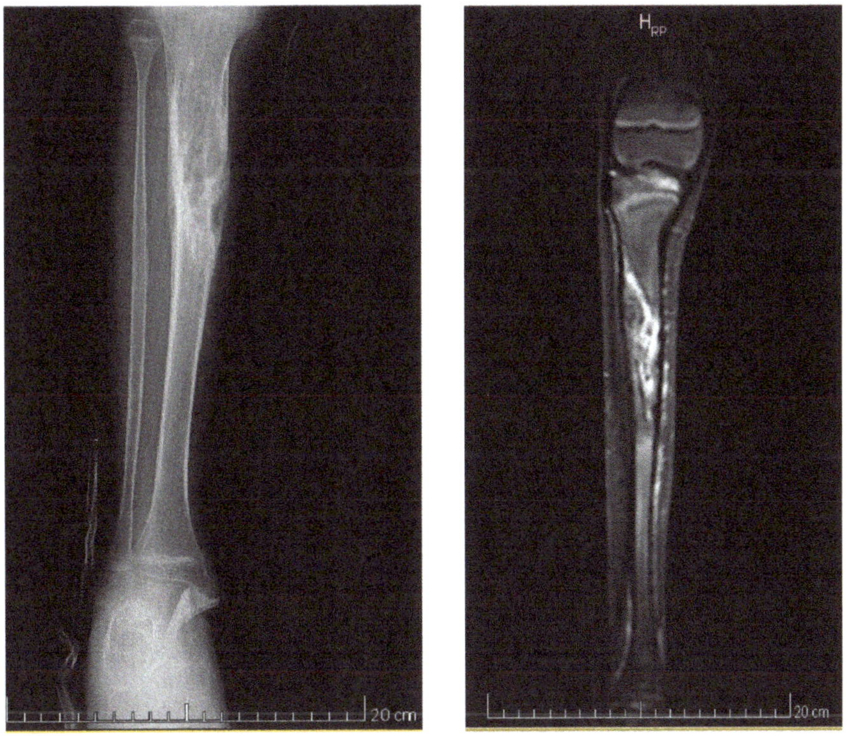

(c) (d)

Figure 2: (a) X-ray at diagnosis, (b) MRI pretreatment, (c) X-ray posttreatment, and (d) MRI posttreatment.

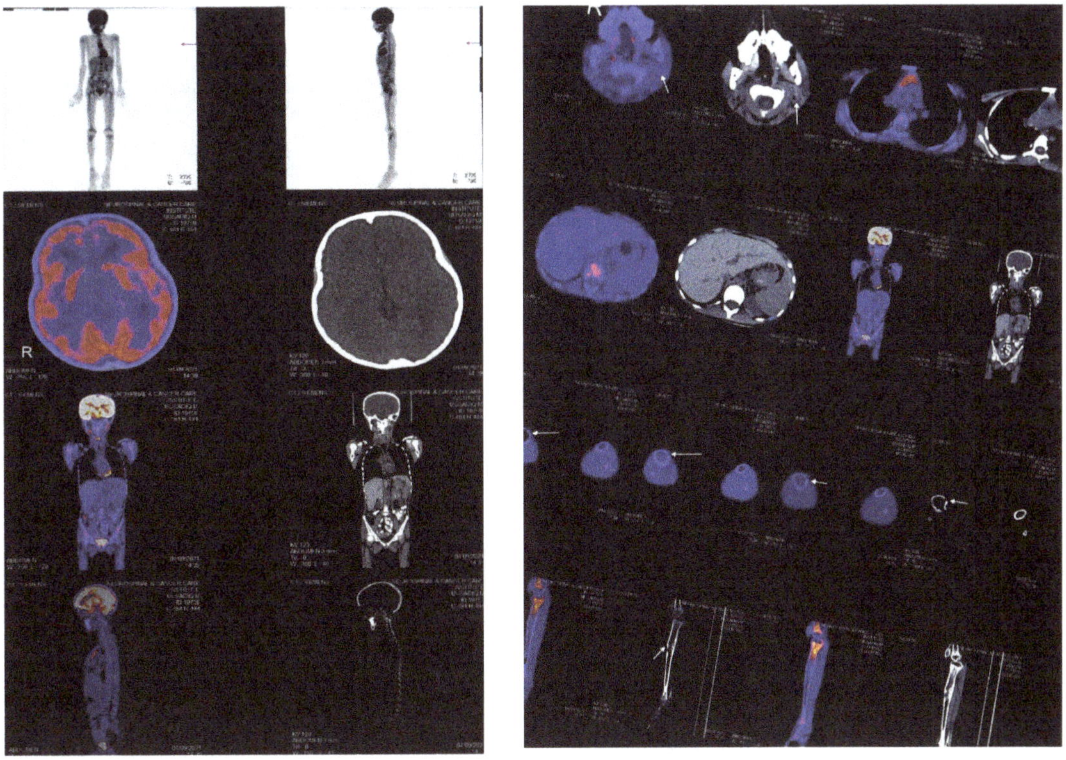

(a) (b)

Figure 3: (a) PET-CT posttreatment and (b) PET-CT posttreatment.

cases of both genders and a wide age group, but the rate of recurrence was high with the prognosis subpar. Components such as sex, lymphoma stage, primary site of involvement, CD4+ count, viral load, EBV status, and use of CHOP do not appear to foretell the survival rate in HIV-associated PBL. Improved and vigorous therapy regimes are suggested for future cases [17]. Another study also concurred with the low incidence of PBL and no appropriate protocol for this special subtype of NHL. This emphasises the need for newer therapies independent of HIV status [18] (see Figures 1–3).

4. Conclusion

Plasmablastic lymphoma is a NHL that most commonly arises in HIV-positive adults. Its diagnosis poses a serious challenge due to its similarities with DLBCL; hence, performing detailed immunophenotypic studies for establishing the diagnosis of PBL is pertinent. Furthermore, it is an aggressive malignancy with a relatively poor outcome and therefore requires a belligerent multimodality treatment.

Consent

Written informed consent was obtained.

Acknowledgments

Akbar Ahmed, Yameena Noman Khan, and Ali Mala are the authors as well as the funders of this research.

References

[1] S. Pather, D. MacKinnon, and R. S. Padayachee, "Plasmablastic lymphoma in pediatric patients: clinicopathologic study of three cases," *Annals of Diagnostic Pathology*, vol. 17, no. 1, pp. 80–84, 2013.

[2] J. Goedhals, K. David, and M. C Botha, "Plasmablastic lymphoma in childhood: a report of two cases," *South African Journal of Child Health*, vol. 8, no. 1, pp. 39-40, 2014.

[3] H.-J. Delecluse, I. Anagnostopoulos, F. E. Dallenbach et al., "Plasmablastic lymphomas of the oral cavity: a new entity associated with the human immunodeficiency virus infection," *Blood*, vol. 89, no. 4, pp. 1413–1420, 1997.

[4] E. Campo, N. Lee, E. S. Jaffe et al., *WHO Classification of Tumours of Haematopoietic and Lymphoid Tissues*, S. H. Swerdlow, Ed., International Agency for Research on Cancer, Lyon, France, 2008.

[5] X. Han, M. Duan, L. Hu, D. Zhou, and W. Zhang, "Plasmablastic lymphoma: review of 60 Chinese cases and prognosis analysis," *Medicine*, vol. 96, Article ID e5981, 2017.

[6] J. J. Liu, L. Zhang, E. Ayala et al., "Human immunodeficiency virus (HIV)-negative plasmablastic lymphoma: a single institutional experience and literature review," *Leukemia Research*, vol. 35, no. 12, pp. 1571-1577, 2011.

[7] M. I. Liu, B. A. I. L. O. Liu, B. I. Liu et al., "Human immunodeficiency virus-negative plasmablastic lymphoma: a comprehensive analysis of 114 cases," *Oncology Reports*, vol. 33, no. 4, pp. 1615–1620, 2015.

[8] Y.-J. Li, J.-W. Li, K.-L. Chen et al., "HIV-negative plasmablastic lymphoma: report of 8 cases and a comprehensive review of 394 published cases," *Blood research*, vol. 55, no. 1, pp. 49–56, 2020.

[9] P. Chabay, E. De Matteo, M. Lorenzetti et al., "Vulvar plasmablastic lymphoma in a HIV-positive child: a novel extraoral localisation," *Journal of Clinical Pathology*, vol. 62, no. 7, pp. 644–646, 2009.

[10] C. Hernandez, A. S. Cetner, and E. L. Wiley, "Cutaneous presentation of plasmablastic post-transplant lymphoproliferative disorder in a 14-month-old," *Pediatric Dermatology*, vol. 26, no. 6, pp. 713–716, 2009.

[11] M. Brahmania, T. Sylwesterowic, and H. Leitch, "Plasmablastic lymphoma in the ano-rectal junction presenting in an immunocompetent man: a case report," *Journal of Medical Case Reports*, vol. 5, no. 1, pp. 168–175, 2011.

[12] C. Y. Adrian Hui and D. Kearney, "Gastric plasmablastic lymphoma–case report," *Pathology*, vol. 47, p. S64, 2015.

[13] Z. Fadoo, A. Belgaumi, M. Alam, I. Azam, and A. Naqvi, "Pediatric lymphoma: a 10-year experience at a tertiary care hospital in Pakistan," *Journal of pediatric hematology/oncology*, vol. 32, no. 1, pp. e14–e18, 2010.

[14] Ji E. Kim, Y. A. Kim, W. Y. Kim et al., "Human immunodeficiency virus-negative plasmablastic lymphoma in Korea," *Leukemia and Lymphoma*, vol. 50, no. 4, pp. 582–587, 2009.

[15] M. A. Scheper, N. G. Nikitakis, J. J. Sauk, C. D. Gocke, and R. A. Ord, "Oral plasmablastic lymphoma in an HIV-negative patient: a case report and review of the literature," *Oral Surgery, Oral Medicine, Oral Pathology, Oral Radiology & Endodontics*, vol. 100, no. 2, pp. 198–206, 2005.

[16] J. I. Vaubell, Y. Sing, A. Ramburan et al., "Pediatric plasmablastic lymphoma: a clinicopathologic study," *International Journal of Surgical Pathology*, vol. 22, no. 7, pp. 607–616, 2014.

[17] J. Castillo, L. Pantanowitz, and B. J. Dezube, "HIV-associated plasmablastic lymphoma: lessons learned from 112 published cases," *American Journal of Hematology*, vol. 83, no. 10, pp. 804–809, 2008.

[18] D. Hansra, N. Montague, S. Alexandra et al., "Oral and extraoral plasmablastic lymphoma: similarities and differences in clinicopathologic characteristics," *American Journal of Clinical Pathology*, vol. 134, no. 5, pp. 710–719, 2010.

27

The Effects of Fecal Donors with Different Feeding Patterns on Diarrhea in a Patient Undergoing Hematopoietic Stem Cell Transplantation

Jianping Zhang,[1] Guangxu Ren,[2] Minghua Li,[1] Peihua Lu,[1] and Suqin Yi[2]

[1]*Bone Marrow Transplantation (BMT) Unit, Hebei Yanda Ludaopei Hospital, Sanhe, China*
[2]*Institute of Food and Nutrition Development, Ministry of Agriculture, Beijing, China*

Correspondence should be addressed to Guangxu Ren; renguangxu@caas.cn

Jianping Zhang and Guangxu Ren contributed equally to this work.

Academic Editor: Håkon Reikvam

Almost 90% of patients undergoing hematopoietic stem cell transplantation (HSCT) experience diarrheal episodes, which represent a severe, often life-threatening complication for these patients. Although fecal microbiota transplantation (FMT) represents an alternative treatment option for infection-related diarrhea, the application of FMT in HSCT patients is greatly restricted for safety reasons. Furthermore, the therapeutic outcomes of FMT as a diarrhea treatment are somewhat related to the choice of the FMT donor. Here, we comprehensively profiled the dynamic changes in the intestinal microbiota after FMT from two donors with different feeding patterns and the same severely diarrheal recipient undergoing HSCT via a 45-day clinical observation. Importantly, no adverse events attributed to FMT were observed. The stool volume and frequency of the patient were reduced when we used feces from donor #1 (mixed feeding), but these changes were not observed after FMT from donor #2 (exclusive breastfeeding). Interestingly, no obvious differences in overall diversity (Shannon) or richness (Chao1) between the two donors were observed. Additionally, *Bifidobacterium* accounted for 29.9% and 18.1% of OTUs in the stools of donors #1 and #2, respectively. *Lactobacillus* accounted for 16.3% and 2.9% of the stools of donors #1 and #2, respectively. Furthermore, through longitudinal monitoring of the patient, we identified 6 OTUs that were particularly sensitive to the different FMT complements. Together, we present a case report suggesting that the overall diversity of the intestinal microbiota may not be the only important element in the selection of an effective FMT donor.

1. Introduction

Almost 90% of patients undergoing hematopoietic stem cell transplantation (HSCT) [1–4] experience diarrheal episodes during the first 3 months after transplantation [1] and can represent a severe and even life-threatening complication in these HSCT patients [3, 4]. Although the etiology of diarrhea in these patients is often difficult to ascertain, the causes can be roughly divided into infectious events (bacterial and viral gastroenteritis) and noninfectious events [1] (conditioning therapy and acute graft-versus-host disease (GVHD)). Currently, some antidiarrheal agents have been approved to mitigate the symptoms of diarrhea [5], but these drugs do not manage diarrhea for some patients undergoing HSCT in some clinical situations.

The gut microbiome plays important roles in regulating diarrhea-related functions, including as a protective barrier to incoming pathogens by colonization competition [6] and in the development of the immune system. Meanwhile, diarrheal episodes are also associated with the composition of the intestinal microbiota [7–10]. An overall decrease in the phylogenetic diversity of the intestinal microbiota has been observed during diarrheal episodes [7, 8, 11, 12]. For patients undergoing HSCT, the most common causes of diarrhea are intestinal infection and GVHD from day 20 to day 100 posttransplant [13]. Interestingly, loss of microbiota diversity has been associated with increased infections and GVHD [14–18]. Thus, the reversal of this intestinal dysbiosis using fecal microbiota transplantation (FMT) has increasingly been used in clinical practice as treatment for diarrhea caused by *Clostridium difficile* infection that cannot be eliminated with antibiotics alone [19].

Given that FMT carries a potential risk of infection [20, 21], the application of FMT in patients with leukemia, especially in patients undergoing HSCT, has been greatly restricted until recently, when some studies evaluated the safety of FMT in patients with leukemia [22, 23]. In cases where diarrhea could not be mitigated with medicine, FMT has commonly been used to treat HSCT patients. However, we found that the outcomes of FMT were to some extent related to the stool sample donors, which raised the question of how to select appropriate donors. To more precisely address the role of stool donors in the outcomes of diarrhea in HSCT patients, we comprehensively profiled the dynamic changes in the intestinal microbiota between donors with different feeding patterns and the same recipient.

2. Case Presentation

Patient #A14, a 56-year-old male subject, was diagnosed with acute myeloid leukemia (AML-M4) in October 2016. A decision was made for haploidentical HSCT with his son as the donor on 28 March 2017. He received grafts from 5/10 HLA-matched peripheral blood stem cells (PBSCs) and bone marrow (BM) stem cells. The conditioning regimen was modified BUCY (busulfan: 3.2 mg/kg, iv days −9 to −6; cyclophosphamide: 1.8 g/m^2, days −5 to −4); GVHD prophylaxis consisted of antithymocyte globulin (ATG), cyclosporin A (CSA), mycophenolate mofetil (MMF), and short-term methotrexate (sMTX). ATG (thymoglobulin, rabbit; Genzyme Europe B.V., Naarden, the Netherlands) was given at a dose of 10 mg/kg from days −5 to −2. CsA (3 mg/kg, iv every 12 h) was administered starting on day −10, and the trough concentration was adjusted to 150–300 ng/ml. MMF was administered orally starting on day −10 (0.5 g, every 12 h) and was withdrawn on day +45 for haploidentical donor (HID) HSCT. sMTX was administered intravenously at 15 mg/m^2 on day +1 and 10 mg/m^2 on days +3, +6, and +11. Neutrophil and platelet engraftment occurred on days +15 and +23, respectively.

One month later, on day +27, the patient developed abdominal tenderness and diarrhea. In addition to abdominal pain, diarrhea, and fever, patient #A14 had no GVHD-related symptoms and no impaired liver function (alanine aminotransferase, aspartate aminotransferase, total bilirubin, and direct bilirubin were normal). Because of insufficient evidence of GVHD, neither enteroscopy (sigmoidoscopy and colonoscopy) nor glucocorticoid therapy was performed for this patient. Virological tests showed that cytomegalovirus (CMV) DNA and Epstein–Barr virus (EBV) DNA were not present in the blood. Antiviral therapy was given acyclovir (0.4 Po Bid) to prevent herpes virus infection. Although the patient's temperature returned to normal and abdominal pain relieved after anti-infection treatment, the diarrhea did not alleviate. Stool screening showed no *Clostridium difficile* infection. Fecal neutrophils were not found in stained smears of diarrheal stools. We did not observe obvious improvement after we treated the patient with Smecta combined with sulperazone for three days. The ratio of cocci to bacilli was 9 : 1 by stool smear. One week after cessation of medical treatment, we attempted to use FMT to treat the diarrhea.

3. Methods

3.1. Study Design. The first stage of FMT (FMT^{1st}) was performed on day 2 after cessation of diarrhea treatment (Figure 1(a)). Fecal samples were obtained from a 1-year-old female infant (donor #1) who had a mixed feeding pattern (formula feeding and complementary food). Doses of 60 mL of fecal suspension were administered for 7 consecutive days via a nasoduodenal tube. Then, we suspended the FMT operation and continually observed the dynamic changes in the intestinal microbiota. However, one week after cessation of FMT, diarrhea recurred in this patient. Unfortunately, stool samples from donor #1 were not available on that occasion. Thus, we used fecal samples from another 1-year-old male infant (donor #2) who had an exclusive breastfeeding pattern. After 3 consecutive days of FMT^{2nd}, we did not observe any improvement in the diarrhea, and we terminated FMT on day 4 (Figure 1(a)). Two days later, we obtained additional stool samples from donor #1 and conducted the third FMT (FMT^{3rd}) for another 7 consecutive days. Afterward, we similarly suspended FMT and continually observed the dynamic changes in the intestinal microbiota for one week. A standardized protocol for donor screening and FMT administration developed by infectious disease and BM transplant specialists was approved by the hospital quality and safety officer. This study was approved by the hospital ethics committee. Informed consent was obtained from both the parents of the stool donors and the FMT recipient. The study was conducted in accordance with the Declaration of Helsinki.

3.2. Donor Characteristics. Donor #1, a 1-year-old female infant, was born term at gestational age 39 weeks via C-section, and her birth weight was 2700 g. Donor #2 was a 1-year-old male infant who was delivered though C-section at gestational age 42 weeks, and his birth weight was 3900 g. Donor #1 received mixed feeding from the fifth month after birth to the start of this study. The mixed-fed donor was predominantly fed complementary food and received formula feedings twice a day (the total dietary nutrient intake is shown in Table 1). Donor #2 was exclusively breastfed from birth to the start of this study. Both donors were healthy, without any gastrointestinal pathology or history of antibiotic usage. All donors tested negative for anti-HIV (human immunodeficiency virus), anti-HTLV-1 (human T-lymphotropic virus type I), and antihepatitis A, B, and C. No symptoms of infectious gastroenteritis, such as fever, abdominal pain, nausea, vomiting, or diarrhea, were present on the day of FMT.

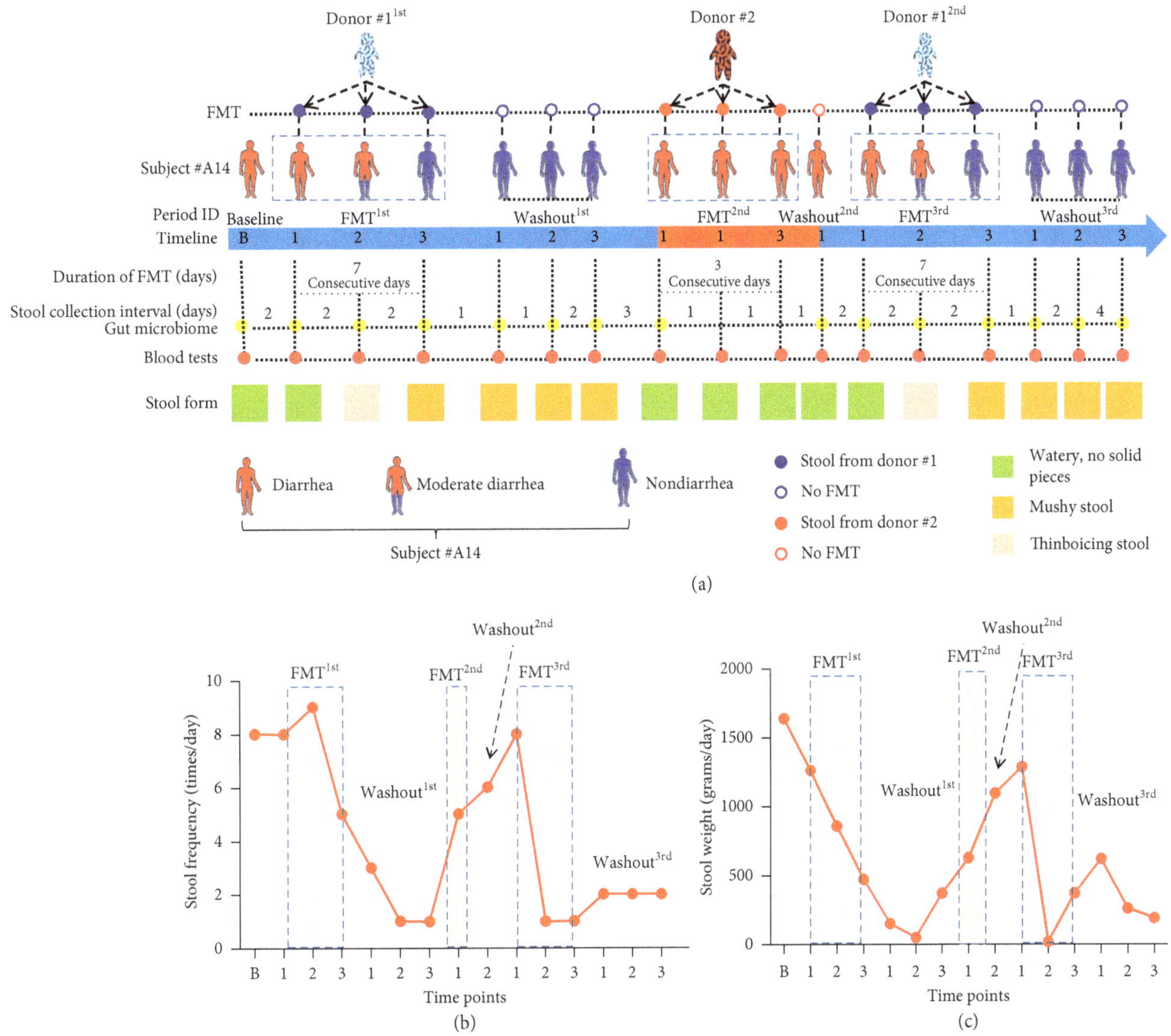

FIGURE 1: Differences in the effects of stools from donors with two feeding patterns on outcomes of diarrhea treatment via FMT in the same recipient. (a) Illustration of this study design, which was a longitudinal observation comparing the effects of stool samples from two donors with different feeding patterns (donor #1 was mixed fed, and donor #2 was exclusively breastfed) on the therapeutic outcomes of diarrhea via FMT in the same recipient (subject #A14). Thinboicing stool is the transitional form between watery stool and musy stool. The stool frequency (b) and weight (c) of the recipient were continuously recorded during the entire study.

TABLE 1: Characteristics and dietary patterns.

Subjects	Items						
	Age (years)	Gender	Body weight (kg)	Dietary pattern	Total dietary nutrient intake (mean ± SD)		
					Calories (kcal/kg/day)	Protein (g/kg/day)	Fat (g/kg/day)
A14 (recipient)	56	Male	58	Rice paste (50 g rice/meal) and egg (1/meal)	$11.5 \pm 2.3^*$	0.38 ± 0.3	0.4 ± 0.2※
Donor #1	1	Female	10	Mixed fed (formula feeding + complementary food※)	65.6 ± 4.2	2.3 ± 0.7	1.2 ± 0.8
Donor #2	1	Male	11	Exclusively breastfeeding	100 ± 1.2	2 ± 0.5	5.3 ± 1.5

Note. The Kruskal–Wallis test was used to calculate the significant differences among A14, donor #1 and donor #2. *A14 vs. donor #1, $p > 0.05$; donor #1 vs. donor #2, $p > 0.05$; A14 vs. donor #2, $p < 0.05$. ※Complementary food includes rice paste, formula and yolk.

3.3. FMT Preparation. Fresh stool samples from healthy donors were collected using sterile bags and immediately transported to the laboratory within 5 h of collection. For each specimen, 5 g of the stool sample was stored in a liquid nitrogen tank for future microbiota analysis. The remaining sample was used for FMT according to the protocol described by Lee et al. [24] with minor modification. Briefly, approximately 60 g of the stool sample was diluted with 60 mL of physiological saline solution and emulsified using a sterile glass rod. After filtering out the solids via a medical gauze, 50 mL of the liquid slurry was aspirated into 60 mL syringes and then used to perform FMT within 6 h.

3.4. Sequencing Methods. DNA was extracted from thawed stool samples using the E.Z.N.A. Stool DNA kit (Omega Bio-Tek, Norcross, GA, US) according to the manufacturer's instructions. The quality of the DNA was evaluated by 2% agarose gel electrophoresis and spectrophotometry. The V3-V4 region of the 16S rRNA gene was amplified using FastPfu DNA Polymerase (TransStart^{TM}, TransGen Biotech). The primers were used as follows: 338F, 5′-ACTCCTACGG-GAGGCAGCAG-3' and 806R, 5′-GGAC-TACHVGGGTWTCTAAT-3'. The PCR cycling conditions were as follows: 95°C for 5 min; 28 cycles of 45 s at 95°C, 50 s at 55°C, 45 s at 72°C, and a final extension at 72°C for 10 min. Purified amplicons were pooled in equimolar amounts and paired-end sequenced (2 × 300) on an Illumina MiSeq platform according to the standard protocols. The sequence data were compiled and filtered for quality. The unique sequence set was classified into operational taxonomic units (OTUs) under a threshold of 97% identity using UCLUST. Chimeric sequences were identified and removed using USEARCH (version 8.0.1623). The taxonomy of each 16S rRNA gene sequence was analyzed by UCLUST against the Silva 119 16S rRNA database using a confidence threshold of 90%. Taxonomic assignments of each OTU were made by similarity using the GLSEARCH program. Alpha diversity values were calculated using Faith's phylogenetic diversity [25].

3.5. Statistical Analysis. Data were analyzed using a combination of the software programs R and Mothur. Heat maps, principal coordinates analysis (PCoA), and bar plots were created in R. The nonparametric Kruskal–Wallis test was performed using GraphPad Prism 4.0 software (GraphPad Inc., San Diego, California, USA). *P* values less than 0.05 were considered significant.

4. Case Outcomes

4.1. Effects of Different Infants' Feces on Diarrhea in a Leukemia Patient. Patient #A14 developed sustained abdominal tenderness and diarrhea after allo-HSCT. Given that both Smecta and sulperazone had no effect on diarrhea status in this case, FMT was recommended and then accepted by the subject. Diarrhea status was routinely monitored via frequency, weight, and shape of bowel movements each day during the entire study period (Figures 1(a)–1(c)). During the B phase (the baseline time point: on day 2 after cessation of medical treatment for diarrhea), patient #A14 had 8 liquid bowel movements a day, and the wet weight of the stool reached 1640 g in 24 h (Figures 1(b) and 1(c)). During the first stage of FMT (FMT^{1st}), in which stool samples were obtained from donor #1, although the frequency of liquid stools was increased at the beginning of FMT^{1st}, the number of bowel movements began to decline significantly from the third sample collection point (3FMT^{1st}) onward. Meanwhile, the patient stool mass was dramatically decreased from 1260 g (1FMT^{1st}) to 470 g (3FMT^{1st}). During the 7-day follow-up after cessation of the first FMT, the shape of the feces was obviously improved (Figure 1(a)), and the frequency of bowel movements gradually decreased from 5 times at 3FMT^{1st} to once at the third sampling time point of the first washout phase (3Washout^{1st}, Figure 1(b)). However, after the 3Washout^{1st} phase, the patient developed serious diarrhea again. Next, we used donor #2's stool to perform FMT^{2nd}, but we did not observe any improvement during the 3-day FMT process. Following a 3-day washout period (Washout^{2nd}), we returned to stool samples from donor #1 to conduct the third FMT (FMT^{3rd}). Similarly, during the 7-day FMT period, we found significant improvements in both the shape and frequency of the patient's stool (Figures 1(a) and 1(b)). After cessation of FMT, we continuously observed for another seven days and found no recurrence of diarrhea in patient #A14.

4.2. Patterns of Diversity and Richness in the Intestinal Microbiome during FMT. To assess the dynamic changes in the gut microbiome during FMT, we sequenced DNA from stool samples collected at the baseline (B point) and the indicated time points (Figure 1(a)) with 16S rRNA gene sequencing. During allo-HSCT, patients normally undergo dramatic alterations of their intestinal microbiota [26]. In this study, we also found that the overall bacterial diversity (Shannon a-diversity = 0.47) and richness (Chao1 index = 26.75) of patient #A14 were significantly reduced at the beginning of FMT (Figures 2(a) and 2(c)). Although we observed that stool samples from donor #1 were more effective for the treatment of diarrhea than those from donor #2, there were no obvious differences in diversity (Shannon) or richness (Chao1) between the two donors (Figures 2(a) and 2(c)). During the entire FMT process, we observed significantly increased bacterial diversity in the patient after the introduction of stool from either donor (FMT^{1st}, FMT^{2nd}, and FMT^{3rd}; Figures 2(b) and 2(d)). Notably, most bacteria tended not to be retained in the patient's intestine after the cessation of a 1-week-long FMT period, regardless of which stool we used (Chao1 index at Washout^{1st}, Washout^{2nd}, and Washout^{3rd} time points; Figures 2(b) and 2(d)). We next asked whether the diversity of bacteria affected the occurrence of diarrhea. To this end, we classified the overall samples we sequenced into three different levels based on the inverse Simpson index and correlated diarrhea status with bacterial diversity (Figure 2(e)). In samples with high diversity (inverse Simpson index > 3), diarrhea was observed in 40% (2/5) of samples. Interestingly, these samples shared the same dominant genera, including *Lactobacillus*, *Veillonella*, and *Enterobacter*. Only one sample of the 4 samples with the middle level of diversity presented signs of diarrhea (inverse Simpson index 2.0–2.9). However, the dominant genera were different among these samples. In samples with low diversity (inverse Simpson index < 2), signs of diarrhea were found in 42.8% (3/7) of samples. *Enterobacter* was the dominant genus in 71.4% (5/7) of the samples.

4.3. Composition of the Intestinal Microbiome during FMT. Based on OTU abundance, we outlined the top 20 genera for each sample (Figure 3(a)). During the baseline measurement, we found that the core microbiome of the patient was *Streptococcus*, which accounted for 94.3% of the sampled OTUs, while *Bifidobacterium* and *Enterococcus* accounted for only 2% and 1.2%, respectively. For the donors, we observed that *Bifidobacterium* (29.8%) and *Faecalibacterium* (28.8%) were the dominant genera in donors #1 and #2, respectively. Other highly represented genera in both donors included *Lactobacillus* (donor #1 = 16.3%, donor #2 = 2.9%), *Veillonella* (donor #1 = 15%, donor #2 = 4.6%), *Streptococcus* (donor #1 = 6.6%, donor #2 = 4.8%), *Haemophilus* (donor #1 = 4.6%, donor #2 = 6.2%), and *Escherichia-Shigella* (donor #1 = 11.3%, donor #2 = 0.6%). Notably, similar compositions were observed in the samples from donor #1 in both FMT^{1st} and FMT^{2nd} procedures (Figure 3(a)). Sequences were assigned to 114 OTUs in patient #A14, and we followed the dynamic changes in each OTU during the entire FMT process. When the patient received the first FMT from donor #1, he showed favorable recovery from diarrhea, and the microbiota composition was dominated by *Streptococcus* (72.2%) and *Bifidobacterium* (18.6%). During the second FMT from donor #2, the microbiota mainly comprised *Enterobacter* (76.5%), *Lactobacillus* (7.8%), and *Veillonella* (7.0%). When the patient received the final FMT from the second donor #1 sample, *Lactobacillus* (23.8%), *Escherichia-Shigella* (19.9%), and *Enterobacter* (23.3%) were the core OTUs of the microbiome. Meanwhile, we identified 6 OTUs that were more sensitive to changes during FMT (OTU_01: *Enterobacter* spp., OTU_29: *Lactobacillus* spp., OTU_52: *Campylobacter* spp., OTU_104: *Ezakiella* spp., OTU_80: *Edwardsiella* spp., and OTU_86: *Luteibacter* spp.) among the 114 recognized OTUs (Figures 3(b)–3(g)).

4.4. Comparison of Diarrhea and Nondiarrhea Stages. A PCoA of unweighted UniFrac values identified significant differences in the patient stool microbiome according to whether diarrhea was occurring or not. The samples from time points with normal stool status (Washout^{1st}: 1, 2, and 3; Washout^{3rd}: 2 and 3) segregated from the other samples (Figure 4(a)). We noted that these samples from the same patient clustered closely and continuously together. To further understand the differences in the microbial communities between diarrhea and nondiarrhea (normal) stages, we also performed linear discriminant analysis effect size (LEfSe) analyses with a logarithmic (LDA) value of 2.0. A total of 7 genera (*Morganella*, *Dysgonomonas*, *Prevotella*, *Fusobacterium*, *Luteibacter*, *Lactococcus*, and *Pyramidobacter*; Figure 4(b)) were found to be significantly different between samples with signs of diarrhea and normal samples. However, no apparent biomarker genera were identified in the nondiarrhea stage.

4.5. Dietary Patterns of Subjects. Given that diet has an important influence on the composition of the human intestinal microbiota [27], we closely monitored the daily dietary intake of all subjects using a 24-h dietary recall questionnaire that was used to calculate the total dietary nutrient intake. We noted no significant differences between donor #1, who received mixed feeding (formula feeding + complementary food), and donor #2, who received exclusive breastfeeding, in total dietary nutrient intake, including calories (donor #1 vs. #2: 65.6 ± 4.2 kcal/kg/day vs. 100 ± 1.2 kcal/kg/day), protein (donor #1 vs. #2: 2.3 ± 0.7 g/kg/day vs. 2 ± 0.5 g/kg/day), and fat (donor #1 vs. #2: 1.2 ± 0.8 g/kg/day vs. 5.3 ± 1.5 g/kg/day) (Table 1). For patient #A14, we found that rice paste (50 g rice/meal) and egg (1 egg/meal) were the main daily foods during the whole study (Table 1).

5. Discussion

Diarrhea induced by unclear factors including infectious events and noninfectious events in patients undergoing HSCT is common [28], frequently causes notable morbidity and mortality and is often persistent, profuse, and incompletely responsive to symptomatic management [3, 28]. Given that the mechanisms inducing diarrhea in these cases remain poorly understood, its treatment can be challenging, especially for patients undergoing HSCT. The introduction of intestinal microbiota from a healthy donor to restore the indigenous gut microbiota, commonly known as FMT, has been successfully used to treat recurrent *C. difficile*-associated diarrhea when standard therapy fails [29, 30]. Because FMT carries a potential risk of infectious disease transmission [21], the application of FMT has been used with caution in HSCT patients, who have a severely immunosuppressed status.

Recently, Bilinski et al. found that FMT in patients with blood disorders promotes eradication of antibiotic-resistant bacteria (ARB) from the gastrointestinal tract [31]. A pilot study administering FMT by oral capsules early after bone marrow transplantation (BMT) showed that third-party FMT could restore intestinal microbiome diversity after allo-HSCT [32]. Furthermore, a multicenter retrospective series investigated the use of FMT in immunocompromised (IC) patients with *Clostridium difficile* infection [33]. This study found that there were no related infectious complications in these IC patients. Therefore, FMT can still be applied to HSCT patients on the premise of strict control of the FMT operation process. In the clinic, we found that the residues of some irritating foods can induce GVHD in patients undergoing HSCT (data not shown). As we know, adults have a more complex diet than that of 1-year-old infants. Thus, for safety reasons, we used feces from infants instead of adults to perform FMT. Infants 1 year of age have more *Bifidobacteria* than do individuals of other age groups [34]. Several trials have suggested that Bifidobacterial preparations have efficacy in the prevention and treatment of pediatric antibiotic-associated diarrhea [35]. Importantly, the infant intestinal microbiome is significantly associated with the feeding method [36]. This raises the question of what types of infant donors are better suited for FMT. Our study

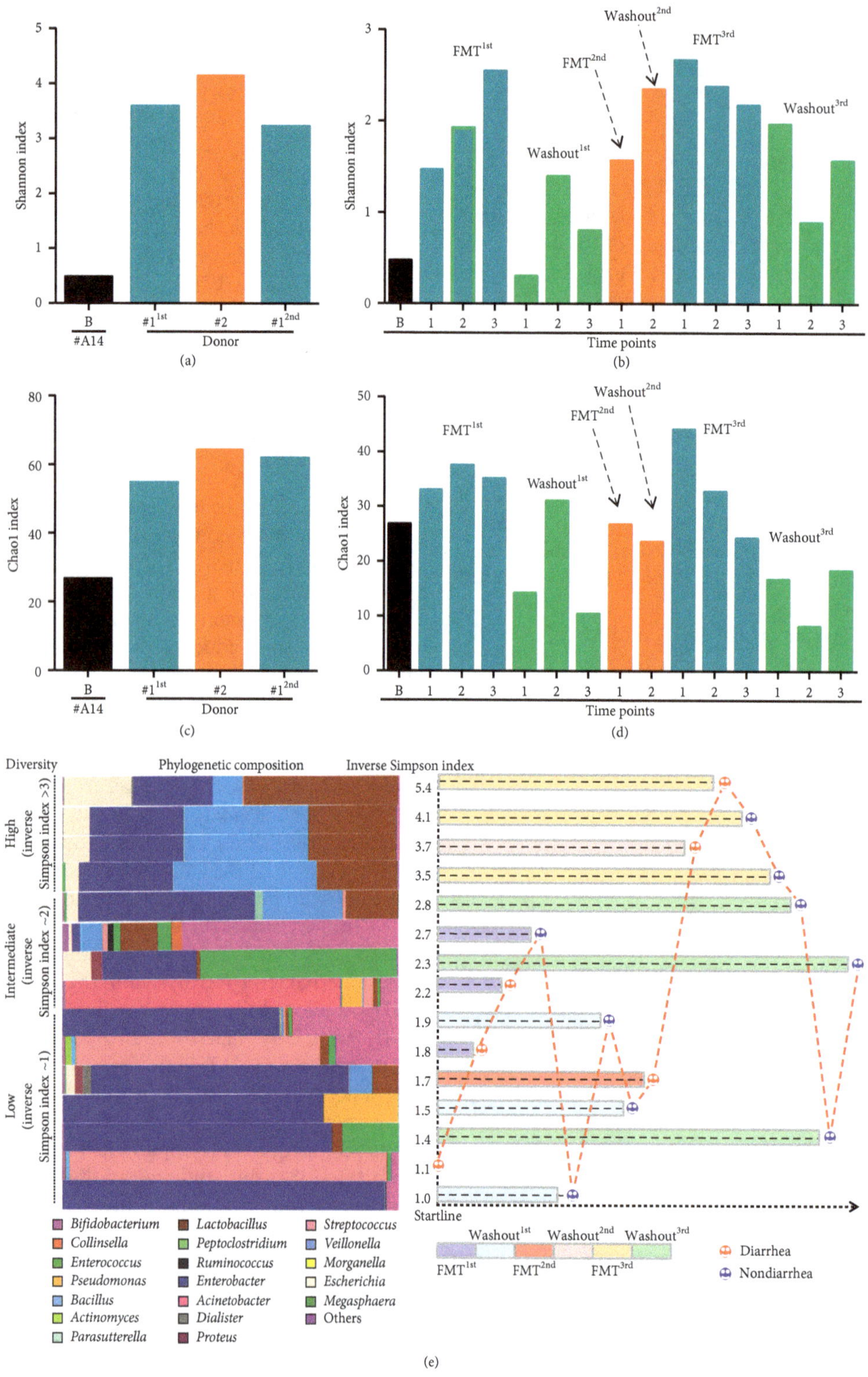

FIGURE 2: Dynamic changes in microbial diversity and richness during the entire FMT process. Microbial diversity was measured by the Shannon index at baseline (a) and the indicated time points (b) for both the FMT donors and the FMT recipient. Microbial richness was evaluated via the Chao1 index at baseline (c) and the indicated time points (d) during the entire FMT process. Recipient specimen collection points were rearranged according to the level of microbial diversity, and diarrhea status is labeled on the right. (e) The horizontal stacked bars on the left side represent the phylogenetic composition of the recipient at each sample collection time point. The hierarchy of microbial diversity was determined by the inverse Simpson index. Time bars are shown in the columns; the length of the time bar depends on the sequence of specimen collection.

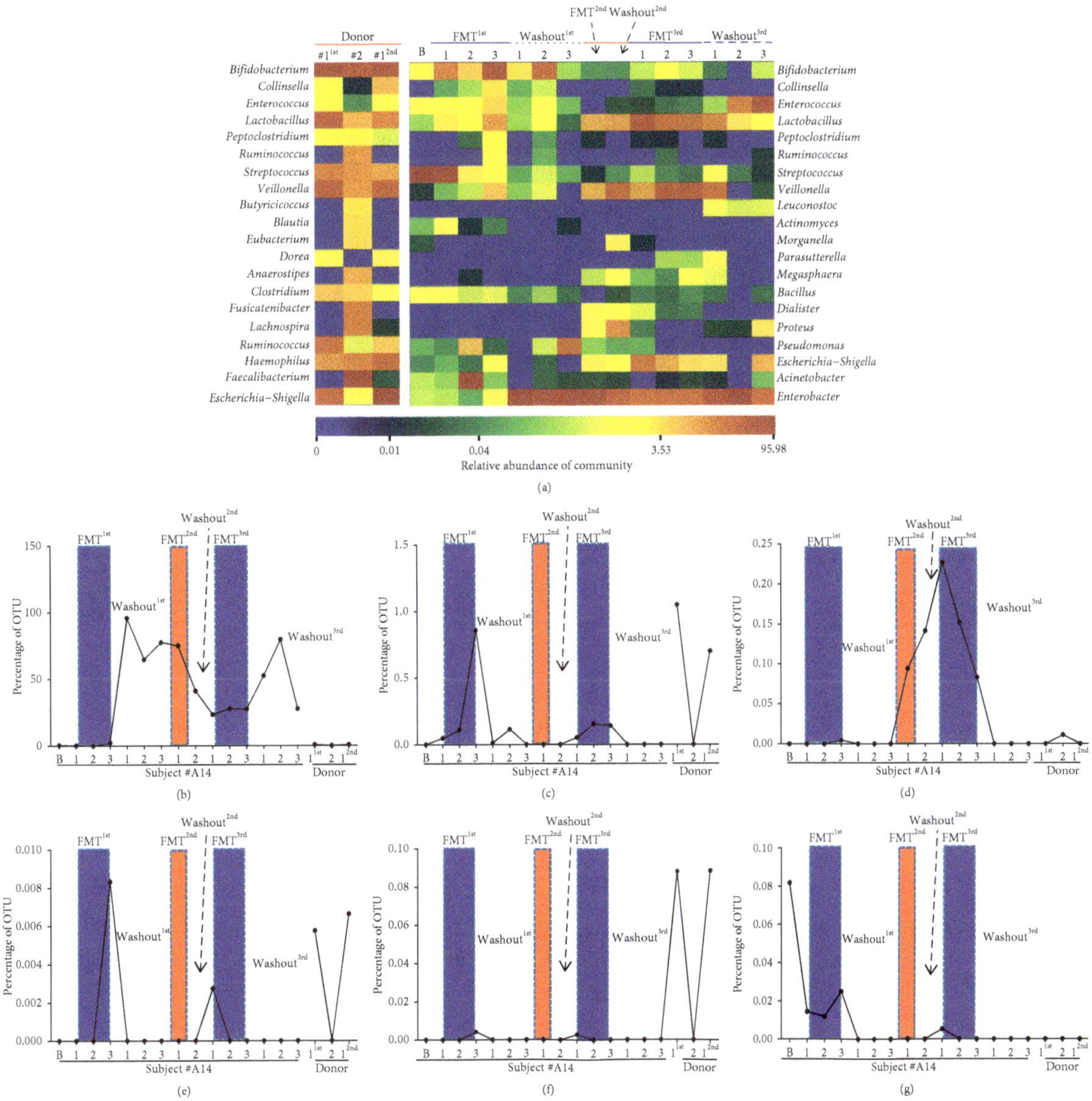

FIGURE 3: Dynamic changes in composition in the intestinal microbiota. (a) OTU heatmap of all the samples from both donors and the recipient during the entire FMT process. The thermal analysis shows the top 20 OTUs based on their relative abundances. The names on the left are the species annotations for each outlined OTU, and the color value of each square in each row indicates the relative abundance of that OTU. Dynamic changes in 6 OTUs were selected (b–g) from the 114 identified OTUs of patient #A19 based on their sensitivity to FMT.

attempts to solve this problem by using feces from two infants with different dietary patterns.

The community of microorganisms within the human gut is critical to health and functions with a level of complexity comparable to that of an organ system [37]. Therefore, dysbiosis of the intestinal microbiome has been implicated in a number of diarrheal diseases [38, 39]. Alterations in the intestinal microbial community have been observed in recurrent *C. difficile*-associated diarrhea [39]. Although *C. difficile* infection was not found in this HSCT patient, the diversity and fitness levels of the fecal microbiome were extremely low at baseline compared with those of a healthy person. Thus, we tried to use feces from healthy donors to rebuild the intestinal microecology of this severe diarrheal patient undergoing HSCT. As we assumed, the diversity and richness of the patient's microbiome were significantly improved after FMT, regardless of the donor that we used. In accordance with previous reports [40, 41], we also found that the bacteria of the two infant donors were largely restricted to a small subset of the bacterial world, namely, *Bifidobacteria*, *Streptococci*, and *Lactobacillus* spp. Increasing evidence has now demonstrated that some microbial species (e.g., *Lactobacilli* and *Streptococcus*) can restore the disrupted gut epithelium that causes the diarrhea commonly experienced by HSCT patients through upregulation or phosphorylation of tight junction proteins [42–44]. Despite this, there was an obvious difference in diarrhea treatment outcomes between these two FMT donors. Through a small FMT substitution, we observed that stool volume and frequency were reduced when we used feces from donor #1, but these effects were not observed after the transplant from donor #2. Our and previous studies have

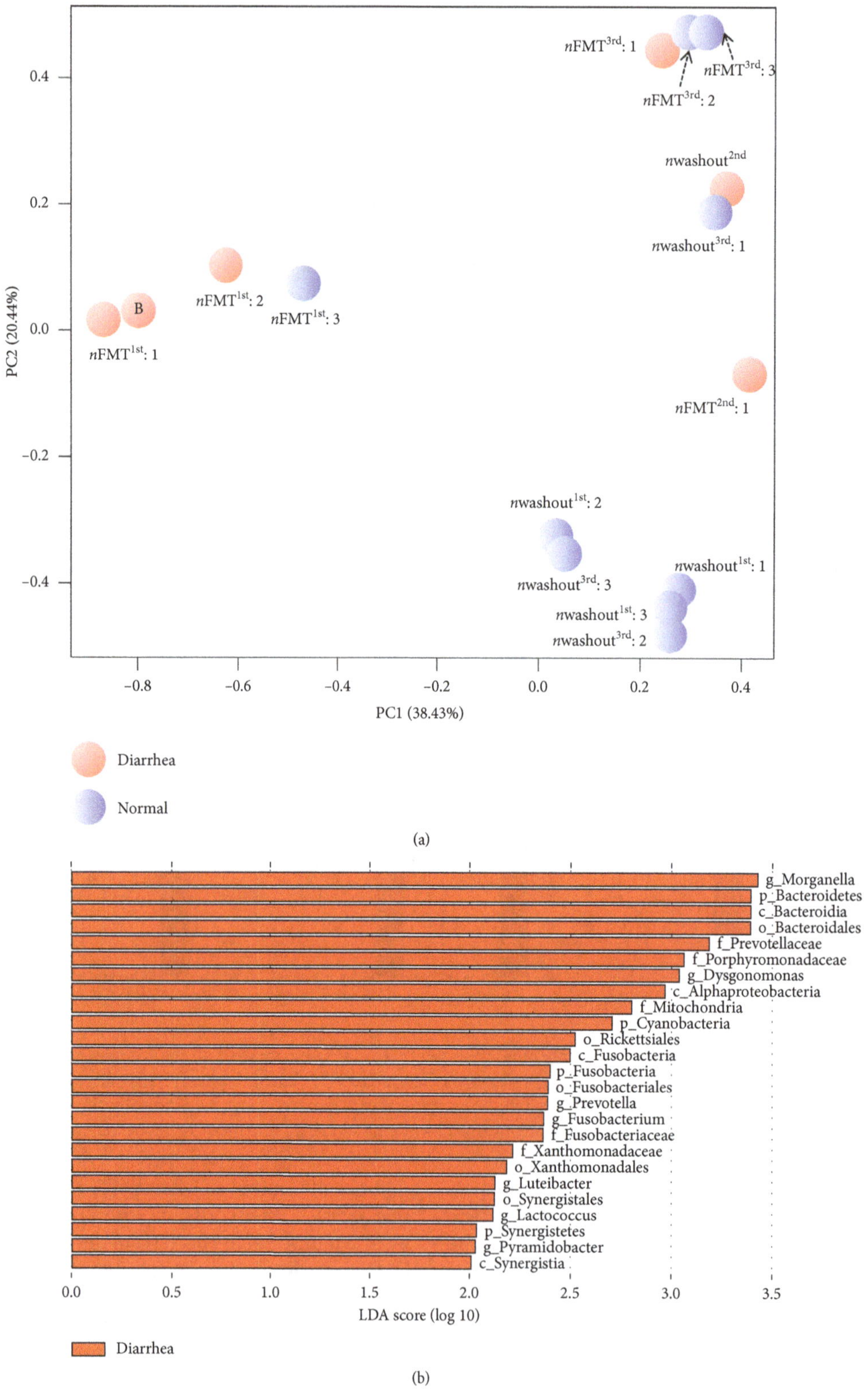

Figure 4: The differences in microbiota species between diarrhea and nondiarrhea stages. (a) Principal coordinates analysis of microbiota species composition of all samples during the whole study. Principal coordinate 1 (PC1, x-axis) explains 38.43% of the variance, and principal coordinate 2 (PC2, y-axis) explains 20.44% of the variation in Bray–Curtis dissimilarity between samples grouped by diarrhea status (pink circle = diarrhea, blue circle = normal). (b) LDA coupled with effect size measurements identifies the most differentially abundant taxa between diarrhea and normal status. Diarrhea-enriched taxa are indicated with a positive LDA score (red). No obvious differentially abundant taxa were observed in samples with normal status (not shown). Only taxa meeting an LDA significance threshold of >2 are shown.

shown that not all FMT is fully effective. Thus, choosing an appropriate FMT donor is particularly important for clinicians when they use FMT to treat diarrhea. However, the mechanisms underlying the beneficial role of FMT in diarrhea have been poorly understood until now, especially for noninfectious diarrhea.

To more precisely address the roles of stool donors in the outcomes of diarrhea in HSCT patients, we comprehensively profiled the dietary patterns of the donors and recipient and the dynamic changes in the intestinal microbiota using a small FMT substitution. Given that HSCT is an intensely immunosuppressive procedure, for safety reasons, we chose two 1-year-old infants whose feeding patterns were relatively simple as FMT donors. During the first year of life, the human infant intestinal microbiome undergoes rapid maturation [45] and is similar to that of an adult in some regions [46]. Importantly, feeding pattern has been shown to influence the structure and function of the intestinal microbiota in infants [45]. Consistent with a previous study [47], we identified Bifidobacteriaceae and *Faecalibacterium* as the dominant taxa in the stool of the exclusively breastfed donor #2 (Figure 3(a)). In contrast, the introduction of solid foods has been associated with increased populations of *Bacteroides* [48] and decreased populations of *Bifidobacteria*, *Enterobacteria*, and some *Clostridium* species [49]. Although the predominant bacterial families in mixed-fed infants have not been well characterized [45], here we found that the microbiome of the mixed-fed infant (donor #1) was more diverse, with greater proportions of *Bifidobacterium*, *Lactobacillus*, *Streptococcus*, *Veillonella*, *Clostridium*, *Ruminococcus*, *Haemophilus*, and *Escherichia-Shigella* (Figure 3(a)). The mixed feeding pattern exposes infants to nondigestible plant carbohydrates, animal protein, and fats, providing new substrates for the survival and dominance of bacterial species not supported by breast milk [49]. The different microbial configurations were also associated with functional shifts, as the increased abundance of *Bacteroides* promoted by the introduction of solid foods has been correlated with increased short-chain fatty acid levels [48].

Antibiotic-associated diarrhea can be reduced to 8% in patients with the administration of *Lactobacillus casei* ssp. *rhamnosus* (*Lactobacillus GG*) [50]. Animal experiments have also confirmed that prophylactic administration of VSL #3 (a mixture of four species of *Lactobacilli*, three species of *Bifidobacteria*, and *Saccharomyces boulardii*) can prevent irinotecan-related diarrhea, and *Lactobacillus GG* can reduce the frequency of severe diarrhea caused by 5FU-based chemotherapy [51]. In our case, *Bifidobacterium* accounted for 29.9% of the OTUs in the stool of donor #1 and 18.1% in the stool of donor #2 (Figure 3(a)); meanwhile, *Lactobacillus* accounted for 16.3% and 2.9% in the stools of donor #1 and donor #2, respectively (Figure 3(a)). Interestingly, the microbiota of donor #1 was characterized as having greater proportions of *Escherichia-Shigella* (11.3%) than that of donor #2 (0.6%). Furthermore, through longitudinal monitoring of the patient, we outlined 6 OTUs that were more sensitive to changes caused by FMT (OTU_01: *Enterobacter* spp., OTU_29: *Lactobacillus* spp., OTU_52: *Campylobacter* spp., OTU_104: *Ezakiella* spp., OTU_80: *Edwardsiella* spp., and OTU_86: *Luteibacter* spp.) among the 114 recognized OTUs (Figures 3(b)–3(g)). According to the outcomes of diarrhea, *Lactobacillus* spp. (OTU_29) might have been one of the possible factors, reducing the incidence of diarrhea when we used stool from donor #1.

Overall, we report the confirmation of the safety of FMT for treating an HSCT patient with diarrhea. FMT offers promise as a potential treatment option for noninfectious diarrhea after HSCT. Importantly, the therapeutic outcomes of diarrhea were somewhat related to the choice of FMT donors. Here, we found that 1-year-old infants can serve as safe FMT donors for treating diarrhea in HSCT patients. Furthermore, the overall diversity of the intestinal microbiota may not be the only important element in the selection of an effective FMT donor. The richness of probiotics, including *Lactobacillus*, *Bifidobacteria*, and *Saccharomyces boulardii*, might be the key factor in choosing the right FMT donor when clinicians treat noninfectious diarrhea. Because this was a small FMT substitution, we are expanding this work by building a larger cohort and using a machine learning method to predict the effects of FMT on diarrhea treatment in leukemia patients by analyzing the intestinal microbiota of FMT donors and recipients.

Abbreviations

HSCT:	Hematopoietic stem cell transplantation
FMT:	Fecal microbiota transplant
GVHD:	Graft-versus-host disease
PCoA:	Principal coordinates analysis
OTUs:	Operational taxonomic units
LEfSe:	Linear discriminant analysis effect size
LDA:	Linear discriminant analysis
FMT^{1st}:	The first FMT
FMT^{2nd}:	The second FMT
FMT^{3rd}:	The third FMT
$Washout^{1st}$:	The first washout
$Washout^{2nd}$:	The second washout
$Washout^{3rd}$:	The third washout
$nFMT^{1st}$, $nFMT^{2nd}$, and $nFMT^{3rd}$:	*n* is the time of sample collection during the FMT phase
$nwashout^{1st}$, $nwashout^{2nd}$, and $nwashout^{3rd}$:	*n* is the time of sample collection during the washout phase.

Authors' Contributions

G. R. and J. Z. were involved in the conception of this study. G. R. designed and funded the study. J. Z. recruited subjects and provided clinical information. M. L. conducted FMT and collected samples. G. R. analyzed the data and wrote the manuscript. P. L. and S. Y. were involved in study coordination.

Acknowledgments

This study was supported by the National Natural Science Foundation of China (81703221 to G. R.), Beijing Natural Science Foundation (no. 7192241 to G. R.), and the Special Fund for Basic Scientific Research (nos. 1610422016003 to G. R. and 1610422017007 to G. R.). The authors are very grateful to the patient and the FMT donors who participated in this study.

References

[1] M. G. van KraaijA. W. Dekker et al., "Infectious gastroenteritis: an uncommon cause of diarrhoea in adult allogeneic and autologous stem cell transplant recipients," *Bone Marrow Transplantation*, vol. 26, no. 3, pp. 299–303, 2000.

[2] D. Bobak, L. M. Arfons, R. J. Creger, and H. M. Lazarus, "Clostridium difficile-associated disease in human stem cell transplant recipients: coming epidemic or false alarm?," *Bone Marrow Transplantation*, vol. 42, no. 11, pp. 705–713, 2008.

[3] R. Avery, B. Pohlman, K. Adal et al., "High prevalence of diarrhea but infrequency of documented Clostridium difficile in autologous peripheral blood progenitor cell transplant recipients," *Bone Marrow Transplantation*, vol. 25, no. 1, pp. 67–69, 2000.

[4] M. Tomblyn, L. Gordon, S. Singhal et al., "Rarity of toxigenic Clostridium difficile infections after hematopoietic stem cell transplantation: implications for symptomatic management of diarrhea," *Bone Marrow Transplantation*, vol. 30, no. 8, pp. 517–519, 2002.

[5] L. R. Schiller, "Antidiarrheal drug therapy," *Current Gastroenterology Reports*, vol. 19, no. 5, p. 18, 2017.

[6] V. Buccigrossi, E. Nicastro, and A. Guarino, "Functions of intestinal microflora in children," *Current Opinion in Gastroenterology*, vol. 29, no. 1, pp. 31–38, 2013.

[7] S. Monira, S. A. Shabnam, N. H. Alam, H. P. Endtz, A. Cravioto, and M. Alam, "16S rRNA gene-targeted TTGE in determining diversity of gut microbiota during acute diarrhoea and convalescence," *Journal of Health, Population and Nutrition*, vol. 30, no. 3, pp. 250–256, 2012.

[8] G. Solano-Aguilar, K. P. Fernandez, H. Ets et al., "Characterization of fecal microbiota of children with diarrhea in 2 locations in Colombia," *Journal of Pediatric Gastroenterology and Nutrition*, vol. 56, no. 5, pp. 503–511, 2013.

[9] D. Vandeputte, G. Falony, S. Vieira-Silva, R. Y. Tito, M. Joossens, and J. Raes, "Stool consistency is strongly associated with gut microbiota richness and composition, enterotypes and bacterial growth rates," *Gut*, vol. 65, no. 1, pp. 57–62, 2016.

[10] G. Falony, M. Joossens, S. Vieira-Silva et al., "Population-level analysis of gut microbiome variation," *Science*, vol. 352, no. 6285, pp. 560–564, 2016.

[11] M. Pop, A. W. Walker, J. Paulson et al., "Diarrhea in young children from low-income countries leads to large-scale alterations in intestinal microbiota composition," *Genome Biology*, vol. 15, no. 6, p. R76, 2014.

[12] C. Ma, X. Wu, M. Nawaz et al., "Molecular characterization of fecal microbiota in patients with viral diarrhea," *Current Microbiology*, vol. 63, no. 3, pp. 259–266, 2011.

[13] G. J. Cox, S. M. Matsui, R. S. Lo et al., "Etiology and outcome of diarrhea after marrow transplantation: a prospective study," *Gastroenterology*, vol. 107, no. 5, pp. 1398–1407, 1994.

[14] W. Huang, A. Bush, N. J. Chao, B. J. Chen, and A. D. Sung, "Syngeneic fecal microbiota transplant effectively attenuated graft-versus-host disease after bone marrow transplantation in mice," *Blood*, vol. 130, p. 4435, 2017.

[15] R. R. Jenq, Y. Taur, S. M. Devlin et al., "Intestinal blautia is associated with reduced death from graft-versus-host disease," *Biology of Blood and Marrow Transplantation*, vol. 21, no. 8, pp. 1373–1383, 2015.

[16] Y. Taur, J. B. Xavier, L. Lipuma et al., "Intestinal domination and the risk of bacteremia in patients undergoing allogeneic hematopoietic stem cell transplantation," *Clinical Infectious Diseases*, vol. 55, no. 7, pp. 905–914, 2012.

[17] Y. Shono, M. D. Docampo, J. U. Peled et al., "Increased GVHD-related mortality with broad-spectrum antibiotic use after allogeneic hematopoietic stem cell transplantation in human patients and mice," *Science Translational Medicine*, vol. 8, no. 339, article 339ra371, 2016.

[18] E. Holler, P. Butzhammer, K. Schmid et al., "Metagenomic analysis of the stool microbiome in patients receiving allogeneic stem cell transplantation: loss of diversity is associated with use of systemic antibiotics and more pronounced in gastrointestinal graft-versus-host disease," *Biology of Blood and Marrow Transplantation*, vol. 20, no. 5, pp. 640–645, 2014.

[19] A. Khoruts and M. J. Sadowsky, "Understanding the mechanisms of faecal microbiota transplantation," *Nature Reviews Gastroenterology & Hepatology*, vol. 13, no. 9, pp. 508–516, 2016.

[20] Y. Ma, J. Liu, C. Rhodes, Y. Nie, and F. Zhang, "Ethical issues in fecal microbiota transplantation in practice," *American Journal of Bioethics*, vol. 17, no. 5, pp. 34–45, 2017.

[21] J. Carmo, S. Marques, I. Chapim et al., "Leaping forward in the treatment of Clostridium difficile infection: update in 2015," *GE Portuguese Journal of Gastroenterology*, vol. 22, no. 6, pp. 259–267, 2015.

[22] K. Kakihana, Y. Fujioka, W. Suda et al., "Fecal microbiota transplantation for patients with steroid-resistant acute graft-versus-host disease of the gut," *Blood*, vol. 128, no. 16, pp. 2083–2088, 2016.

[23] W. Spindelboeck, E. Schulz, B. Uhl et al., "Repeated fecal microbiota transplantations attenuate diarrhea and lead to sustained changes in the fecal microbiota in acute, refractory gastrointestinal graft-versus-host-disease," *Haematologica*, vol. 102, no. 5, pp. e210–e213, 2017.

[24] C. H. Lee, T. Steiner, E. O. Petrof et al., "Frozen vs fresh fecal microbiota transplantation and clinical resolution of diarrhea in patients with recurrent clostridium difficile infection: a randomized clinical trial," *JAMA*, vol. 315, no. 2, pp. 142–149, 2016.

[25] D. P. Faith and A. M. Baker, "Phylogenetic diversity (PD) and biodiversity conservation: some bioinformatics challenges," *Evolutionary Bioinformatics Online*, vol. 2, pp. 121–128, 2007.

[26] T. Andermann, J. U. Peled, C. Ho et al., "Microbiome-host interactions in hematopoietic stem cell transplant recipients," *Biology of Blood and Marrow Transplantation*, vol. 24, no. 7, pp. 1322–1340, 2018.

[27] D. Graf, R. D. Cagno, F. Fåk et al., "Contribution of diet to the composition of the human gut microbiota," *Microbial Ecology in Health & Disease*, vol. 26, article 26164, 2015.

[28] J. Andreyev, P. Ross, C. Donnellan et al., "Guidance on the management of diarrhoea during cancer chemotherapy," *Lancet Oncology*, vol. 15, no. 10, pp. e447–e460, 2014.

[29] M. J. Hamilton, A. R. Weingarden, M. J. Sadowsky, and A. Khoruts, "Standardized frozen preparation for trans-

plantation of fecal microbiota for recurrent Clostridium difficile infection," *American Journal of Gastroenterology*, vol. 107, no. 5, pp. 761–767, 2012.

[30] C. P. Kelly, "Current strategies for management of initial Clostridium difficile infection," *Journal of Hospital Medicine*, vol. 7, no. 3, pp. S5–S10, 2012.

[31] J. Bilinski, P. Grzesiowski, N. Sorensen et al., "Fecal microbiota transplantation in patients with blood disorders inhibits gut colonization with antibiotic-resistant bacteria: results of a prospective, single-center study," *Clinical Infectious Diseases*, vol. 65, no. 3, pp. 364–370, 2017.

[32] Z. DeFilipp, J. U. Peled, S. Li et al., "Third-party fecal microbiota transplantation following allo-HCT reconstitutes microbiome diversity," *Blood Advances*, vol. 2, no. 7, pp. 745–753, 2018.

[33] C. R. Kelly, C. Ihunnah, M. Fischer et al., "Fecal microbiota transplant for treatment of Clostridium difficile infection in immunocompromised patients," *American Journal of Gastroenterology*, vol. 109, no. 7, pp. 1065–1071, 2014.

[34] T. Odamaki, K. Kato, H. Sugahara et al., "Age-related changes in gut microbiota composition from newborn to centenarian: a cross-sectional study," *BMC Microbiology*, vol. 16, no. 1, p. 90, 2016.

[35] H. B. Xu, R. H. Jiang, and H. B. Sheng, "Meta-analysis of the effects of Bifidobacterium preparations for the prevention and treatment of pediatric antibiotic-associated diarrhea in China," *Complementary Therapies in Medicine*, vol. 33, pp. 105–113, 2017.

[36] J. C. Madan, A. G. Hoen, S. N. Lundgren et al., "Association of cesarean delivery and formula supplementation with the intestinal microbiome of 6-week-old infants," *JAMA Pediatrics*, vol. 170, no. 3, pp. 212–219, 2016.

[37] C. R. Kelly, S. Kahn, P. Kashyap et al., "Update on fecal microbiota transplantation 2015: indications, methodologies, mechanisms, and outlook," *Gastroenterology*, vol. 149, no. 1, pp. 223–237, 2015.

[38] J. Halfvarson, C. J. Brislawn, R. Lamendella et al., "Dynamics of the human gut microbiome in inflammatory bowel disease," *Nature Microbiology*, vol. 2, no. 5, p. 17004, 2017.

[39] J. Y. Chang, D. A. Antonopoulos, A. Kalra et al., "Decreased diversity of the fecal Microbiome in recurrent clostridium difficile-associated diarrhea," *Journal of Infectious Diseases*, vol. 197, no. 3, pp. 435–438, 2008.

[40] P. L. Stark and A. Lee, "The microbial ecology of the large bowel of breast-fed and formula-fed infants during the first year of life," *Journal of Medical Microbiology*, vol. 15, no. 2, pp. 189–203, 1982.

[41] C. Palmer, E. M. Bik, D. B. DiGiulio, D. A. Relman, and P. O. Brown, "Development of the human infant intestinal microbiota," *PLoS Biology*, vol. 5, no. 7, article e177, 2007.

[42] A. Seth, F. Yan, D. B. Polk, and R. K. Rao, "Probiotics ameliorate the hydrogen peroxide-induced epithelial barrier disruption by a PKC- and MAP kinase-dependent mechanism," *American Journal of Physiology-Gastrointestinal and Liver Physiology*, vol. 294, no. 4, pp. G1060–1069, 2008.

[43] S. Resta-Lenert and K. E. Barrett, "Live probiotics protect intestinal epithelial cells from the effects of infection with enteroinvasive *Escherichia coli* (EIEC)," *Gut*, vol. 52, pp. 988–997, 2003.

[44] S. Resta-Lenert and K. E. Barrett, "Probiotics and commensals reverse TNF-alpha- and IFN-gamma-induced dysfunction in human intestinal epithelial cells," *Gastroenterology*, vol. 130, no. 3, pp. 731–746, 2006.

[45] A. L. Thompson, A. Monteagudo-Mera, M. B. Cadenas, M. L. Lampl, and M. A. Azcarate-Peril, "Milk- and solid-feeding practices and daycare attendance are associated with differences in bacterial diversity, predominant communities, and metabolic and immune function of the infant gut microbiome," *Frontiers in Cellular and Infection Microbiology*, vol. 5, p. 3, 2015.

[46] F. Backhed, J. Roswall, Y. Peng et al., "Dynamics and stabilization of the human gut microbiome during the first year of life," *Cell Host & Microbe*, vol. 17, no. 6, p. 852, 2015.

[47] G. W. Tannock, B. Lawley, K. Munro et al., "Comparison of the compositions of the stool microbiotas of infants fed goat milk formula, cow milk-based formula, or breast milk," *Applied and Environmental Microbiology*, vol. 79, no. 9, pp. 3040–3048, 2013.

[48] J. E. Koenig, A. Spor, N. Scalfone et al., "Succession of microbial consortia in the developing infant gut microbiome," *Proceedings of the National Academy of Sciences*, vol. 108, no. 1, pp. 4578–4585, 2011.

[49] M. Fallani, S. Amarri, A. Uusijarvi et al., "Determinants of the human infant intestinal microbiota after the introduction of first complementary foods in infant samples from five European centres," *Microbiology*, vol. 157, no. 5, pp. 1385–1392, 2011.

[50] J. A. Vanderhoof, "Lactobacillus GG in the prevention of antibiotic-associated diarrhea in children," *Journal of Pediatrics*, vol. 135, pp. 564–568, 1999.

[51] P. Osterlund, T. Ruotsalainen, R. Korpela et al., "Lactobacillus supplementation for diarrhoea related to chemotherapy of colorectal cancer: a randomised study," *British Journal of Cancer*, vol. 97, no. 8, pp. 1028–1034, 2007.

28

A Rare Co-Occurrence of Triple Mutations in *JAK2*, *CALR* and *MPL* in the Same Patient with Myelofibrosis

Sherine J. Thomas[1] **and D. P. Dash**[2]

[1]*Hematology and Oncology, Northside Hospital Cancer Institute, Georgia Cancer Specialists, Atlanta, GA, USA*
[2]*Molecular Oncology & Genetics (MOGL), Versiti Wisconsin (Formerly Known as Blood Center Wisconsin), Milwaukee, WI, USA*

Correspondence should be addressed to Sherine J. Thomas; sherine.thomas@gacancer.com

Academic Editor: Tatsuharu Ohno

Background. The diagnosis and prognostication of myeloproliferative neoplasm rely on the presence of driver mutations in JAK2, calreticulin (CALR), and MPL mutations. In the past, the presence of these mutations was thought to be mutually exclusive. Since then, there have been multiple reports of the presence of dual mutations. The presence of all three driver mutations in the same patient with myelofibrosis has not been previously described. Case. A 73-year-old female underwent a hematological workup in our facility after a routine hemogram performed prior to complex ophthalmological surgery revealed severe thrombocytosis. A comprehensive workup including an NGS panel for MPN driver mutations demonstrated that she had a calreticulin type-1 mutation, a JAK2 exon 14 (JAK2L611S) mutation, and an abnormal hotspot variant for MPL with VAF1%. A bone marrow biopsy confirmed a myeloproliferative neoplasm with grade 2 reticulin fibrosis suggesting primary myelofibrosis. Molecular profiling of bone marrow confirmed the previously noted mutations and an MPLW515R mutation. The patient was started on treatment with hydroxyurea and aspirin with improvement in platelet count and resolution of anemia. Discussion. The clinical significance of the presence of multiple driver mutations in the same patient is not well understood at this time. There have been 11 publications between 2014 and 2020 that have described dual mutations of JAK2V617F, MPL, and CALR mutations. The JAK2 exon 14 mutation noted, in this case, is JAK2L611S which has not previously been reported in MPN and only reported in 5 cases in the COSMIC database. The JAK2 exon 14 mutation identified in this case is not an established driver mutation for myeloproliferative neoplasm, and its clinical implication remains unknown. Conclusions. The above case in addition to recent case reports and case series supports the use of broader NGS sequencing panels for diagnosis and prognostication of MPN. These mutations should not be considered mutually exclusive. The clinical behavior and prognosis of the subgroup with multiple mutations need to be studied in larger series.

1. Introduction

The molecular basis of myeloproliferative neoplasms (MPNs) came into the limelight in 2005 with the identification of *JAK2* mutations in almost all cases of polycythemia vera and most essential thrombocythemia (ET) [1–4]. In 2006, somatic mutations in myeloproliferative leukemia virus oncogene (*MPL*) provided additional mechanistic understanding of the JAK-STAT pathway activation in MPN [5]. In 2013, somatic mutations in calreticulin (*CALR*) were reported as a driver mutation of essential thrombocythemia [6].

In clinical practice, these three driver mutations serve as diagnostic and prognostic markers during workup of myeloproliferative neoplasms. JAK2 mutations are present in most cases of polycythemia vera. Somatic mutation of codon 515 in exon 10 of the "myeloproliferative leukemia virus oncogene" (*MPL*) is found in an estimated 3-4% of patients with essential thrombocythemia (ET) and 7% of patients with primary myelofibrosis (PMF). Somatic mutations in calreticulin (CALR) are present in 25–30% of patients with essential thrombocytosis (ET) and primary myelofibrosis (PMF). CALR mutations have rarely been described in polycythemia vera. Importantly, mutations in *CALR* have previously been reported to be mutually exclusive with *JAK2* or *MPL* mutations [6–8].

More recently, several case reports and case series have reported the coexistence of two driver mutations in Philadelphia chromosome-negative MPN, but these are known to be rare events. The presence of triple mutations in *JAK2*, *CALR*, and *MPL* in the same patient with MPN has not been previously reported, and therefore, here, we intend to present this unique case report.

2. Case

A 73-year-old African American female with a medical history of glaucoma and cataracts presented for hematology evaluation after routine hemogram performed before eye surgery demonstrated thrombocytosis and anemia. Her hemogram demonstrated hemoglobin of 9.9 g/dL and hematocrit of 31.1%. WBC count was normal at 9300/mcL, absolute neutrophil count was 5952 mcg/dL, basophils were 3% with absolute basophil count 279/mcL, monocytes were 14%, and absolute monocyte count was 1302/microliter. Platelet count was elevated to 750,000/mcL. She underwent workup for iron deficiency which showed a normal iron panel. Evaluation for myeloproliferative disorder (MPN) driver mutations was also performed.

The patient's peripheral blood sample was obtained for targeted gene sequencing. DNA extracted from peripheral blood was amplified via PCR with primers specific for gene targets—*ABL1, ASXL1, BCOR, BRAF, CLAR, CDKN2A, CBL, CEBPA, CSF3R, DNMT3A, ETV6, EZH2, FLT3, GATA2, HRAS, IDH1, IDH2, FBXW7, IKZF1, JAK2, KIT, KRAS, MPL, MYD88, NF1, NPM1, NRAS, PHF6, PTEN, PTPN11, PRPF8, RB1, RUNX1, SETBP1, SF3B1, SH2B3, SRSF2, STAG2, TET2, TP53, UAF1, WT1,* and *ZRSR2.* Specific genomic regions were targeted using a customized AmpliSeq Myeloid Next-Generation Sequencing (NGS) panel (Illumina), and sequencing by synthesis chemistry with paired-end 201 base pair read was performed. Bioinformatics sequence analysis pipeline was customized to limit analysis for only MPN gene targets.

Gene targets analyzed included all exons for *CALR* and selected exons with a high prevalence for the presence of pathogenic variants *JAK2* (exons 12–15) and *MPL* (exons 3, 4, 10, and 12).

The following abnormal gene alterations were identified:

(1) *CALR* p.(Leu367ThrfsTer46) with a variant allele frequency of 46.5% (c.1099_1150delCTTAAGGAG GAGGAAGACAAGAAACGCAAAGAGGAGGAG GAGGCAGAGG) (52 bp deletion, type 1).

(2) She was also found to have *JAK2* p.(Leu611Ser) with variant allele frequency 23.2% (c.1832T > C).

(3) In addition to the above, abnormal testing for hotspot variant *MPL* p. Trp515Arg was detected with VAF 1%, which is below the level of detection for that test (1.75%): variant depth 56 and total depth 5554. Confirmatory testing with higher sensitive PCR-based locked nucleic acid (LNA) demonstrated the same *MPL* mutation (p. Trp515Arg (W515R)) (tier I variant: NM_005373.2). The confirmatory testing for *MPL* exon 10 mutation analysis is validated based on locked nucleic acid (LNA) methods for the *MPL* W515R codon which offers a higher sensitivity than traditional Sanger sequencing assays. Based on the LNA methods of detection, the higher sensitive MPL assay can detect mutation at the *MPL* W515R codon with low allele burden as low as 2% or below.

Given the unusual genetic mutation profile, a bone marrow biopsy was undertaken to quantify bone marrow fibrosis.

Flow cytometry on the bone marrow aspirate specimen failed to identify any unique cell populations of myeloid or lymphoid origin. A small population of cells identified by surface markers, CD13, CD22, low-density CD20 5, moderate CD33, bright CD38, moderate CD45, bright CD123, and negative for CD19, and by side scatter properties as basophils were noted to comprise 2% of the total nucleated sample. Monocytes were 6% of the nucleated sample, granulocytes 59%, and lymphocytes 25%.

Morphologically, the core biopsy demonstrated a hypercellular marrow (95% cellularity) with trilineage hematopoiesis, myeloid-to-erythroid ratio >5 : 1, with atypical megakaryocytic hyperplasia, moderately increased fibrosis, but no increase in blasts (Figures 1 and 2). Karyotype was noted to be normal-46, XX [20].

Based on the above workup, the patient was diagnosed with chronic myeloproliferative neoplasm-primary myelofibrosis.

The patient was started on treatment with hydroxyurea for cytoreduction and on aspirin for thromboprophylaxis, with improvement in the platelet count (Figure 3). She had improvement and normalization of hemoglobin (Figure 4).

Peak platelet count was 976,000/mcL at the time of initiation of cytoreductive therapy with hydroxyurea. Within 4 months of starting cytoreduction with hydroxyurea, the patient was noted to have normalization of the platelet count to 220,000/mcL. WBC count and neutrophils remained stable, and anemia resolved. The patient remained stable and continued to tolerate hydroxyurea therapy. She has remained on aspirin for thromboprophylaxis.

3. Discussion

The presence of driver mutations has diagnostic, prognostic, and therapeutic implications in myeloproliferative disorders. To our knowledge, this is the first case of a patient with ET identified to have triple mutations *JAK2* L611S, *CALR* type 1, and tier 1, *MPL* W515R, co-occurring in the same patient.

As mentioned above, the presence of multiple driver mutations in patients with MPN is well described, but they are rare events. For example, in a study evaluating the prevalence of MPN driver mutations in 928 Chinese patients, the *JAK2* V617F and *CALR* exon 9 dual mutation was identified in six (0.6%) patients, and the coexistence of *JAK2* V617F and *MPL* exon 10 was even more uncommon, occurring in two (0.2%) patients [9].

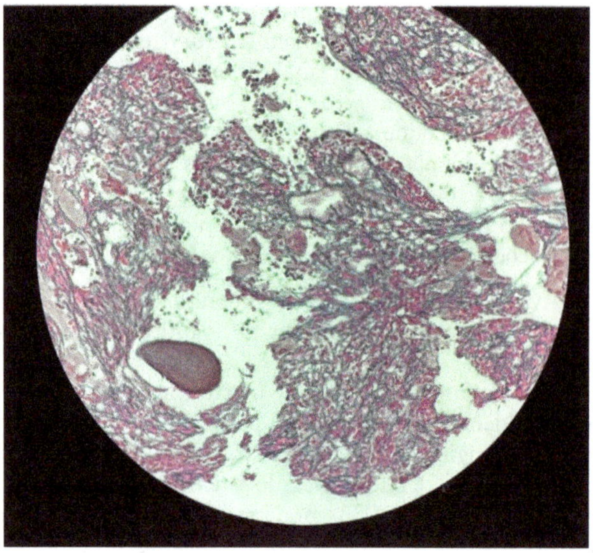

Figure 1: Reticulin-stained bone marrow core biopsy showing increased reticulin fibrosis. WHO* classification MF2 (*World Health Organization).

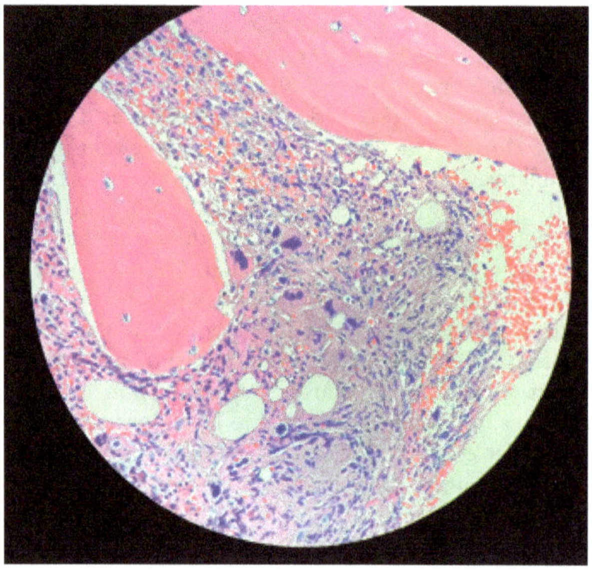

Figure 2: H&E-stained section of bone marrow core biopsy showing atypical megakaryocytic hyperplasia.

JAK2 V617F mutation was the first and the most well-characterized driver mutation in myeloproliferative neoplasm. The patient described in this report had a less common *JAK2* p.L611S mutation. We note that *JAK2* p.L611S mutation is not a recognized driver mutation in MPN. However, given the clinical relevance of *JAK2* mutations in MPN, we feel that this patient's less common *JAK2* mutation profile should be described.

3.1. JAK2 p.L611S Mutation. Janus kinase 2 (*JAK2*) helps in modulating response to extracellular cytokine signalling. While *JAK2* is a nonreceptor TKI, it needs a cognate receptor for response. Activated *JAK2* signalling is necessary for normal hematopoiesis including erythropoiesis and thrombopoiesis. Once activated, *JAK2* triggers recruitment and phosphorylation of downstream molecules such as STAT3/5 and MAP kinase which in turn allows the translocation of signalling molecules to the nucleus and thereby activates transcription of functional proteins.

JAK2 p.L611S is a missense mutation in exon 14 of the *JAK2* gene in chromosome 9. It results in the replacement of amino acid leucine to serine at codon 611 (p.L611S). This variant represents a hotspot mutation within the JAK2-JH1 interface including one in the JH2 domain (L611S) and is supposed to destabilize JH2-JH1 interaction and enhance *JAK2* signalling.

JAK2 p.L611S has been reported in the COSMIC database (COSV67633764, legacy identifier: COSM21361) for a total of 4 cases including PV (with comutation in *JAK2* V617F), AML in conjunction with Down syndrome myeloid disorder (DS-AMKL) (comutated with *GATA* and *NIPBL* and 7qdel, B-ALL, and squamous cell carcinoma (COSM21361, February 2021). *JAK2* p.L611S has been shown to be associated with tumorigenesis in animal models [10]. Although *JAK2* p.L611S mutation has not been reported with myelofibrosis or essential thrombocytosis, it has been reported in a child with congenital thrombocytosis.

3.2. Coexistence of Multiple Driver Mutations. Most cases of myeloproliferative neoplasm are known to harbour driver mutations *JAK2*, *MPL*, or *CALR* in a mutually exclusive manner [11]. However, there have been cases of rare patients with 2 coexisting mutations.

Co-occurrence of *CALR* and *MPL* has been reported in one patient from India [12]. Similarly, a case report from South Korea of 123 MPN patients reported the presence of *JAK2* and *CALR* mutations in 7 (4%) patients [13]. Another case from Korea in 2021 reported a case of comutation of *JAK2* V617F and MPL mutation [14].

A case series of 11 MPN patients published in 2018 with multiple driver mutations (including *BCR-ABL*) had 8 patients positive for *BCR-ABL* and *JAK2* V617F mutations, 1 patient positive for *BCR-ABL* and *CALR* type 2 mutations, and 2 patients (referenced in Table 1) negative for Philadelphia chromosome, and one each among them had *JAK2* V617F + *MPL*, *JAK2* V617F, and *CALR* mutations [22].

The clinical behaviour of patients with these rare comutations is not well understood because of the rarity of these events. The limited case reports regarding these comutations have provided some insights.

A previous case series has suggested that the presence of *JAK2* and *CALR* did not appear to affect the prognosis or clinical features of ET, thereby suggesting that the disease phenotype is dictated primarily by the *JAK2* mutation. They also noted that ET patients harboring mutations in the *JAK2* gene had inferior progression-free survival (PFS) regardless of the presence of a mutation in *CALR*. They also suggested that response to therapy was superior in patients bearing *JAK2* mutations as compared to patients with *CALR* mutations [16].

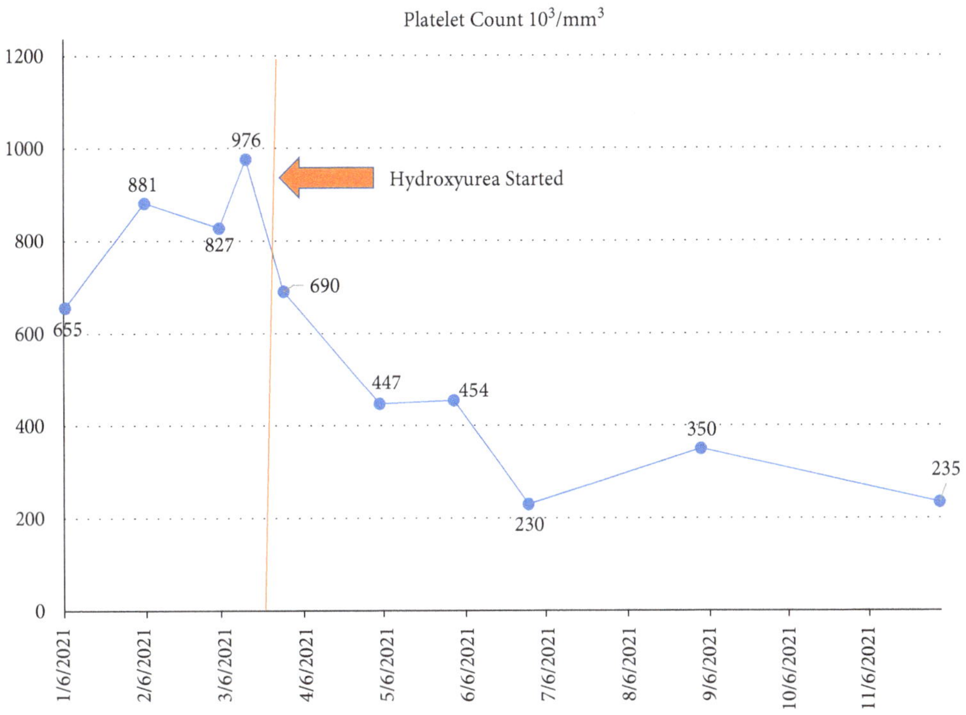

FIGURE 3: Graph of the platelet count at presentation and response to hydroxyurea.

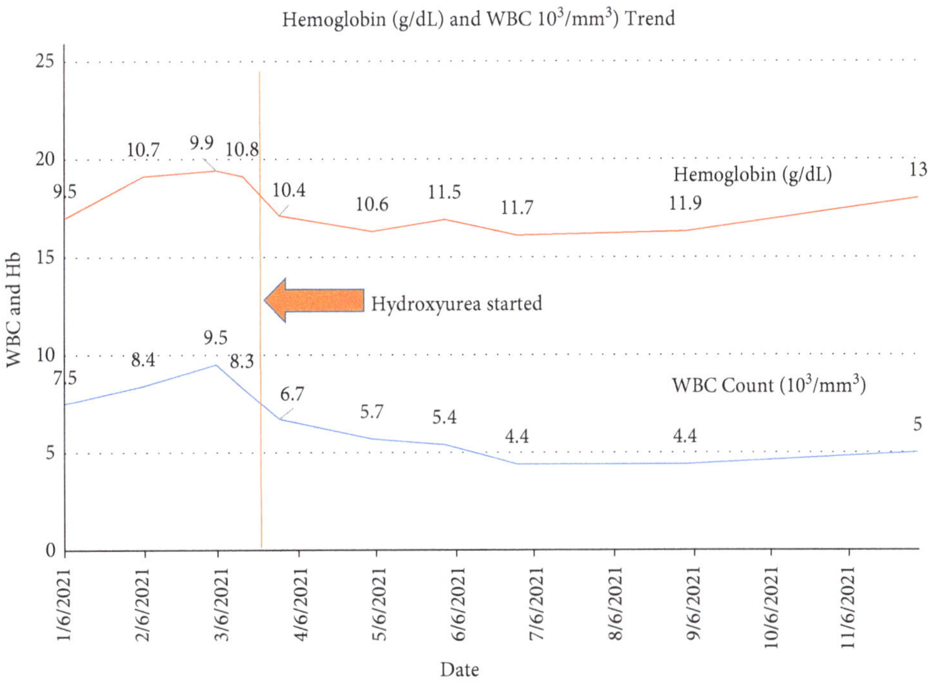

FIGURE 4: Graph of hemoglobin and white blood cell count trend and response to hydroxyurea.

Authors from a separate series suggested that the double mutated phenotype has a different clinical course compared to those with a single driver mutation [15].

Another larger case series of 40 double mutated patients with essential thrombocythemia showed that these patients with multiple mutations have a male predominance, the advanced age of onset, lower hemoglobin, and higher platelet count compared to the patients with a single mutation. However, the incidence of thrombosis was not different compared to patients with a single driver mutation [23].

The *JAK2* p.L611S mutation identified in this case has not been recognized as a driver mutation of myeloproliferative neoplasm. However, given the seminal role of *JAK2*

Table 1: A summary of case reports and case series with multiple driver mutations present in patients with ET and PMF.

No.	Author	N	MPN	JAK2 exon 14	JAK2 exon 12	MPL	CALR	Year
1	McGaffin et al. [15]	1	—	V617F	—	—	Type 6 (48 bp del)	2014
2	Kang et al. [16]	7	ET	V617F	—	—	All types (1, 2, and3)	2016
3	Rashid et al. [17]	1	ET	V617F	—	—	Type 1 (52 bp del)	2016
4	Cleyrat et al. [18]	1	ET	—	—	p.W515R	Type 1 (52 bp del)	2017
		12	—	V617F	—	Type not reported	—	2017
5	Jeromin et al. [19]	6	—	V617F	—	—	Type unreported	
		1	—	—	—	Type not reported	Type unreported	
		3	ET	V617F	—	W515L	—	2017
6	Usseglio et al. [20]	1	ET	V617F	—	W515R	—	
		4	ET	V617F	—	—	Type 1 (52 bp del)	
7	Boddu et al. [21]	1	ET	V617F (VAV <1%)	—	—	Type 1 (52 bp del)	
8	De Roeck et al. [22]	1	ET	V617F	—	p.W515R	—	2018
		1	PMF	V617F	—	—	Type 1 (52 bp del)	
		5	—	V617F (VAF <5%)	—	—	Type unreported	2018
		32	—	V617F	—	—	Type unreported	
9	Mansier et al. [23]	11	—	V617F	—	Type not reported	—	
		2	—	—	—	Type not reported	Type unreported	
		1	—	V617F	Type not reported	—	2 CALR mutations	
10	Ramanan et al. [12]	1	—	—	—	p.W515R (VAF 9.8%)	Type 1 52 bp deletion (VAF 13%)	2019
11	Zhou et al. [13]	1	PMF	—	—	p.X636W	CALR-p.364fs	2020

Table 1 is modified from Table 1 of Ramanan et al. [12].

mutations in these diseases, this patient's mutation profile is of interest.

4. Conclusion

To the best of our knowledge, this represents the first reported case of the coexistence of *JAK2* p.L611S, *CALR* type 1, and tier 1 *MPL* mutation in the same patient with essential thrombocythemia. It is also the first reported case of *JAK2* p.L611S in an adult with myelofibrosis. This case report highlights the increased recognition of cases with multiple mutations in *JAK2*, *MPL*, and *CALR*. Longer-term follow-up of patients with these comutations will lead to a greater understanding of their clinical behaviour and prognosis.

References

[1] C. James, V. Ugo, J. -P. Le Couédic et al., "A unique clonal *JAK2* mutation leading to constitutive signalling causes polycythaemia vera," *Nature*. vol. 434, no. 7037, pp. 1144–1148, 2005.

[2] R. Kralovics, F. Passamonti, A. S. Buser et al., "A gain-of-function mutation of *JAK2* in myeloproliferative disorders," *New England Journal of Medicine*, vol. 352, pp. 1779–1790, 2005.

[3] R. L. Levine, M. Wadleigh, J. Cools et al., "Activating mutation in the tyrosine kinase *JAK2* in polycythemia vera, essential thrombocythemia, and myeloid metaplasia with myelofibrosis," *Cancer Cell*, vol. 7, pp. 387–397, 2005.

[4] E. J. Baxter, L. M. Scott, P. J. Campbell et al., "Acquired mutation of the tyrosine kinase *JAK2* in human myeloproliferative disorders," *Lancet*, vol. 365, pp. 1054–1061, 2005.

[5] Y. Pikman, B. H. Lee, T. Mercher et al., "*MPL* W515L is a novel somatic activating mutation in myelofibrosis with myeloid metaplasia," *PLoS Medicine*, vol. 3, p. e270, 2006.

[6] T. Klampfl, H. Gisslinger, A. S. Harutyunyan et al., "Somatic mutations of calreticulin in myeloproliferative neoplasms," *New England Journal of Medicine*, vol. 369, no. 25, pp. 2379–2390, 2013.

[7] J. Nangalia, C. E. Massie, E. J. Baxter et al., "Somatic *CALR* mutations in myeloproliferative neoplasms with nonmutated *JAK2*," *New England Journal of Medicine*, vol. 369, no. 25, pp. 2391–2405, 2013.

[8] E. Rumi, D. Pietra, V. Ferretti et al., "*JAK2* or *CALR* mutation status defines subtypes of essential thrombocythemia with substantially different clinical course and outcomes," *Blood*, vol. 123, no. 10, pp. 1544–1551, 2014.

[9] Y. Lin, E. Liu, Q. Sun et al., "The Prevalence of *JAK2, MPL,* and *CALR* Mutations in Chinese Patients With *BCR-ABL1*-Negative Myeloproliferative Neoplasms," *American Journal of Clinical Pathology*, vol. 144, no. 1, pp. 165–171, 2015.

[10] M. Funakoshi-Tago, K. Tago, K. Sumi et al., "The acute lymphoblastic leukemia-associated *JAK2* L611S mutant induces tumorigenesis in nude mice," *Journal of Biological Chemistry*, vol. 284, no. 19, pp. 12680–12690, 2009.

[11] T. Ayalew and T. Barbui, "Polycythemia Vera and essential thrombocythemia: 2021 update on diagnosis, risk-stratification, and management," *American Journal of Hematology*, vol. 95, no. 12, pp. 1599–1613, Article ID 3297493920, 2020.

[12] V. Ramanan, K. Kelkar, S. Ranade et al., "The clinical utility of a custom-developed targeted next-generation sequencing assay for detection of mutations associated with Philadelphia negative journal of hematopathology (2019) 12:163-168-167 chronic myeloproliferative neoplasms: two case examples with *CALR* exon 9 mutations," *The International Journal of Molecular and Immuno Oncology*, vol. 1, pp. 28–34, 2016.

[13] F. P. Zhou, C. C. Wang, H. P. Du, S. B. Cao, and J. Zhang, "Primary myelofibrosis with concurrent *CALR* and *MPL* mutations: a case report," *World Journal of Clinical Cases*, vol. 8, no. 22, pp. 5618–5624, 2020.

[14] M. Jang, M. Y. Seo, K. J. Choi, and D. -S. Hong, "A rare case of ET with coexisting *JAK2* and *MPL* driver mutations," *Journal of Korean Medical Science*, vol. 35, 2020.

[15] G. McGaffin, K. harper, D. Stirling, and L. McLintock, "*JAK2* V617F and *CALR* mutations are not mutually exclusive, findings from retrospective analysis of a small patient cohort," *British Journal of Haematology*, vol. 167, pp. 276–278, 2014.

[16] M. G. Kang, H. -W. Choi, J. H. Lee et al., "Co-existence of *JAK2* and *CALR* mutations and their clinical implications in patients with ET.2016 Oncotarget, vol.7, no.35 57036-57049 Jang M.-A., M. Y. Seo, K. J. Choi and D. -S. Hong a rare case of ET with co-existing JAK2 and MPL driver mutations," *Journal of Korean Medical Science*, vol. 35, no. 23, 2020.

[17] M. Rashid, Z. Ahmed, S. Ahmed, M. Nadeem, N. Ahmed, and T. S. Shams, "Coexisting *JAK2* V617F and *CALR* exon 9 mutation in essential thrombocythaemia," *Indian Journal of Hematology and Blood Transfusion*, vol. 32, pp. 112–116, 2016.

[18] C. Cleyrat, D. S. Chabot-Richards, D. T. Lynch et al., "Leukemic transformation of post-essential thrombocythemia myelofibrosis: a unique case presenting with double MPL and CALR mutations," *Blood*, vol. 130, no. 1, p. 4215, 2017.

[19] S. Jeromin, M. Meggendorfer, and A. Fasan, "Frequency of concurrent BCR-ABL1, JAK2, CALR and MPL mutations in a cohort of 5,545 cases with suspected MPN by a deep sequencing approach," *EHA Learn Center*, vol. 2017, Article ID 181088, 2017.

[20] F. Usseglio, N. Beaufils, A. Calleja, S. Raynaud, and J. Gabert, "Detection of *CALR* and *MPL* mutations in low allelic burden JAK2 V617F essential thrombocythaemia," *Journal of Molecular Diagnostics*, vol. 91, pp. 92–98, 2017.

[21] P. Boddu, D. Chihara, L. Masarova, N. Pemmaraju, K. P. Patel, and S. Verstovsek, "The co-occurrence of driver mutations in chronic myeloproliferative neoplasms," *Annals of Hematology*, vol. 97, pp. 2071–2080, 2018.

[22] L. De Roeck, L. Michaux, K. Debackere, E. Lierman, P. Vandenberghe, and T. Devos, "Coexisting driver mutations in MPN: clinical and molecular characteristics of a series of 11 patients," *Hematology*, vol. 23, pp. 785–792, 2018.

[23] O. Mansier, D. L. Paz, J. C. Lanotto et al., "Clinical and biological characterization of MPN patients harboring two driver mutations, a French intergroup of myeloproliferative neoplasms (FIM) study," *American Journal of Hematology*, vol. 93, pp. E84–E109, 2018.

29

Sigmoid Venous Thrombosis in JAK2 V617F Mutated Polycythemia Vera

Cilomar Martins De Oliveira Filho and Alexander Gavralidis

Mass General Brigham, Salem Hospital, Salem, MA, USA

Correspondence should be addressed to Cilomar Martins De Oliveira Filho; cmartins5@mgb.org

Academic Editor: Stephen E. Langabeer

A 60-year-old female presented with headaches, blurry vision, diplopia, and dizziness for six weeks. Her workup revealed an elevated hematocrit, thrombocytosis, high ferritin, and normal erythropoietin. She was diagnosed with polycythemia vera with the JAK2 V617F mutation. The patient underwent magnetic resonance venography, which showed left-sided sigmoid venous thrombosis. She was placed on low-molecular-weight heparin, with a plan to transition to oral anticoagulation after four weeks and repeat imaging in three months to assess for resolution. Thrombotic events may occur in patients with polycythemia vera, and a JAK2 mutation further heightens that risk. Even so, intracranial venous thrombosis is not among the most common events, and it should be kept in the differential for any patient with myeloproliferative neoplasms presenting with new neurological symptoms.

1. Introduction

The risk of venous thromboembolism in myeloproliferative neoplasms (MPN), including polycythemia vera, is well established and not uncommon. However, primary venous thromboembolism occurring intracranially is rare. A large retrospective study found a disease-specific frequency of 1.2% for cerebral venous thrombosis (CVT) in patients with polycythemia vera [1]. Women seem to be at higher risk for those events, as are patients with the Janus kinase 2 (JAK2) mutation, and those presenting with leukocytosis [2–4]. Headaches are the leading symptom, but visual disturbances, nausea and vomiting, hemiparesis, seizures, and vertigo have also been reported [1, 5].

Here we report a case of sigmoid venous thrombosis in a patient recently diagnosed with polycythemia vera with the JAK2 V617F mutation, causing headaches and diplopia.

2. Case Presentation

A 60-year-old female with a past medical history of ductal carcinoma in situ after lumpectomy and radiation and currently on hormonal therapy with an aromatase inhibitor presented with six weeks of pinpoint frontal headaches, blurry vision, diplopia, and dizziness. Her symptoms worsened over the past two weeks prior to her presentation. Her past medical history is also remarkable for tremors, for which she was seeing a neurologist, obesity, and obstructive sleep apnea on CPAP (continuous positive airway pressure). There are no additional cardiovascular risk factors in her past medical history, and she has never smoked. She is a frequent blood donor, as she claims that her blood counts are always on the higher side.

She started taking topiramate and a trial of indomethacin for the headaches, with only modest improvement. As an outpatient, her hematocrit was found to be elevated at 49.8% (Table 1), and she was referred to a hematologist. Her erythropoietin level was 4.4 mIU/mL (reference range 2.6–18.5). She was found to have a mutation on JAK2 V617F, measured at 16% of total JAK2 DNA (Table 2). Retrospectively, it was discovered that the patient has a sister with polycythemia vera.

The patient was scheduled to initiate phlebotomy treatment with a plan to start hydroxyurea afterwards. She underwent one session of phlebotomy without complications.

Table 1: Baseline complete blood count.

Hemoglobin	16.6 g/dL
Hematocrit	49.8%
RBCs	5.28 M/uL
MCV	94.3 fL
MCH	31.4 pg
MCHC	33.3 g/dL
Platelets	497 K/uL
MPV	10.7 fl
RDW	13.8%
WBC	10.17 K/uL

RBC: red blood cell; MCV: mean corpuscular volume; MCH: mean corpuscular hemoglobin; MCHC: mean corpuscular hemoglobin concentration; MPV: mean platelet volume; RDW: red cell distribution width; WBC: white blood cell.

Table 2: Hematology workup.

Ferritin	263 ug/L
Iron	119 ug/dL
Iron saturation	51%
TIBC	234 ug/dL
PT	13 sec
PT-INR	1.0
PTT	26.1 sec
EPO	4.4 mIU/mL
$JAK2^{V617F}$	Positive; 16%

TIBC: total iron binding capacity; PT: prothrombin time; INR: international normalized ratio; PTT: partial thromboplastin time; EPO: erythropoietin; JAK2: Janus kinase 2.

On arrival at the hospital, the patient's vital signs were normal. On physical examination, she was awake, alert, and oriented. Extraocular movements were intact with no nystagmus. There was no rest tremor, no dysmetria, and no intention tremor on finger-nose-finger testing. Ambulation was normal. No lymphadenopathy was found. There was no pruritus, no erythromelalgia, no ecchymosis, petechiae, or rash. Respiratory, cardiovascular, and abdominal exams were also unremarkable.

A brain magnetic resonance imaging was ordered and failed to reveal an acute change or finding to explain her symptoms. Consequently, magnetic resonance venography (MRV) was obtained, revealing *T1* hyperintensity with a lack of enhancement in the lateral aspect of the left proximal sigmoid sinus, compatible with dural venous sinus thrombosis, with likely extension to the left jugular bulb (Figure 1).

The patient was admitted and started on low-molecular-weight heparin. It was suggested that her double vision might have been a partial CN VI palsy secondary to increased intracranial pressure, and a trial of IV acetazolamide (250 mg BID) was given. The patient's headaches and visual disturbances gradually improved, and she was discharged on enoxaparin for four weeks, planning to transition to oral anticoagulation with either direct oral agents or warfarin for three to twelve months, at the discretion of her hematologist. There was also a plan to repeat the MRV in three months to assess its resolution. She had a follow-up two weeks after discharge, and the patient was still experiencing some symptoms, even though they were now milder.

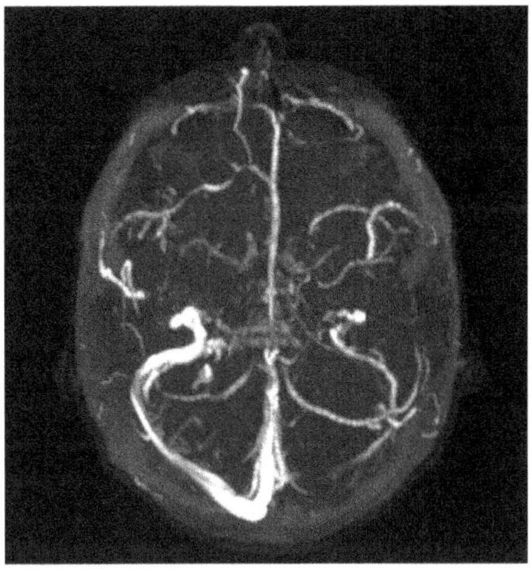

Figure 1: Magnetic resonance venography: *T1* hyperintensity with lack of enhancement in the lateral aspect of the left proximal sigmoid sinus.

3. Discussion

The most common venous thrombotic events in patients with MPNs are deep vein thrombosis, pulmonary embolism, splanchnic vein thrombosis, and superficial thrombophlebitis. Those events are usually found shortly after the diagnosis of either polycythemia vera (PV) or essential thrombocythemia (ET) is made [6]. Patients at risk for thrombosis are those over 60 years of age with a previous history of thrombosis and the $JAK2^{V617F}$ mutation. Additionally, patients with severe thrombocytosis may be at risk for bleeding, as it can be associated with acquired von Willebrand syndrome [7]. Our patient also has a sister with a diagnosis of PV, which raises the possibility of familial MPNs. This is of importance because in patients with either familial PV or ET, the $JAK2^{V617F}$ mutation has been associated with a higher risk of thrombotic events than in those with nonfamilial MPNs, despite bearing a similar prognosis [8]. Finally, in our case, the patient was prescribed an aromatase inhibitor for the treatment of breast cancer. Those agents are not usually associated with thrombotic events, and hence there is a less likely chance that this therapy is associated with the patient's current presentation [9].

3.1. Pathogenesis. The pathogenesis leading up to thrombotic events in polycythemia vera is not entirely clear. Blood hyperviscosity is thought to be one of the causes of thrombotic events both in neoplastic and in nonclonal exaggerated erythropoiesis [10]. However, there are likely other implicating factors, given that polycythemia itself would not explain higher rates of thrombosis seen in other MPNs such as essential thrombocythemia. It is postulated that patients with PV present with higher prothrombotic gene expression, including F3, IL10, VEGFA, LDHA, and SLC2A1. These genes were found to correlate positively with a JAK2 mutation in PV [11]. Leukocytosis may also be an implicating cause. The biological plausibility lies in the fact that patients with PV express higher levels of beta-2 integrin, CD11b, and leukocyte alkaline phosphatase, ultimately leading to increased activation of neutrophils. These activated polymorphonuclear cells interact with platelets, impairing normal hemostasis [12]. A meta-analysis confirmed that leukocytosis is associated with increased thrombotic events in PV, but a subgroup analysis revealed that this was true for arterial rather than venous events. Furthermore, the study could not establish a cutoff for white blood cell counts that portended a higher risk for thrombosis [13].

3.2. Epidemiology, Clinical Manifestations, and Diagnosis. A large observational study found the prevalence of venous thrombotic events, regardless of location, in patients with polycythemia vera to be 9% [2]. Another study identified a prevalence of 1.2% for CVT in patients with PV. The most common sites for cerebral sinus thrombosis in this series of cases were the transverse sinus, the sagittal sinus, and the sigmoid sinus, respectively [1] (Figure 2). Headache and blurry vision are among the leading symptoms; however, nausea and vomiting, diplopia, and seizures have also been reported [1, 5]. CVT should also raise concern for signs and symptoms of intracranial hypertension, such as associated papilledema [14]. Most recent guidelines recommend screening oncologic patients for cerebral venous thrombosis. Furthermore, they state that either magnetic resonance or computed tomography angiography are the tests of choice to diagnose CVT [15].

3.3. Management and Prognosis. Few studies address treatment of CVT, specifically in the subgroup of patients with MPNs. In general, low molecular weight heparin (LMWH) seems to be a better option for acute anticoagulation than unfractionated heparin (UFH) when considering adverse events such as major bleeding and thrombotic complications [16]. Heparin should be used in the acute setting, defined as a period short after the diagnosis, when intracranial hypertension and brain herniation may occur [17]. There is no high-quality evidence assessing the duration of anticoagulation. Hence, it is reasonable to maintain oral therapy for a period of 3 to 12 months [15]. The use of direct oral anticoagulants (DOACs) in CVT appears to be a safe choice when compared to coumarins [18, 19]. A large multicenter retrospective study assessed DOACs for treatment of CVT of any cause. It showed no statistically significant difference between DOACs and warfarin regarding outcomes such as recurrence, death, and venous recanalization. It also showed a higher risk of major hemorrhage with warfarin when compared to DOACs [19]. Even though cerebral sinus thrombosis does not seem to affect mortality rates, it might be associated with morbidity as some patients may present persistent neurological symptoms [1]. As for both arterial and venous thromboembolic episodes in the MPN population, observational studies suggest that DOACs seem both effective and safe when compared with vitamin K antagonists [20].

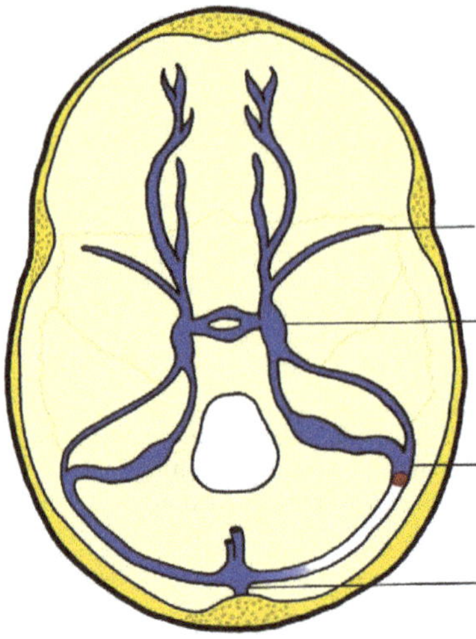

FIGURE 2: Anatomy of the cerebral venous system and sigmoid sinus thrombosis.

This is a case of cerebral sinus thrombosis in a patient with the JAK2 V617F mutation of polycythemia vera. Even though thrombosis is a well-established complication of myeloproliferative neoplasms, sigmoid thrombosis is not particularly common. The patient presented with headaches and diplopia, signs of intracranial hypertension, and was diagnosed using the gold-standard method, a magnetic resonance venography. Patients with CVT should be treated with anticoagulation for three to 12 months, starting with a heparinoid product in the acute setting and transitioning to oral anticoagulation for the long-term outpatient treatment. This case reinforces that CVT should be kept on the differential for patients with MPNs and new neurological symptoms.

Abbreviations

CVT: Cerebral venous thrombosis
DOAC: Direct oral anticoagulant
JAK2: Janus kinase 2
LMWH: Low-molecular-weight heparin
MPN: Myeloproliferative neoplasm
MRV: Magnetic resonance venography
PV: Polycythemia vera
UFH: Unfractionated heparin.

References

[1] N. Gangat, P. Guglielmelli, S. Betti et al., "Cerebral venous thrombosis and myeloproliferative neoplasms: a three-center study of 74 consecutive cases," *American Journal of Hematology*, vol. 96, no. 12, pp. 1580–1586, 2021.

[2] A. Tefferi, E. Rumi, G. Finazzi et al., "Survival and prognosis among 1545 patients with contemporary polycythemia vera: an international study," *Leukemia*, vol. 27, no. 9, pp. 1874–1881, 2013.

[3] R. Landolfi, L. Di Gennaro, T. Barbui et al., "Leukocytosis as a major thrombotic risk factor in patients with polycythemia vera," *Blood*, vol. 109, no. 6, pp. 2446–2452, 2007.

[4] A. Carobbio, J. Thiele, F. Passamonti et al., "Risk factors for arterial and venous thrombosis in WHO-defined essential thrombocythemia: an international study of 891 patients," *Blood*, vol. 117, no. 22, pp. 5857–5859, 2011.

[5] H. X. Shen, X. Q. Huang, C. Q. Fan, Y. X. Cao, H. Zhao, and J. G. Duan, "Cerebral venous sinus thrombosis in polycythemia vera patients with JAK2V617F mutation," *Chinese Medical Journal*, vol. 134, no. 10, pp. 1251–1253, 2021.

[6] M. Griesshammer, J. J. Kiladjian, and C. Besses, "Thromboembolic events in polycythemia vera," *Annals of Hematology*, vol. 98, no. 5, pp. 1071–1082, 2019.

[7] A. Tefferi and T. Barbui, "Polycythemia vera and essential thrombocythemia: 2021 update on diagnosis, risk-stratification and management," *American Journal of Hematology*, vol. 95, no. 12, pp. 1599–1613, 2020.

[8] S. Malak, M. Labopin, C. Saint-Martin, C. Bellanne-Chantelot, A. Najman, and French Group of Familial Myeloproliferative Disorders, "Long term follow up of 93 families with myeloproliferative neoplasms: life expectancy and implications of JAK2V617F in the occurrence of complications," *Blood Cells, Molecules, and Diseases*, vol. 49, no. 3-4, pp. 170–176, 2012.

[9] P. Dombernowsky, I. Smith, G. Falkson et al., "Letrozole, a new oral aromatase inhibitor for advanced breast cancer: double-blind randomized trial showing a dose effect and improved efficacy and tolerability compared with megestrol acetate," *Journal of Clinical Oncology*, vol. 16, no. 2, pp. 453–461, 1998.

[10] R. Marchioli, G. Finazzi, G. Specchia et al., "Cardiovascular events and intensity of treatment in polycythemia vera," *New England Journal of Medicine*, vol. 368, no. 1, pp. 22–33, 2013.

[11] R. Gangaraju, J. Song, S. J. Kim et al., "Thrombotic, inflammatory, and HIF-regulated genes and thrombosis risk in polycythemia vera and essential thrombocythemia," *Blood Advances*, vol. 4, no. 6, pp. 1115–1130, 2020.

[12] R. Landolfi, L. Di Gennaro, and A. Falanga, "Thrombosis in myeloproliferative disorders: pathogenetic facts and speculation," *Leukemia*, vol. 22, no. 11, pp. 2020–2028, 2008.

[13] A. Carobbio, A. Ferrari, A. Masciulli, A. Ghirardi, G. Barosi, and T. Barbui, "Leukocytosis and thrombosis in essential thrombocythemia and polycythemia vera: a systematic review and meta-analysis," *Blood Advances*, vol. 3, no. 11, pp. 1729–1737, 2019.

[14] V. Biousse, A. Ameri, and M. G. Bousser, "Isolated intracranial hypertension as the only sign of cerebral venous thrombosis," *Neurology*, vol. 53, no. 7, pp. 1537–1542, Article ID 10534264, 1999.

[15] J. M. Ferro, M. G. Bousser, P. Canhão et al., "European stroke organization guideline for the diagnosis and treatment of cerebral venous thrombosis—endorsed by the European academy of neurology," *European Journal of Neurology*, vol. 24, no. 10, pp. 1203–1213, 2017.

[16] S. M. Silvis, D. A. de Sousa, J. M. Ferro, and J. M. Coutinho, "Cerebral venous thrombosis," *Nature Reviews Neurology*, vol. 13, no. 9, pp. 555–565, 2017.

[17] L. Ulivi, M. Squitieri, H. Cohen, P. Cowley, and D. J. Werring, "Cerebral venous thrombosis: a practical guide," *Practical Neurology*, vol. 20, no. 5, pp. 356–367, 2020.

[18] J. M. Ferro, J. M. Coutinho, F. Dentali et al., "Safety and efficacy of dabigatran etexilate vs. dose-adjusted warfarin in patients with cerebral venous thrombosis: a randomized clinical trial," *JAMA Neurology*, vol. 76, no. 12, pp. 1457–1465, 2019.

[19] S. Yaghi, L. Shu, E. Bakradze et al., "Direct oral anticoagulants versus warfarin in the treatment of cerebral venous thrombosis (ACTION-CVT): a multicenter international study," *Stroke*, vol. 53, no. 3, pp. 728–738, 2022.

[20] E. N. Hamulyák, J. G. Daams, F. W. G. Leebeek et al., "A systematic review of antithrombotic treatment of venous thromboembolism in patients with myeloproliferative neoplasms," *Blood Advances*, vol. 5, no. 1, pp. 113–121, 2021.

30

Acute Myelogenous Leukemia with the t(7;7)(p15;p22) Translocation, a Novel Simple Variant of t(7;11)(p15;p15) Translocation: First Description

Motoharu Shibusawa

IMS Group, Shinmatsudo Central General Hospital, Department of Hematology, Chiba, Japan

Correspondence should be addressed to Motoharu Shibusawa; m_sibusawa@hotmail.com

Academic Editor: Kazunori Nakase

The t(7;11)(p15;p15) translocation is a recurrent genetic abnormality associated with acute myelogenous leukemia (AML). The translocation results in a fusion between the nucleoporin 98 and homeobox genes. We describe a case of AML with t(7; 7)(p15; p22) translocation, which is a novel simple variant of the t(7;11)(p15;p15) translocation. A 66-year-old woman presented with subcutaneous hemorrhage in both forearms. Laboratory test revealed hyperleukocytosis (white blood cell count: 97,800 cells/μL (blasts, 51.0%)), anemia (hemoglobin level: 7.6 g/dL), thrombocytopenia (platelet count: $6.5 \times 10^4/\mu$L), and hyperfibrinolysis (elevated d-dimer level: 12.4 μg/mL; fibrin/fibrinogen degradation products: 26.9 μg/mL). The patient was diagnosed with AML; the blast morphology was unclassifiable according to the French-American-British classification. Flow cytometry CD45 gating revealed that the blasts expressed CD34, CD13, CD33, and CD117. G-banding of tumor cells revealed the t(7;7)(p15;p22) translocation [20/20]. The patient underwent chemotherapy. At 48 days of admission, the patient died of multiple organ failure. The t(7;7)(p15;p22) translocation involved chromosome 7p15, indicating its association with the homeobox genes. To the best of our knowledge, this is the first report of a patient with AML with the t(7;7)(p15;p22) translocation, which is a simple novel variant of the t(7;11)(p15;p15) translocation.

1. Introduction

The recurrent genetic abnormalities in acute myeloid leukemia (AML) are associated with distinct clinicopathological characteristics and have prognostic significance. Most of these structural chromosomal rearrangements lead to the creation of a fusion gene encoding a chimeric protein. Many diseases that result from such alterations have characteristic morphological and immunophenotypic characteristics [1]. The t(7;11)(p15;p15) translocation is a recurrent genetic abnormality associated with AML. The translocation results in a fusion between the nucleoporin 98 (NUP98) and homeobox (HOX) genes [2]. The frequency of AML with this translocation is only 2.2% [3], with most cases often reported in Asian countries [3–5]. Compared with patients with AML without the t(7;11)(p15;p15) translocation, the clinicopathological characteristics of those with the translocation are as follows: younger age, predominance in women, and M2-subtype according to the French-American-British (FAB) classification. Moreover, the overall survival (OS) and disease-free survival (DFS) of the latter patient group are poorer than those of the former patient group [3]. A simple variant of the t(7;11)(p15;p15) translocation has been reported [6, 7]. This article describes a novel case of AML with the t(7; 7)(p15;p22) translocation and a literature review of the t(7;11)(p15;p15) translocation.

2. Case Presentation

A 66-year-old Japanese woman visited a local hospital with the chief complaint of malaise for two days. She presented with subcutaneous hemorrhage in both forearms; therefore, she was referred to the hematology department of our hospital. She had no remarkable medical history except pneumonia. Physical examination revealed a body temperature of 37.1°C, blood pressure of 136/86 mmHg, pulse rate of 85 beats per minute, and oxygen saturation of 99% in ambient air. She had no palpable lymphadenopathy, and chest auscultation revealed no rales or murmur. Her abdomen was soft, without palpable hepatosplenomegaly. Laboratory test results were as follows: hyperleukocytosis (white blood cell count: 97,800 cells/μL), differential count (blasts, 51.0%; neutrophils, 31.5%; monocytes, 2.5%; metamyelocytes, 5.5%; lymphocytes, 5.0%; basophils, 4.5%), anemia (hemoglobin level: 7.6 g/dL), thrombocytopenia (platelet count: $6.5 \times 10^4/\mu$L), and hyperfibrinolysis (elevated d-dimer level: 12.4 μg/mL; fibrin/fibrinogen degradation products: 26.9 μg/mL; elevated lactate dehydrogenase level, 1,398 IU/L). According to the bone marrow examination, blasts accounted for 30.4% of cells and presented with delicate nuclear folds and a high nucleus-to-cytoplasm ratio. The size of the blasts ranged from medium to large, and some presented with cytoplasmic nucleoli and granules. Most blasts were myeloperoxidase negative, although some were positive (Figure 1). We were unable to morphologically classify blasts using the FAB classification. Flow cytometry CD45 gating revealed that the blasts expressed CD34, CD13, CD33, and CD117. G-banding of tumor cells and T cells in peripheral blood samples revealed the t(7;7)(p15;p22) translocation [20/20] (Figure 2) and 46, XX [20/20], respectively; thus, the novel translocation was observed. She was diagnosed with AML and the t(7;7)(p15;p22) translocation. She was first treated with cytoreductive therapy with hydroxyurea. However, hydroxyurea failed to improve hyperleukocytosis, and on hospital day 25, she presented with subcutaneous bleeding around both eyelids secondary to severe disseminated intravascular coagulation (DIC). On day 26, she developed sudden dyspnea and hypoxia. Chest computed tomography revealed bilateral shadows in the lung, which was highly suggestive of leukostasis of the lungs. She required a respirator. On day 27, chemotherapy comprising idarubicin and cytarabine was started, but on the following day, she developed oliguria, which was suggestive of renal failure due to tumor lysis syndrome (TLS) and sepsis. She required hemodialysis. On day 37, hematological remission was confirmed by bone marrow examination. On day 48 of her hospital stay, she died of multiple organ failure secondary to severe infection and gastrointestinal bleeding.

3. Review of Literature and Discussion

The t(7;11)(p15;p15) translocation has been reported to occur not only in AML but also in the acute phase of chronic myelogenous leukemia, chronic myelomonocytic leukemia, and myelodysplastic syndrome [2, 8]. AML-associated translocation is often reported in Asian countries [3–5]. Chou et al. analyzed 493 adult patients with AML in Taiwan and found 11 patients (2.2%) to have the t(7;11)(p15;p15) translocation [3].

As mentioned earlier, the t(7;11)(p15;p15) translocation results in a fusion between NUP98 and HOX [2]. NUP98 is located on chromosome 11p15.5 [9] and belongs to the nucleoporin protein family and forms multisubunit channels in nuclear membranes. These nuclear pore complexes facilitate the transfer of metabolites and molecules between the cytoplasm and the nucleus. NUP98 oncogenes are fused to one of the eight HOX partners, HOXA9, leading to the upregulation of additional HOX genes (HOXA5, HOXA7, HOXA9, and HOXA10) and thereby contributing to leukemogenesis [10, 11]. HOXA9 genes are located on chromosome 7q15 [2]. HOXA9 is a homeodomain-containing transcription factor that plays an important role in hematopoietic stem cell expansion. HOXA9 directly regulates critical downstream genes such as B-cell lymphoma-2 and Ink4a/ARF/Ink4b, which are linked to poor outcomes [10]. Moreover, patients with AML harbor the NUP98-HOXA9 fusion that has been shown to be strongly associated with KRAS and WT1 mutations [3].

The clinical characteristics of patients with AML with the t(7;11)(p15;p15) translocation are reported [3, 4]. In total, 17 patients with the t(7;11)(p15;p15) translocation have been reported, with most patients being relatively young (median age 34 years, range 18–67) and the majority being women (13 of 17 patients). Moreover, most patients presented with the M2-subtype, according to the FAB classification (M2, nine patients; M4, four patients; M5, three patients; M6, one patient). Flow cytometry revealed CD33 ($n = 17$ patients), CD13 and CD117 ($n = 15$ patients), and HLR-DR and CD34 ($n = 12$ patients) antigens [4]. All patients were treated with conventional chemotherapeutic drugs, including anthracycline, cytarabine, and homoharringtonine. The rate of complete remission (CR) was 88.2% (15/17 patients). Two patients underwent allogeneic hematopoietic stem cell transplantation (HSCT) (1 patient was after first remission and the other after relapse) [4]. AML patients with the translocation had poorer OS (median: 13.5 vs. 20 months) and DFS (median: 6 vs. 12 months) than those without the translocation [3].

Harada et al. analyzed 91 AML patients with the t(7;11)(p15;p15) translocation from 1986 to 2014. The 3-year OS and DFS rates after allogeneic HSCT were 40.1% and 37.8%, respectively. Patients who underwent allogeneic HSCT after the second CR were more likely to relapse than those who underwent allogeneic HSCT in the first CR. The 2-year OS and DFS rates of AML patients with the translocation who underwent allogeneic HSCT after the first CR were 60.6% and 56.1%, respectively. These rates were higher than those observed in patients who underwent allogeneic HSCT after the second CR (OS, 37.3%; DFS, 25.0%) [12].

Simple variants of the t(7;11)(p15;p15) translocation have been reported [6, 7]. A 52-year-old man with AML (FAB classification M2) had the t(1;11)(q23;p15), add (7)(q22) karyotype [6]. This case involved chromosome 11p15, indicating its association with NUP98. A 76-year-old woman was diagnosed with AML (FAB classification M2) whose karyotype was a complex t(7;11)-variant, i.e., t(7;11;13;17)(p15;p15;p?;p1?2); this case involved NUP98 [7].

The patient in the present report was a 66-year-old woman with AML; the blast morphology was unclassifiable according to the FAB classification. G-banding of blasts revealed the t(7;7)(p15;p22) translocation, whereas that of T cells revealed a normal karyotype. These findings indicated translocation, which involved chromosome 7p15, indicating

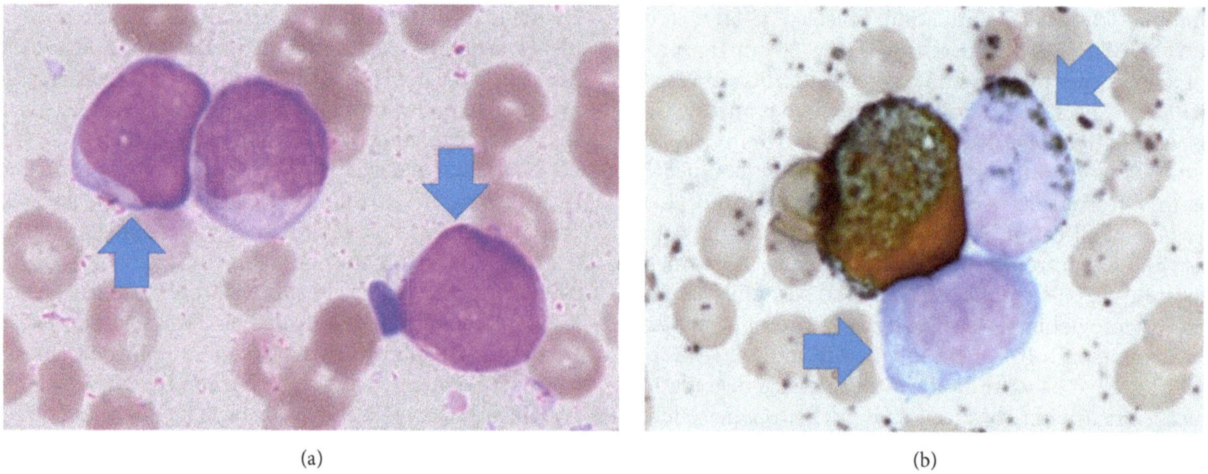

Figure 1: Bone marrow aspiration. (a) Wright–Giemsa staining (×1,000) and (b) myeloperoxidase staining (×1,000). Arrows indicate blasts. Blasts presented with loose reticular chromatin and a high nucleus-to-cytoplasm ratio. Their size ranged from medium to large, and some showed cytoplasmic nucleoli and granules. Most blasts were myeloperoxidase negative.

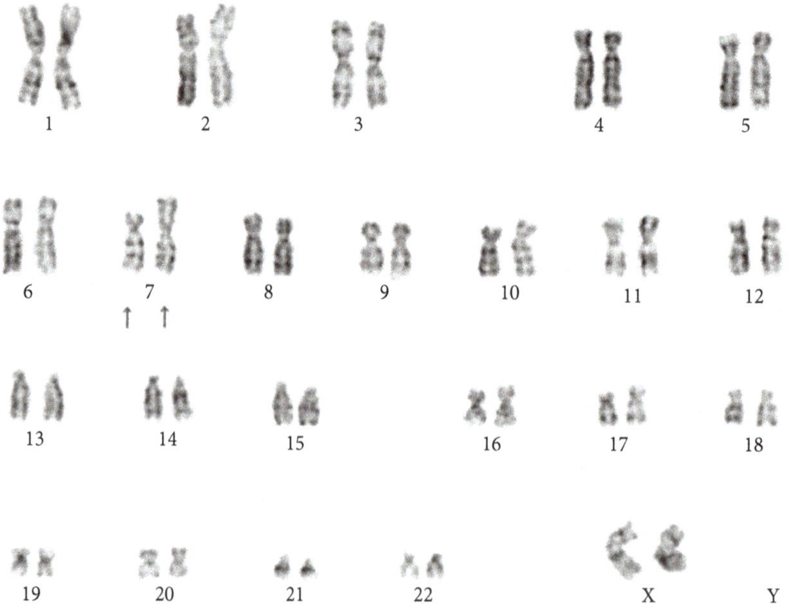

Figure 2: G-banding: translocation t(7;7)(p15;p22).

its association with HOX. The white blood cell count at the presentation of the present case was high at 97,800 cells/μL. Previous studies have reported that hyperleukocytosis leads to leukostasis, DIC, and TLS, which are associated with early death after the diagnosis of leukemia [13–15]. It is speculated that in the present case, the translocation caused rapid leukemic cell expansion, resulting in hyperleukocytosis, which led to severe DIC, leukostasis of the lungs, and renal failure due to TLS. These complications affected the patient's survival, which was very short: 48 days after admission. Based on this history, the t(7;7)(p15;p22) translocation may cause a rapid expansion of leukemic cells, leading to leukocytosis. This translocation may also be associated with poorer OS as well as t(7;11)(p15;p15) translocation.

4. Conclusion

To the best of our knowledge, this is the first report of a patient with the AML with t(7;7)(p15;p22) translocation, a simple novel variant of the t(7;11)(p15;p15) translocation.

Authors' Contributions

M. S treated the patient and wrote the article.

Acknowledgments

The author would like to thank Dr. Tetsuya Tanimoto for constructive advice on this article.

References

[1] D. A. Arber, R. D. Brunning, M. M. L. Beau et al., "Acute myeloid leukaemia with recurrent genetic abnormalities," in *WHO Classification of Tumours of Haematopoietic and Lymphoid Tissues*, H. S. StevenC. Elias et al., Eds., International Agency for Research on Cancer, Lyon, France, 2017.

[2] S. M. Gough, C. I. Slape, and P. D. Aplan, "NUP98 gene fusions and hematopoietic malignancies: common themes and new biologic insights," *Blood*, vol. 118, no. 24, pp. 6247–6257, 2011.

[3] W.-C. Chou, C.-Y. Chen, H.-A. Hou et al., "Acute myeloid leukemia bearing t (7;11)(p15;p15) is a distinct cytogenetic entity with poor outcome and a distinct mutation profile: comparative analysis of 493 adult patients," *Leukemia*, vol. 23, no. 7, pp. 1303–1310, 2009.

[4] S. Wei, S. Wang, S. Qiu et al., "Clinical and laboratory studies of 17 patients with acute myeloid leukemia harboring t (7; 11)(p15;p15) translocation," *Leukemia Research*, vol. 37, no. 9, pp. 1010–1015, 2013.

[5] S. Y. Huang, J. L. Tang, Y. J. Liang, C. H. Wang, Y. C. Chen, and H. F. Tien, "Clinical, haematological and molecular studies in patients with chromosome translocation t (7;11): a study of four Chinese patients in Taiwan," *British Journal of Haematology*, vol. 96, no. 4, pp. 682–687, 1997.

[6] Y. Hatano, I. Miura, M. Kume, and A. B. Miura, "Translocation (1;11) (q23;p15), a novel simple variant of translocation (7;11)(p15;p15), in a patient with AML (M2) accompanied by non-Hodgkin lymphoma and gastric cancer," *Cancer Genetics and Cytogenetics*, vol. 117, no. 1, pp. 19–23, 2000.

[7] I. Lahortiga, E. Belloni, I. Vázquez et al., "NUP98 is fused to HOXA9 in a variant complex t (7;11;13;17) in a patient with AML-M2," *Cancer Genetics and Cytogenetics*, vol. 157, no. 2, pp. 151–156, 2005.

[8] Y. Hatano, I. Miura, T. Nakamura, Y. Yamazaki, N. Takahashi, and A. B. Miura, "Molecular heterogeneity of the NUP98/HOXA9 fusion transcript in myelodysplastic syndromes associated with t (7;11)(p15;p15)," *British Journal of Haematology*, vol. 107, no. 3, pp. 600–604, 1999.

[9] C. Slape and P. D. Aplan, "The role of NUP98 gene fusions in hematologic malignancy," *Leukemia & Lymphoma*, vol. 45, no. 7, pp. 1341–1350, 2004.

[10] C. T. Collins and J. L. Hess, "Role of HOXA9 in leukemia: dysregulation, cofactors and essential targets," *Oncogene*, vol. 35, no. 9, pp. 1090–1098, 2016.

[11] R. L. Novak, D. P. Harper, D. Caudell, C. Slape, S. H. Beachy, and P. D. Aplan, "Gene expression profiling and candidate gene resequencing identifies pathways and mutations important for malignant transformation caused by leukemogenic fusion genes," *Experimental Hematology*, vol. 40, no. 12, pp. 1016–1027, 2012.

[12] K. Harada, N. Doki, J. Aoki et al., "Outcomes after allogeneic hematopoietic stem cell transplantation in patients with acute myeloid leukemia harboring t (7;11)(p15;p15)," *Haematologica*, vol. 103, pp. e69–e72, 2018.

[13] U. Y. Malkan, G. Gunes, E. Eliacik et al., "The factors affecting early death after the initial therapy of acute myeloid leukemia," *International Journal of Clinical and Experimental Medicine*, vol. 8, no. 12, pp. 22564–22569, 2015.

[14] C. Röllig and G. Ehninger, "How I treat hyperleukocytosis in acute myeloid leukemia," *Blood*, vol. 125, no. 21, pp. 3246–3252, 2015.

[15] C. Ganzel, J. Becker, P. D. Mintz, H. M. Lazarus, and J. M. Rowe, "Hyperleukocytosis, leukostasis and leukapheresis: practice management," *Blood Reviews*, vol. 26, no. 3, pp. 117–122, 2012.

31

A Chinese Child Presented with Early T Cell Precursor Lymphoblastic Lymphoma

Xiangyang Pu,[1,2] Shengyong Deng,[1,2] Nange Yin,[1,3] Lin Song,[3,4,5] Xiangling He,[6] and Jianwen Xiao [1,7,8]

[1]*Ministry of Education Key Laboratory of Child Development and Disorders, Chongqing, China*
[2]*Department of Pediatric Respiratory Medicine, Qianjiang Central Hospital of Chongqing, Chongqing, China*
[3]*Department of Pharmacy, Children Hospital of Chongqing Medical University, Chongqing, China*
[4]*National Clinical Research Center for Child Health and Disorders, Chongqing, China*
[5]*China International Science and Technology Cooperation Base of Child Development and Critical Disorders, Chongqing 400014, China*
[6]*Department of Pediatric Hematology and Oncology, Children's Medical Center of Hunan Provincial People's Hospital (The First-Affiliated Hospital of Hunan Normal University), Changsha, China*
[7]*Chongqing Key Laboratory of Pediatrics, Chongqing, China*
[8]*Department of Hematology, Children Hospital of Chongqing Medical University, Chongqing, China*

Correspondence should be addressed to Jianwen Xiao; tomahawk6502@sohu.com

Academic Editor: Saveria Capria

T cell lymphoblastic lymphoma (T-LBL) is regarded as the leukemic phase of T cell acute lymphoblastic leukemia (T-ALL). The early T cell precursors ALL/LBL (ETP-LBL/ALL) are derived from thymic cells at the ETP differentiation stage and recognized as a high-risk subgroup of T-ALL/LBL. Most of these cases presented with ALL at the disease onset, but the ETP-LBL phase is uncommon. Here, we report a patient who presented with ETP-LBL at the disease onset. In this case, ALL developed even despite receiving chemotherapy, but the patient achieved a complete remission with intensive chemotherapy.

1. Introduction

T cell lymphoblastic lymphoma (T-LBL) and T cell acute lymphoblastic leukemia (T-ALL) are both hematological tumors that originate from an immature T cell lineage. T-ALL is regarded as the leukemic phase of T-LBL, and a lymphoblast count in bone marrow (BM) < 25% is defined as the cutoff value between T-LBL and T-ALL [1, 2]. The prognosis of T-LBL/ALL remains historically poor. ALL-based chemotherapy and allogenic hematopoietic stem cell transplantation (allo-HSCT) demonstrated effective results, and event-free survival (EFS) in children and adolescents exceeds 80–90% in developed countries [2, 3]. However, the survival of relapsed and/or refractory cases remains poor [2–4]. The early T cell precursors ALL/LBL (ETP-LBL/ALL) are derived from thymic cells at the ETP differentiation stage and are recognized as a high-risk subgroup of T-ALL/LBL [5]. ETP-LBL/ALL occurs in 10–12% or 20–25% of pediatric or adult T-LBL/ALL populations [5–7]. Most of these cases present with ALL, and the LBL phase is uncommon [6–8]. Here, we report a patient who presented with ETP-LBL at disease onset. ALL developed eventhough he subsequently received chemotherapy, and he achieved a complete remission (CR) with intensive chemotherapy.

2. Case Presentation

A 16-year-3-month-old boy was admitted with an irritating dry cough and cervical lymphadenopathy on 28 January 2020. During the physical examination, bilateral cervical lymph node masses were palpable, and signs of pleural effusion were also noted. Laboratory tests showed normal complete blood cell counts (white blood cells 6.22×10^9/L, platelets 295×10^9/L, and hemoglobin 161 g/L) and normal lactate dehydrogenase levels (233 U/L). A computed tomography (CT) scan revealed pericardial and right pleural effusion and lymphadenopathy at the cervical area bilaterally and within the mediastinum (Figure 1(a)). A core needle biopsy and subsequent immunohistochemical (IHC) staining of the mediastinum mass was performed for CD3+, CD20−, PAX5−, CD7+, CD34−, Ki-67+(90%), MPO−, and CD99+(Figure 2). A sample of the pleural effusion was analyzed which showed that the nucleated cell counts were 31×10^9/L, the lymphoblasts were 92%, and there were 55.4% T cell lymphoblasts as detected by flow cytometry (FCM). Positive results for CD7, CD13, and cCD3 and negative results for CD1a, CD4, CD8, CD19, CD20, CD22, CD34, and MPO were confirmed (Figure 3). A diagnosis of ETP-ALL/LBL was considered, and additional IHC samples of the mediastinum mass sample were stained via IHC and were tested. The results showed CD45pro-,CD5-, and CD79a were weak+, CD21 was positive, MUM-1 was negative, CD10 was positive, CK was negative, BCL6 was negative, c-MYC was (40%+), CyclinD1 was negative, ALK was negative, CD30 was negative, and P53 was negative (Figure 2).

A chromosome karyotype of the pleural effusion sample was obtained using the International System of Human Cytogenetic Nomenclature 2009 (ISCN-2009) [2]: 43–50, *X*, *Y*, add(7) (p13), 9,?i(9) (q10), 14, 16, +22,?del(22) (q13), inc [CP8] (Figure 3). BM samples were acquired at the bilateral posterior superior iliac area, and blast cells were not detected by a BM smear, biopsy, or via FCM.

Samples were taken from the mediastinum mass, and whole exome sequencing (WES) and RNA sequencing (RNAseq) were performed. FBXW7 and GATA3 somatic mutations were detectable by WES (Table 1); transcripts of FBXW7, GATA3, JAK1, and NCOR1 were confirmed by RNAseq (Table 2).

A diagnosis of ETP-LBL was given based on previous literature reports [5–8], and the patient was classified as stage III by the revised International Pediatric Non-Hodgkin's Lymphoma Staging System [9]. He was treated with a modified BFM-LBL-95 protocol and was placed in an intermediate-risk (IR) group at the initial diagnosis [10]; the detail of the disease evaluation, risk group classification, treatment courses, dosages, and intrathecal injections had been listed at Supplementary Tables S1–S5, respectively; his treatment response was evaluated by BM, CT, or positron emission tomography/computed tomography (PET/CT) imaging at different time points (TP) as the protocol required. On day 15 and day 33 (TP1 or TP2) during the course of the induction of remission I, the BM smear showed 29.5% and 80% blast cells, FCM had 29% and 55.4% ETP lymphoblasts (Figures 4(a) and 4(b)), and a chest CT scan revealed an unchanged mediastinum mass (Figure 1(b)).

He was considered to have progressive disease (PD) and refractory disease at TP2 [5, 6], and two standard courses A of the HyperCVAD protocol [11] were administered. After the 1st course, lymphoblasts were no longer detected in the BM during the evaluation of the BM smear (Figure 4(c)); the CT scan showed a partial remission (PR) [5, 6], which was subsequently monitored by CT scans (Figure 1(c)). He achieved CR after the 2nd course A, which was monitored by using BM smears (Figure 4(d)) and PET-CT scans (Figure 1(d)). The minimal residual disease (MRD) level was also detected by FCM [12], and a negative result was obtained ($<10^{-4}$). Allo-HSCT was declined by the family, and he was treated with the CCLG-ALL-2008 protocol for the high-risk (HR) group [12]. Up until June 2021, he was alive without any evidence of a relapse.

3. Discussion

ETP-ALL/LBL is a recently described subgroup of T-ALL/LBL according to the World Health Organization criteria from 2016 (WHO 2016) [4]; usually, these cases are aggressive and present with ETP-ALL, whereas pediatric ETP-LBL is uncommon (20–30% in adult T-ALL/LBL, pediatric data are absent). In the presented case, we reported a child who suffered from ETP-LBL without BM infiltration at the onset.

ETP-ALL/LBL patients are distinguished from non-ETPs by FCM and genomic signatures. ETP-ALL/LBL is immunophenotypically defined by weak or absent expression of T cell markers (CD1a, CD5, and CD8) and positive expression of at least one hematopoietic stem cell (HSC) and/or myeloid markers (CD13, CD33, CD34, CD117, and HLA-DR). The diagnosis of T-LBL was based on the pathological results and IHC staining, but not all the T cell, HSC, and myeloid markers were evaluated. Fortunately, the patient was diagnosed with ETP-ALL/LBL by FCM detected in a pleural effusion sample. FCM is an important technique to subclassify T-ALL/LBL, and all these T-ALL/LBL samples should be evaluated if possible.

Genomic signatures of ETP-ALL/LBL patients also exhibit unique genotypes compared with those of non-ETPs patients [7, 8]. Recurrent mutations were not only identified in the genes involved in T-lymphoid development or oncogenesis because myeloid markers were also detectable. Activating mutations encoding cytokine receptors and mediating the RAS signal transduction system (NRAS, KRAS, FLT3, and JAK1), inactivating mutations encoding transcription factors (GATA3, ETV6, and RUNX1) and histone repair (EZH2 and EP300) during hematopoietic stem cell development are common in ETP-ALL/LBL patients [5, 6, 13]. WES and RNAseq of LN samples have been evaluated, common gene mutations and transcripts (FBXW7, NOTCH1, and JAK1) in T-ALL/LBL have been identified, and unique genomic signatures of ETP-ALL/LBL have also been identified. This suggests that gene analysis can assist in the diagnosis of ETPs without using FCM detection.

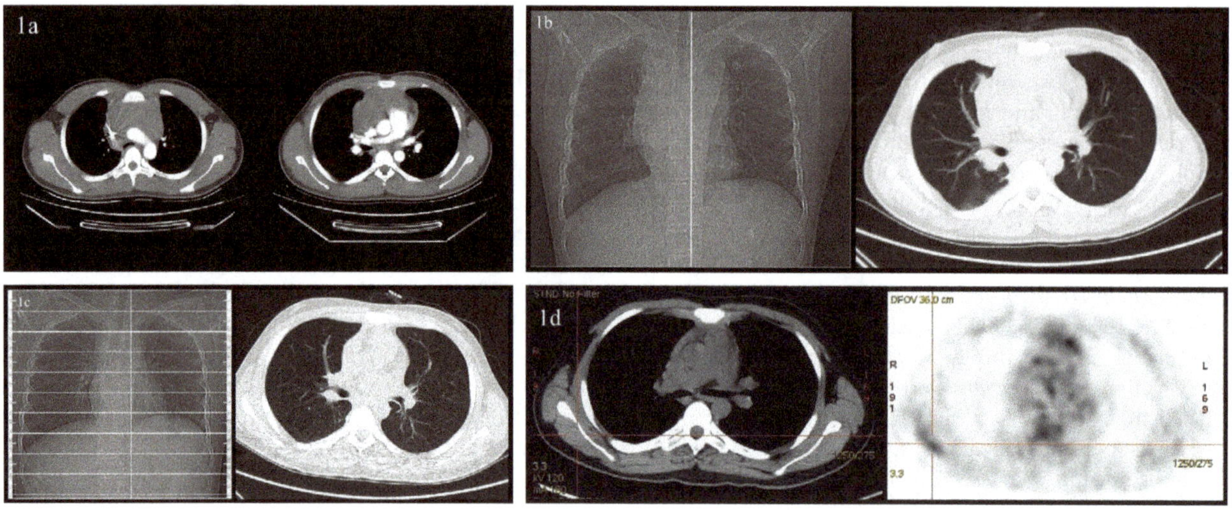

FIGURE 1: Results of chest CT or PET-CT scan.

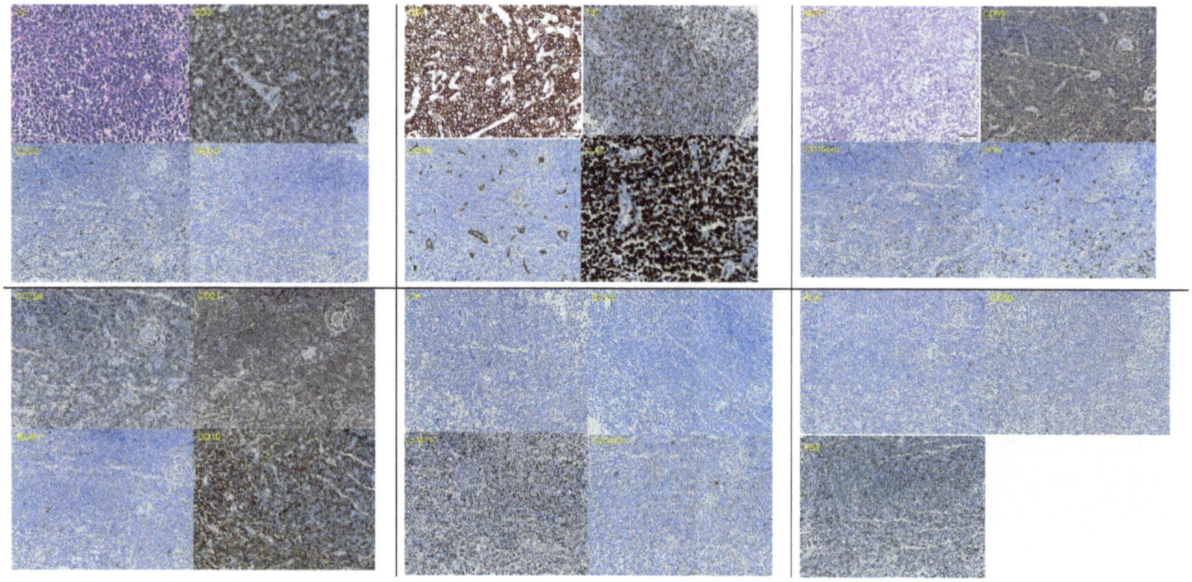

FIGURE 2: Results of mediastinum mass sample.

The best treatment and the prognosis for ETPs patients is unclear. Treatment responses and outcomes for ETP-ALL/LBL patients treated with chemotherapy were poorer than those for non-ETP-ALL/LBL adult patients, and it was reported that these cases benefit from allo-HSCT [4–6]. Although early reports of pediatric ETP-ALL showed a poor prognosis, recent clinical trials of COGAALL0434 and UKALL2003 showed that the prognosis of ETP-ALL was similar to that of other T-ALLs [14, 15]. However, ETP-LBL was uncommon, but the treatment experience was limited. The patient in this case report was treated with a modified BFM-LBL-95 protocol, the ALL-based classic protocol for T-LBL patients, but he was considered to have refractory disease and infiltration into the BM. It was reported that adults benefited from the hyperCVAD protocol [5, 6], and in our patient, two courses A were administered, but course B was omitted due to financial constraints. The patient obtained CR, and chemotherapy was continued.

In conclusion, we reported a case of ETP-LBL that took an aggressive clinical course. Our case revealed that clinicians should pay attention to the possibility of ETP-LBL in common T-LBL cases, and FCM and genomic signatures are important to distinguish ETP-LBL. Further studies are needed to research the most effective treatment for ETP-ALL/LBL patients.

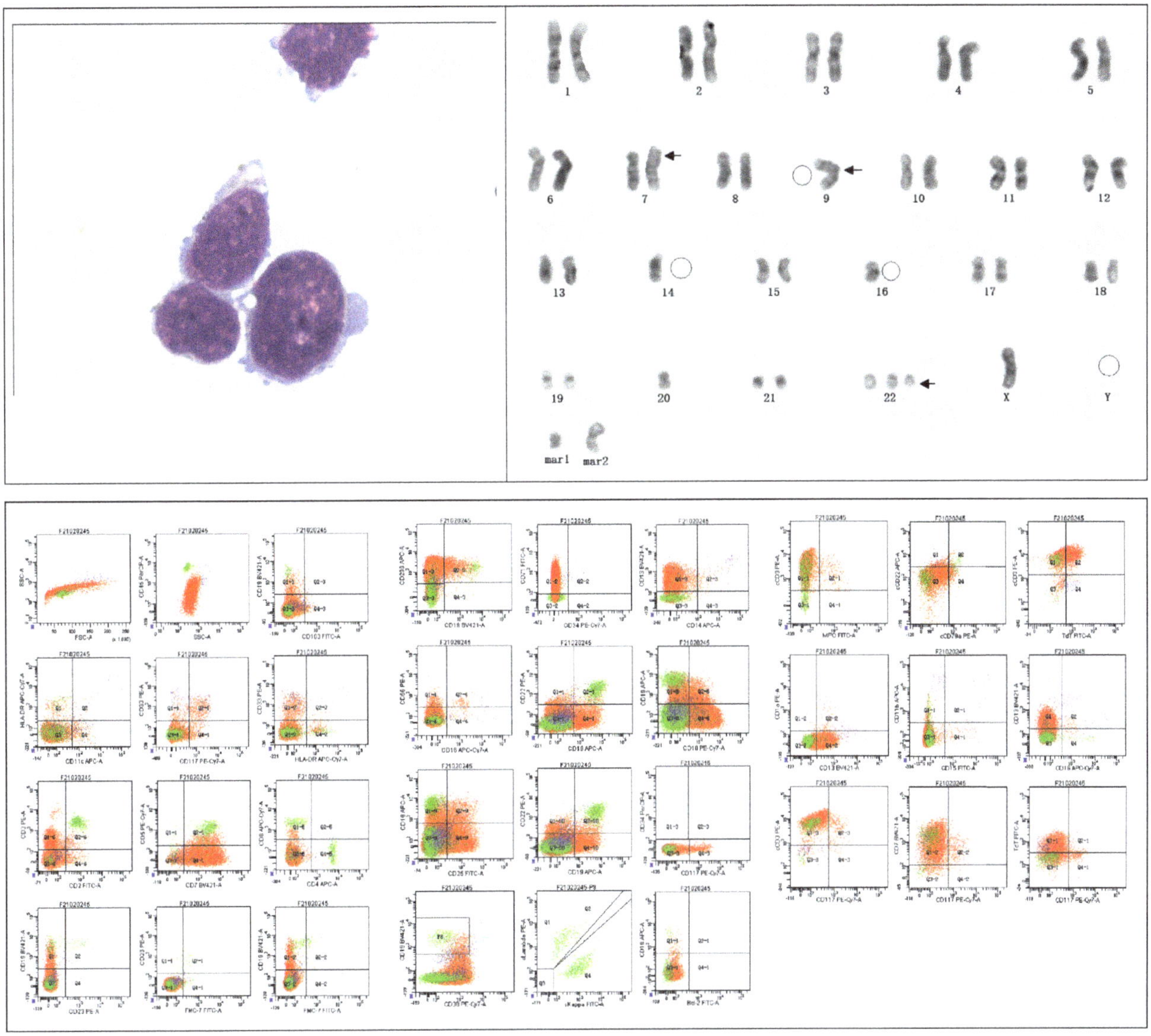

Figure 3: Results of pleural effusion sample.

Table 1: Results of whole exome sequencing.

Genes	Chromosome coordinate	Mutation site	Mutation frequency (%)
FBXW7 (NM_033632)	chr4: 153247366	c.1436G > A (p.Arg479Gln)	38.3
GATA3 (NM_0010022)	chr10: 8106004	c.827G > A (p.Arg276Gln)	38.8
GATA3 (NM_0010022)	chr10: 8105986	c.811_812dup (p.Thr272ArgfsTer24)	26.7

Table 2: Results of RNA sequencing.

Gene mutations	Mutation type	Mutation frequency (%)
FBXW7 R479Q	Missense mutation	51.9
GATA3 R276Q	Missense mutation	68.8
GATA3 T270fs	Frameshift mutation	24.4
JAK1 L783F	Missense mutation	58.5
NCOR1 Y1435*	Truncating mutation	34.6
NOTCH1 V1721E	Missense mutation	34.1

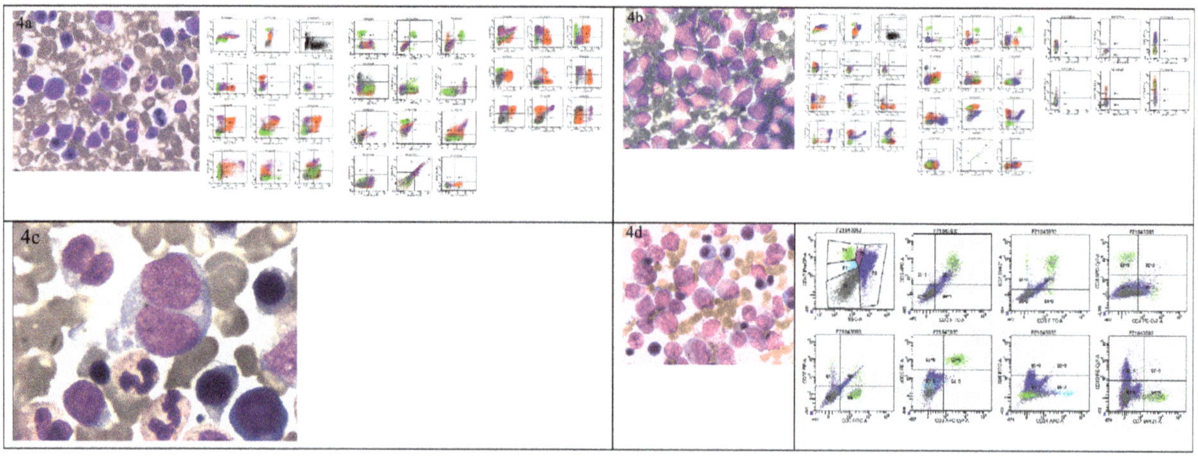

FIGURE 4: Results of bone marrow samples.

Authors' Contributions

JX, XP, and SD prepared the original draft. LS and JX helped with the design of the project. JX treated the patient and supervised the manuscript. All authors reviewed the final version.

Acknowledgments

The authors thank the patient and his family who participated in this study. This research was supported by the National Natural Science Foundation of China (Project no. 81900162) and the Chongqing Science and Technology Commission of PR China (Project no. cstc2018jsyj-jsyjX0015).

References

[1] B. Burkhardt and M. L. Hermiston, "Lymphoblastic lymphoma in children and adolescents: review of current challenges and future opportunities," *British Journal of Haematology*, vol. 185, no. 6, pp. 1158–1170, 2019.

[2] B. Burkhardt, S. Mueller, T. Khanam, and S. L. Perkins, "Current status and future directions of t-lymphoblastic lymphoma in children and adolescents," *British Journal of Haematology*, vol. 173, no. 4, pp. 545–559, 2016.

[3] M. J. You, L. J. Medeiros, and E. D. Hsi, "T-lymphoblastic leukemia/lymphoma," *American Journal of Clinical Pathology*, vol. 144, no. 3, pp. 411–422, 2015.

[4] W. Guan, Y. Jing, L. Dou, M. Wang, Y. Xiao, and L. Yu, "Chidamide in combination with chemotherapy in refractory and relapsed T lymphoblastic lymphoma/leukemia," *Leukemia and Lymphoma*, vol. 61, no. 4, pp. 855–861, 2020.

[5] N. Jain, A. V. Lamb, S. O'Brien et al., "Early T-cell precursor acute lymphoblastic leukemia/lymphoma (ETP-ALL/LBL) in adolescents and adults: a high-risk subtype," *Blood*, vol. 127, no. 15, pp. 1863–1869, 2016.

[6] J. Bond, C. Graux, L. Lhermitte et al., "Early response-based therapy stratification improves survival in adult early thymic precursor acute lymphoblastic leukemia: a group for research on adult acute lymphoblastic leukemia study," *Journal of Clinical Oncology*, vol. 35, no. 23, pp. 2683–2691, 2017.

[7] M. Ma, X. Wang, J. Tang et al., "Early T-cell precursor leukemia: a subtype of high risk childhood acute lymphoblastic leukemia," *Frontiers of Medicine*, vol. 6, no. 4, pp. 416–420, 2012.

[8] Y. Jiang, A. Maiti, and Z. Kanaan, "A young man with a mass: non-early precursor t-cell lymphoblastic lymphoma," *The American Journal of Medicine*, vol. 132, no. 1, pp. 58–60, 2019.

[9] A. Rosolen, S. L. Perkins, C. R. Pinkerton et al., "Revised international pediatric non-hodgkin lymphoma staging system," *Journal of Clinical Oncology*, vol. 33, no. 18, pp. 2112–2118, 2015.

[10] C. Y. Zheng, J. W. Xiao, J. Yu, and Y. G. Chen, "Prognosis and side effects of T-NHL-2009 protocol on treatment of lymphoblastic lymphoma in Children," *Clinics in Laboratory Medicine*, vol. 14, no. 13, pp. 1883–1887, 2017.

[11] C. R. Rausch, E. J. Jabbour, H. M. Kantarjian, and T. M. Kadia, "Optimizing the use of the hyperCVAD regimen: clinical vignettes and practical management," *Cancer*, vol. 126, no. 6, pp. 1152–1160, 2020.

[12] L. Cui, Z.-G. Li, Y.-H. Chai et al., "Outcome of children with newly diagnosed acute lymphoblastic leukemia treated with CCLG-ALL 2008: the first nation-wide prospective multicenter study in China," *American Journal of Hematology*, vol. 93, no. 7, pp. 913–920, 2018.

[13] O. C. Puglianini and N. Papadantonakis, "Early precursor T-cell acute lymphoblastic leukemia: current paradigms and evolving concepts," *Therapeutic Advances in Hematology*, vol. 11, Article ID 2040620720929475, 2020.

[14] S. S. Winter, K. P. Dunsmore, M. Devidas et al., "Improved survival for children and young adults with t-lineage acute lymphoblastic leukemia: results from the children's oncology group AALL0434 methotrexate randomization," *Journal of Clinical Oncology: Official Journal of the American Society of Clinical Oncology*, vol. 36, no. 29, pp. 2926–2934, 2018.

[15] K. Patrick, R. Wade, N. Goulden et al., "Outcome for children and young people with early t-cell precursor acute lymphoblastic leukaemia treated on a contemporary protocol, ukall 2003," *British Journal of Haematology*, vol. 166, pp. 421–4, 2014.

32

Flow Cytometric Test with Eosin-5-Maleimide for a Diagnosis of Hereditary Spherocytosis in a Newborn

Kanda Fanhchaksai,[1] **Suphara Manowong**,[2] **Rungrote Natesirinilkul**,[2] **Lalita Sathitsamitphong**,[2] **and Pimlak Charoenkwan**[2]

[1]*Research Cluster of Thalassemia and Red Blood Cell Disorders, Faculty of Medicine, Chiang Mai University, Chiang Mai 50200, Thailand*
[2]*Department of Pediatrics, Faculty of Medicine, Chiang Mai University, Chiang Mai 50200, Thailand*

Correspondence should be addressed to Kanda Fanhchaksai; kanda.f@cmu.ac.th

Academic Editor: Neelam Giri

A term male newborn born to a mother who had hereditary spherocytosis presented with neonatal jaundice at 20 hours of life. Complete blood count showed hemoglobin 17.1 g/dL, MCV 104.2 fL, MCH 32.9 pg, and MCHC 31.6 g/dL. The patient had indirect hyperbilirubinemia requiring phototherapy. The maximum total bilirubin level was 12.15 mg/dL at 20 hours of life. Peripheral blood smear revealed spherocytes, crenated red cells, and polychromasia. A flow cytometric test with eosin-5-maleimide- (EMA-) labeled RBC was performed in the patient and parents. The fluorescence histograms of EMA-labeled RBC from the patient and mother were shifted to the left, and the fluorescence ratio when compared with normal was 0.69 and 0.84, respectively. The flow cytometric test with EMA is useful in supporting the diagnosis of hereditary spherocytosis during newborn period.

1. Introduction

Hereditary spherocytosis (HS) is an inherited red blood cell (RBC) membrane disorder resulted from deficiencies of cytoskeletal membrane protein involving in the vertical connection between the phospholipid bilayer and structural proteins of the cell membrane [1]. The clinical severity varies from mild to severe anemia [1]. Newborns with HS may present with indirect hyperbilirubinemia requiring phototherapy or exchange transfusion.

HS is generally diagnosed by the significant presence of spherocytes in peripheral blood smear. The diagnosis can be confirmed by osmotic fragility test (OFT), autohemolysis test, acid glycerol lysis test, or pink test [2–5]. However, those tests have low sensitivity to detect cases with mild disease and are affected by several factors unrelated to the defects of red cell cytoskeleton [6]. To establish the diagnosis of HS in newborns by RBC morphology alone is unreliable because spherocytes and hyperdense RBCs may also be seen in normal newborns [7]. OFT may be normal in the presence of iron deficiency and obstructive jaundice, and in the recovery phase of aplastic crisis affected by increased reticulocytes [8]. Neonatal RBCs show different response to OFT than adult RBCs due to high hemoglobin (Hb) F concentration [9]. For the use in newborns, an incubated OFT is a recommended method [1, 9]. More specific tests such as the osmotic gradient ektacytometry and hypertonic cryohemolysis test are not widely available [10, 11].

Flow cytometric analysis with eosin-5-maleimide- (EMA-) labeled RBCs has shown a high sensitivity and specificity for diagnosing HS [12–14]. The fluorescent dye EMA binds to ξ-NH2 group of Lys-430 on band 3 protein which is a predominant protein in the RBC membrane [13]. The deficiency of band 3 protein results in a decrease of fluorescence intensity of EMA binding. Deficiencies of other RBC cytoskeletal proteins including band 4.2 and ankyrin also decrease fluorescence intensity because of the interaction between those proteins with band 3 [1]. The flow cytometric analysis with EMA-labeled RBCs has been recommended for diagnosis of HS in newborns [1, 15].

2. Case Presentation

A term male newborn with gestational age of 38 weeks was born by normal delivery. The birth weight was 2,350 g. His mother's blood type was O, Rh positive, and prenatal thalassemia screening test was negative. His mother and aunt has had mild hemolytic anemia and recently been diagnosed with HS. The patient was noted with jaundice at 20 hours of life. Physical examination showed jaundice without pallor and nonpalpable liver and spleen, while the rest of physical examination was unremarkable. He was investigated for the cause of neonatal hyperbilirubinemia. The peripheral blood smear showed spherocytes, crenated red cells, and polychromasia. The diagnosis of hereditary spherocytosis was suspected, and flow cytometry with EMA-labeled RBCs was performed to support the diagnosis.

3. Materials and Methods

Complete blood count (CBC), peripheral blood smear, and flow cytometric analysis with EMA-labeled RBCs of the patient and his parents were performed. The results are shown in Table 1. A healthy subject with normal hematological parameters and red blood cell morphology was investigated as a normal control. The patient's maximum total bilirubin level was 12.15 mg/dL at 20 hours of life. His blood type was O, Rh positive, and glucose-6-phosphate dehydrogenase (G-6-PD) assay by the fluorescent spot test showed normal result.

3.1. Flow Cytometric Analysis. The flow cytometric analysis with EMA-labeled RBCs was performed as previously described [14]. In brief, 100 μL of whole blood in EDTA from each subject were washed twice with 1 mL of sterile phosphate buffered saline (PBS), pH 7.4, and centrifuged at 1,500 rounds per minute (rpm) for 5 minutes. Five μL of red blood cells were incubated with 25 μL EMA dye or PBS (as an unstained control) at room temperature in the dark for 1 hour. The cell suspension was centrifuged at 1,500 rpm for 1 minute. Then, the unbound dye was removed. The pellet with EMA-labeled RBCs was washed twice with 0.5 mL of sterile 0.5% bovine serum albumin (BSA) solution in PBS. Those EMA-labeled RBCs were suspended in 0.5 mL of 0.5% BSA in PBS. This cell suspension 100 μL was added to 1.4 mL of 0.5% BSA in PBS solution for flow cytometric analysis. Mean fluorescence intensity (MFI) as mean of geometric mean (X-GMean) was determined for 10,000 events in FL1 channel of Beckman Coulter CyAn™ ADP High-speed Analyzer (Beckman Coulter, Fullerton, CA).

4. Results and Discussion

Red blood cell parameters and flow cytometry results of the patient and parents are summarized in Table 1. The peripheral blood smears from the patient and his mother are as shown in Figure 1. The fluorescence histograms of EMA-labeled RBCs of the patient and parents compared with a normal control are shown in Figure 2. The patient had normal Hb level, while the mother had anemia. Spherocytes and crenated red cells were demonstrated in the patient and his mother. The MFI of the patient and mother was low in comparison with that of the father and control. The findings supported the diagnosis of HS in the patient and mother.

Indirect hyperbilirubinemia in newborns is caused by overproduction of bilirubin, impaired bilirubin uptake, or impaired bilirubin conjugation. Hemolysis is an important cause of increased bilirubin production resulting in neonatal indirect hyperbilirubinemia. The common causes of hemolysis in neonates include red blood cell membrane disorders, alpha-thalassemia disease, or G-6-PD deficiency. Impaired bilirubin conjugation could be found in G-6-PD deficiency or other inherited diseases, Gilbert syndrome, or Crigler–Najjar syndrome. HS was the most likely the cause of hyperbilirubinemia in our patient.

The patient was treated phototherapy for indirect hyperbilirubinemia for 2 days. He also received folic acid supplementation. RBC transfusion was not required. After phototherapy, the total bilirubin was reduced from 12.15 mg/dL at hour 20 of life to 9.53 mg/dL at 32 hours of life. The CBC of the last visit at the age of 9 months showed Hb of 11.1 g/dL, MCV of 66.7 fL, and MCHC of 32.9 g/dL with 15% spherocytes. His growth parameters and developmental milestones were normal for his age.

This report demonstrates the usefulness of flow cytometric analysis of EMA-labeled RBCs to diagnose HS in a newborn. The patient and his mother who had HS showed a decreased MFI and fluorescence ratio when compared with a normal control. The findings are consistent with the previous reports of HS in newborns [1, 16, 17]. Of note, in this case report, red cells from a healthy adult were used as a control. The guideline for a diagnosis of HS by EMA-flow cytometry in newborns suggests using red cells from healthy term newborns as controls [1, 7, 16]. However, two previous studies have shown that the EMA-flow cytometry results obtained from healthy newborns or neonatal cord blood red cells are not significantly different to those from adult red cells [18, 19]. These findings suggest that red cells from adults can be used as controls for a newborn study.

The 2011 guideline for diagnosis of HS recommends the flow cytometry with EMA-labeled RBCs for diagnosing HS [15]. This test is also useful for screening of atypical HS with mild severity. The test has been used in newborns with a high sensitivity (92.7–96.6%) and high specificity (99.1%) [14, 20]. The MFI ratio in adults with HS ranges from 59.1–90.1% [5]. The MFI in newborns with HS is distinctly lower than that in normal newborns [16]. The MFI ratios in our patient and his mother were 0.69 and 0.84, comparable to the MFI seen in HS patients.

The main limitation of the flow cytometric analysis with EMA-labeled RBCs is the need of fresh red cells. Alternatively, the red cells can be stored at 4°C for a maximum of 7 days [21–25]. The reproducibility of the results can also be

TABLE 1: Red blood cell parameters and flow cytometry results of the patient and parents.

Red blood cell parameters	Normal control	Patient	Mother	Father
Hemoglobin (g/dL)	12.2	17.1	9.6	15.9
Hematocrit (%)	38.4	54.1	31.6	51.1
Red blood cell count ($\times 10^6/mm^3$)	4.44	5.19	2.94	5.64
MCV (fL)	86.5	104.2	107.5	90.6
MCH (pg)	27.5	32.9	32.7	28.2
MCHC (g/dL)	31.8	31.6	30.4	31.1
RDW (%)	13.1	18.4	24.5	14.8
Reticulocyte (%)	—	4.2	—	—
Fluorescence intensity (X-GMean)	755.92	519.31	636.37	748.07
Fluorescence ratio	1.00	0.69	0.84	0.99

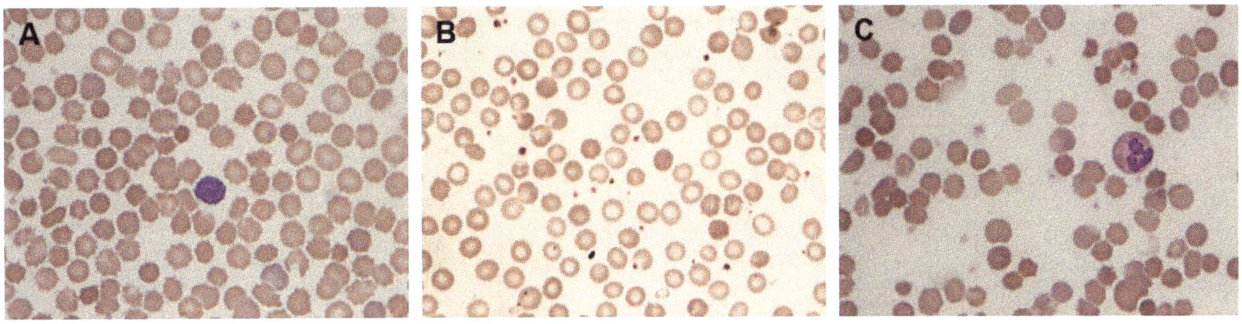

FIGURE 1: The peripheral blood smear (PBS) from the patient and his mother: (A) the patient at the age 2 days showing spherocytes, crenated red cells, and polychromasia; (B) the patient at the age 9 months showing spherocytes; (C) mother showing spherocytes and few crenated red cells.

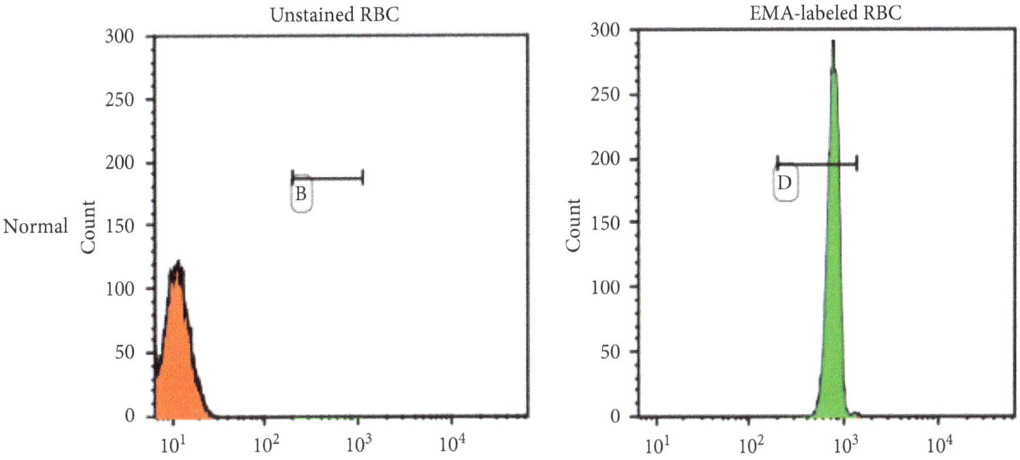

(a)

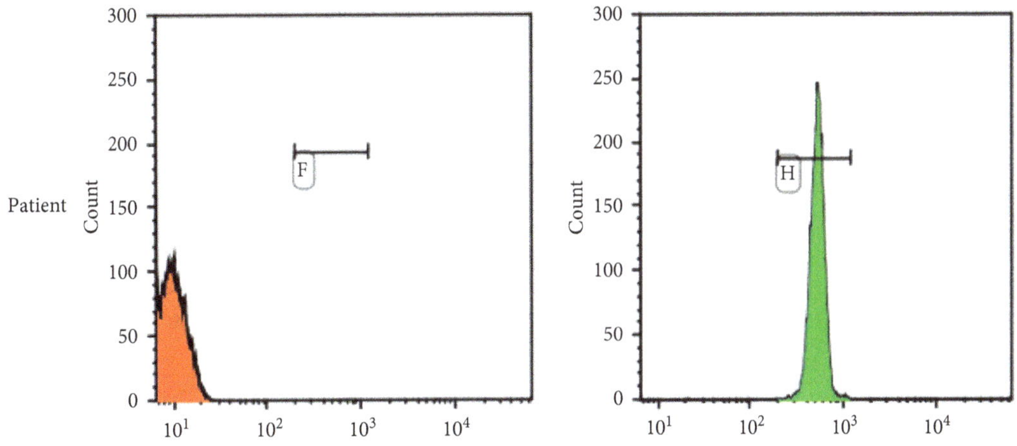

(b)

FIGURE 2: Continued.

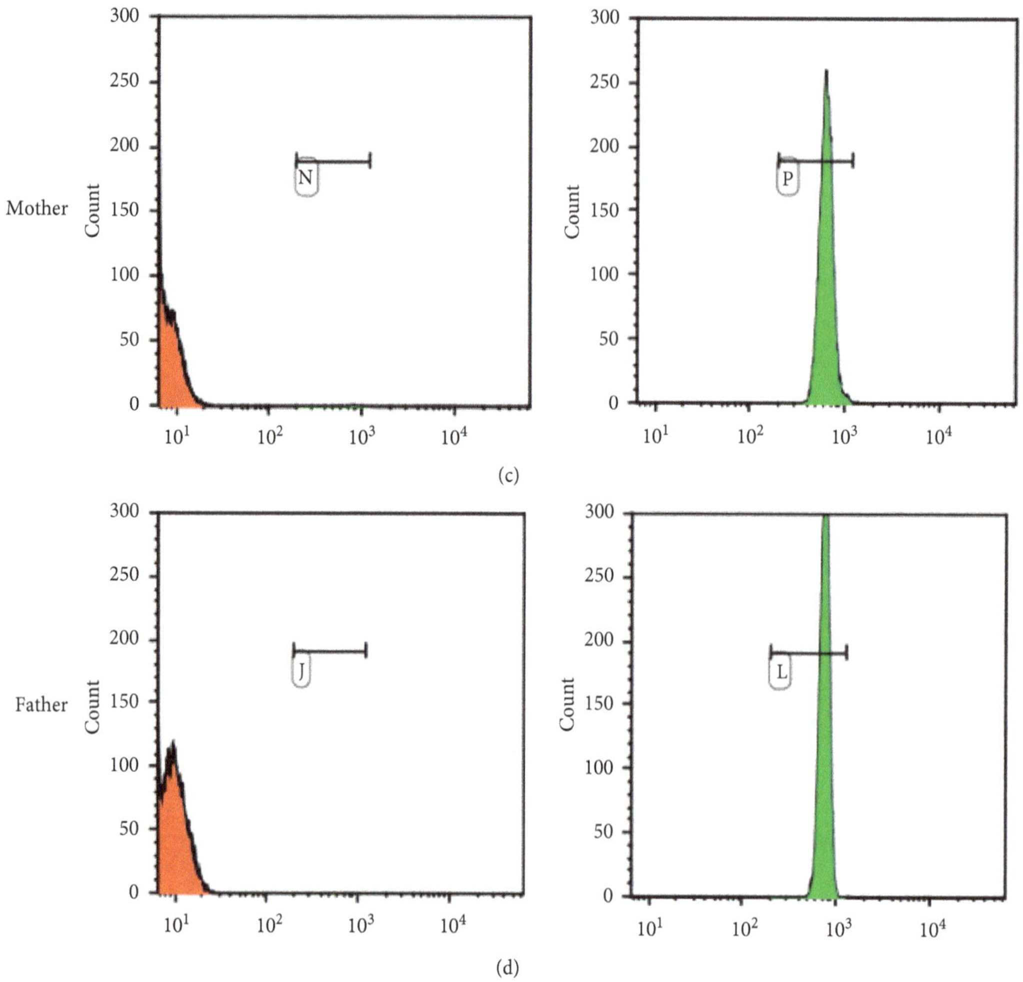

FIGURE 2: Fluorescence histogram of eosin-5-maleimide- (EMA-) labeled red blood cells of the patient and parents compared with a normal control. The unstained red blood cells and EMA-labeled red blood cells are shown in red and green, respectively.

affected by the dye stability and dye concentration [26]. The previous studies recommended reconstitution of the EMA dye every 6 months and storage at −20°C for 4 months [14] or −80°C for 6 months [26] in dark conditions. The test may be tested after a blood transfusion, which will show a double peak of fluorescence, indicating two red cells populations with normal fluorescence intensity and decreased fluorescence intensity [27].

The definite diagnosis of HS can be made by identification of the causative mutation. However, as the information of the involved genes and mutations causing HS remains limited, the current genetic identification technique is usually based on the whole-exome sequencing (WES) method which is costly and not widely available. Using flow cytometry with EMA-labeled RBCs provides a fast and practical diagnostic test which is helpful to identify HS as the cause of neonatal anemia and hyperbilirubinemia.

5. Conclusions

The careful examination of RBC morphology of the newborn and parents is the most crucial step of investigations of RBC disorders in newborns. EMA is a fluorescent dye that binds to band 3 protein. The deficiencies of band 3 and other adjacent proteins, ankyrin and band 4.2 which cause hereditary spherocytosis, result in a decrease of fluorescence intensity of EMA binding. Thus, the flow cytometry with EMA-labeled red blood cells is a practical and useful test for diagnosis of HS in newborn. The test is easily operated, rapid, and requires small amount of blood which is ideal to use in newborns.

Authors' Contributions

KF designed the study, performed the laboratory tests, collected and analyzed the data, and wrote the manuscript. PC supervised the experimental study. SM performed the laboratory tests, and RN collected the clinical data. LS wrote the manuscript. All authors gave critical comments, revised, and approved the final manuscript.

Acknowledgments

The authors would like to thank Pediatrics Laboratory staff for their laboratory supports.

References

[1] R. D. Christensen, H. M. Yaish, and P. G. Gallagher, "A pediatrician's practical guide to diagnosing and treating hereditary spherocytosis in neonates," *Pediatrics*, vol. 135, no. 6, pp. 1107–1114, 2015.

[2] A. K. Parpart, P. B. Lorenz, E. R. Parpart, J. R. Gregg, and A. M. Chase, "The osmotic resistance (fragility) of human red cells," *Journal of Clinical Investigation*, vol. 26, no. 4, pp. 636–640, 1947.

[3] E. L. Gottfried and N. A. Robertson, "Glycerol lysis time of incubated erythrocytes in the diagnosis of hereditary spherocytosis," *Journal of Laboratory and Clinical Medicine*, vol. 84, no. 5, pp. 746–751, 1974.

[4] M. J. Bucx, W. P. Breed, and J. J. M. L. Hoffmann, "Comparison of acidified glycerol lysis test, pink test and osmotic fragility test in hereditary spherocytosis: effect of incubation," *European Journal of Haematology*, vol. 40, no. 3, pp. 227–231, 1988.

[5] S. H. Park, C.-J. Park, B.-R. Lee et al., "Comparison study of the eosin-5′-maleimide binding test, flow cytometric osmotic fragility test, and cryohemolysis test in the diagnosis of hereditary spherocytosis," *American Journal of Clinical Pathology*, vol. 142, no. 4, pp. 474–484, 2014.

[6] R. Kar, P. Mishra, and H. P. Pati, "Evaluation of eosin-5-maleimide flow cytometric test in diagnosis of hereditary spherocytosis," *International Journal of Laboratory Hematology*, vol. 32, no. 1-2, pp. 8–16, 2010.

[7] O. Andres, S. Eber, and C. P. Speer, "Early postnatal diagnosis of hereditary spherocytosis by combining light microscopy, acidified glycerol lysis test and eosin-5'-maleimide binding assay," *Annals of Hematology*, vol. 94, no. 12, pp. 1959–1964, 2015.

[8] D. Korones and H. A. Pearson, "Normal erythrocyte osmotic fragility in hereditary spherocytosis," *Journal of Pediatrics*, vol. 114, no. 2, pp. 264–266, 1989.

[9] M. G. Farias, "Advances in laboratory diagnosis of hereditary spherocytosis," *Clinical Chemistry and Laboratory Medicine (CCLM)*, vol. 55, no. 7, pp. 944–948, 2017.

[10] N. Mohandas, Y. R. Kim, D. H. Tycko et al., "Accurate and independent measurement of volume and hemoglobin concentration of individual red cells by laser light scattering," *Blood*, vol. 68, no. 2, pp. 506–513, 1986.

[11] S. Streichman and Y. Gescheidt, "Cryohemolysis for the detection of hereditary spherocytosis: correlation studies with osmotic fragility and autohemolysis," *American Journal of Hematology*, vol. 58, no. 3, pp. 206–212, 1998.

[12] G. Stoya, B. Gruhn, H. Vogelsang, E. Baumann, and W. Linss, "Flow cytometry as a diagnostic tool for hereditary spherocytosis," *Acta Haematologica*, vol. 116, no. 3, pp. 186–191, 2006.

[13] M.-J. King, J. S. Smythe, and R. Mushens, "Eosin-5-maleimide binding to band 3 and Rh-related proteins forms the basis of a screening test for hereditary spherocytosis," *British Journal of Haematology*, vol. 124, no. 1, pp. 106–113, 2004.

[14] M.-J. King, J. Behrens, C. Rogers, C. Flynn, D. Greenwood, and K. Chambers, "Rapid flow cytometric test for the diagnosis of membrane cytoskeleton-associated haemolytic anaemia," *British Journal of Haematology*, vol. 111, no. 3, pp. 924–933, 2000.

[15] P. H. B. Bolton-Maggs, J. C. Langer, A. Iolascon, P. Tittensor, and M.-J. King, "Guidelines for the diagnosis and management of hereditary spherocytosis—2011 update," *British Journal of Haematology*, vol. 156, no. 1, pp. 37–49, 2012.

[16] R. D. Christensen, A. M. Agarwal, R. H. Nussenzveig, N. Heikal, M. A. Liew, and H. M. Yaish, "Evaluating eosin-5-maleimide binding as a diagnostic test for hereditary spherocytosis in newborn infants," *Journal of Perinatology*, vol. 35, no. 5, pp. 357–361, 2015.

[17] R. D. Christensen and E. Henry, "Hereditary spherocytosis in neonates with hyperbilirubinemia," *Pediatrics*, vol. 125, no. 1, pp. 120–125, 2010.

[18] A. M. Agarwal, M. A. Liew, R. H. Nussenzveig et al., "Improved harmonization of eosin-5-maleimide binding test across different instruments and age groups," *Cytometry Part B: Clinical Cytometry*, vol. 90, no. 6, pp. 512–516, 2016.

[19] P. S. Kedar, R. B. Colah, S. Kulkarni, K. Ghosh, and D. Mohanty, "Experience with eosin-5'-maleimide as a diagnostic tool for red cell membrane cytoskeleton disorders," *Clinical and Laboratory Haematology*, vol. 25, no. 6, pp. 373–376, 2003.

[20] P. Bianchi, E. Fermo, C. Vercellati et al., "Diagnostic power of laboratory tests for hereditary spherocytosis: a comparison study in 150 patients grouped according to molecular and clinical characteristics," *Haematologica*, vol. 97, no. 4, pp. 516–523, 2012.

[21] M.-J. King, P. Telfer, H. MacKinnon et al., "Using the eosin-5-maleimide binding test in the differential diagnosis of hereditary spherocytosis and hereditary pyropoikilocytosis," *Cytometry Part B: Clinical Cytometry*, vol. 74, no. 4, pp. 244–250, 2008.

[22] O. Ciepiela, "Old and new insights into the diagnosis of hereditary spherocytosis," *Annals of Translational Medicine*, vol. 6, no. 17, p. 339, 2018.

[23] L. Da Costa, L. Suner, J. Galimand et al., "Diagnostic tool for red blood cell membrane disorders: assessment of a new generation ektacytometer," *Blood Cells, Molecules, and Diseases*, vol. 56, no. 1, pp. 9–22, 2016.

[24] O. Ciepiela, I. Kotuła, E. Górska et al., "Delay in the measurement of eosin-5'-maleimide (EMA) binding does not affect the test result for the diagnosis of hereditary spherocytosis," *Clinical Chemistry and Laboratory Medicine*, vol. 51, no. 4, pp. 817–823, 2013.

[25] F. Girodon, L. Garçon, E. Bergoin et al., "Usefulness of the eosin-5'-maleimide cytometric method as a first-line screening test for the diagnosis of hereditary spherocytosis: comparison with ektacytometry and protein electrophoresis," *British Journal of Haematology*, vol. 140, no. 4, pp. 468–470, 2008.

[26] S. Mehra, N. Tyagi, P. Dorwal et al., "Stability of eosin-5'-maleimide dye used in flow cytometric analysis for red cell membrane disorders," *Blood Research*, vol. 50, no. 2, pp. 109–112, 2015.

[27] E. Cheli, J. Roze, T. Garrot, S. Tagarist, C. Briandet, and F. Girodon, "Usefulness of the EMA flow cytometric test in the diagnosis of hereditary spherocytosis post-transfusion," *British Journal of Haematology*, vol. 178, no. 2, p. 180, 2017.

33

Immunotherapy- (Blinatumomab-) Related Lineage Switch of *KMT2A/AFF1* Rearranged B-Lymphoblastic Leukemia into Acute Myeloid Leukemia/Myeloid Sarcoma and Subsequently into B/Myeloid Mixed Phenotype Acute Leukemia

Rui R. He,[1] Zacharia Nayer,[2] Matthew Hogan,[3] Raymund S. Cuevo,[4] Kimberly Woodward,[1] David Heyer,[4] Christine A. Curtis,[5] and Jess F. Peterson[6]

[1]*Department of Pathology, Inova Fairfax Hospital, Falls Church, VA, USA*
[2]*School of Medicine, George Washington University, Washington, DC, USA*
[3]*School of Medicine, Virginia Commonwealth University, Richmond, VA, USA*
[4]*Inova Schar Cancer Institute, Inova Fairfax Hospital, Falls Church, VA, USA*
[5]*Department of Cytogenetics, Quest Diagnostics Nichols Institute, Chantilly, VA, USA*
[6]*Division of Laboratory Genetics and Genomics, Department of Laboratory Medicine and Pathology, Mayo Clinic, Rochester, MN, USA*

Correspondence should be addressed to Jess F. Peterson; peterson.jess@mayo.edu

Academic Editor: Kostas Konstantopoulos

The presence of *KMT2A/AFF1* rearrangement in B-lymphoblastic leukemia (B-ALL) is an independent poor prognostic factor and has been associated with higher rate of treatment failure and higher risk of linage switch under therapy. Blinatumomab has shown promising therapeutic results in refractory or relapsed B-ALL; however, it has potential risk of inducing lineage switch, especially in *KMT2A/AFF1* rearranged B-ALL into acute myeloid leukemia and/or myeloid sarcoma. We report a 40-year-old female with *KMT2A/AFF1*-rearranged B-ALL that was refractory to conventional chemotherapy. Following administration of blinatumomab, she developed a breast mass proven to be myeloid sarcoma, in addition to bone marrow involvement by AML. Approximately six weeks after cessation of blinatumomab, a repeat bone marrow examination revealed B/myeloid MPAL.

1. Introduction

Immunotherapy targeted at CD19, either antibody-based (blinatumomab) or T-cell mediated (CAR T cells), represents a promising treatment strategy for patients with refractory B-lymphoblastic leukemia (B-ALL). Early phase clinical trials have shown high rates of complete remission in refractory pediatric B-ALL patients after CD19 CAR-T-cell or blinatumomab therapy [1, 2]. However, a rare event, lineage switch from B-ALL to acute myeloid leukemia (AML) can occur following CD19 targeted therapy, most commonly in *KMT2A*-rearranged B-ALL [3–6]. The *KMT2A* gene is a critical target of chromosomal rearrangements observed in ALL, AML, mixed phenotype acute leukemia (MPAL), and therapy-related myeloid neoplasms [7]. The presence of *KMT2A* rearrangement, especially in B-ALL, has long been associated with a higher risk of lineage switch under therapy and is an independent dismal prognostic factor [8]. However, the exact mechanism and management of linage switch events are unclear. Herein, we report a 40-year-old female with *KMT2A/AFF1*-rearranged B-ALL refractory to conventional chemotherapy. Following administration of blinatumomab, she developed a breast mass proven to be myeloid sarcoma, in addition to bone marrow involvement by AML. Approximately six weeks after cessation of blinatumomab, a repeat bone marrow examination revealed B/myeloid MPAL.

2. Case Description

A 40-year-old female without a past medical history presented with two weeks of easy bruising, fatigue, and muscle aches. A complete blood count revealed leukocytosis (white blood cell count, $71.8 \times 10^3/\mu L$; reference, $3.4–9.6 \times 10^3/\mu L$), anemia (hemoglobin, 12.6 g/dL; reference, 13.2–16.6 g/dL), and thrombocytopenia (platelet count, $77 \times 10^3/\mu L$; reference, $135–317 \times 10^3/\mu L$). Peripheral blood smear revealed numerous small-to-intermediate-sized blasts with high nuclear-to-cytoplasmic (N : C) ratio, fine chromatin, and prominent nucleoli. Flow cytometry performed on peripheral blood sample revealed a large population of blasts in the dim CD45 region expressing CD19 (bright), CD34 (dim), and CD15 (dim) and was negative for CD10. A subset of blasts appeared to be positive for myeloperoxidase (MPO). Bone marrow evaluation revealed a hypercellular bone marrow (90%) composed of numerous small-to-intermediate-sized blasts with similar morphology as the blasts are identified in peripheral blood smear (Figure 1, A1 and A2). Flow cytometry of bone marrow aspirate revealed a large population of blasts immunophenotypically identical to the blasts detected in peripheral blood (Figure 1, F). Since it was questionable for MPO positivity in a subset of blasts, immunohistochemical analysis was performed on the bone marrow biopsy specimen. The blasts were strongly positive for PAX5 (Figure 1, A3), CD19, and CD79a; focally positive for CD34; but were completely negative for MPO (data not shown). Taken together, these findings are consistent with a diagnosis of B-ALL. Chromosomal analysis revealed a complex karyotype including *t*(4; 11)(*q*21; *q*23), while fluorescence *in situ* hybridization (FISH) confirmed *KMT2A* rearrangement (Table 1). The patient received induction chemotherapy with cyclophosphamide, daunorubicin, vincristine, and dexamethasone (HyperCVAD cycle 1A). A month after her blood cell count recovery, she was found to have circulating blasts and was treated with HyperCVAD cycle 1B (with high dose cytarabine and methotrexate) but had resistant disease on day 21 of therapy. She was started on salvage blinatumomab the next day and treated per protocol. The patient developed cytokine release syndrome and was treated transiently. A month into blinatumomab therapy, the patient subsequently developed a painful right breast mass. The biopsy from the mass showed sheets of large-sized blastic cells (Figure 1, B1 andB2) which were positive for lysozyme (B3) but negative for CD19, PAX5, and other B-cell markers (data not shown) by immunohistochemistry, consistent with a diagnosis of myeloid sarcoma. A bone marrow evaluation revealed a hypercellular marrow (90%) composed of sheets of blasts with monocytic features (Figure 1, C1 andC2). Flow cytometry from the bone marrow aspirate detected a population of blasts expressing CD33 and CD64 (dim), but was negative for CD19 and CD34 (Figure 1, G). The blasts were also positive for CD13 and myeloperoxidase and negative for cytoCD79a (data not shown). Immunohistochemical study performed on bone marrow biopsy showed the blasts were positive for lysozyme (Figure 1, C3). Taken together, a diagnosis of AML with monocytic differentiation was rendered. Conventional chromosome analysis from the bone marrow aspirate revealed *t*(4; 11)(*q*21; *q*23) and additional chromosomal abnormalities (Figure 1, E1; Table 1). Six weeks after discontinuation of blinatumomab, a repeat bone marrow biopsy and aspirate demonstrated a hypercellular marrow (80%) with a dimorphic population of blasts composed of mixed small-and large-sized blasts (Figure 1, D1-D2). Flow cytometry and immunohistochemical studies confirmed the presence of two populations of blasts: (1) B-lymphoblasts phenotypically identical to those in the patient's initial bone marrow specimen expressing CD19, CD34 (dim), and cytoCD79a and (2) myeloblasts phenotypically similar to those in her second bone marrow specimen expressing CD33 and CD64 (Figure 1, H). The myeloblasts were also positive for myeloperoxidase (data not shown). These findings indicated a diagnosis of B/myeloid MPAL. Chromosome and FISH studies confirmed the presence of *KMT2A/AFF1* fusion with additional chromosomal abnormalities (Figure 1, E2–E4; Table 1). The patient's leukemia did not respond to mitoxantrone, etoposide, cytarabine (MEC), and fludarabine, cytarabine, and idarubicin with growth factor (FLAG-ida), and she passed away on day 12 of her last regimen.

3. Discussion

We present a case of a 40-year-old female with an initial diagnosis of *KMT2A/AFF1* rearranged B-ALL that subsequently switched to more aggressive types of leukemic events and with extramedullary involvement. The unique features of this case include several clonally related, but phenotypically distinct leukemic events (B-ALL, AML, myeloid sarcoma of the breast, and MPAL) that occurred within a six-month period. The transformed AML/myeloid sarcoma and MPAL were associated with administration and cessation of blinatumomab, respectively, and demonstrated additional cytogenetic abnormalities in addition to *KMT2A/AFF1* fusion. This case provides evidence that two key factors appear to be involved in this lineage switching event: *KMT2A* rearrangement and blinatumomab therapy. *KMT2A*-rearranged acute leukemia represents a heterogeneous group of disease overlapping lymphoid and myeloid with more than 100 different fusion partners identified to date [6]. The presence of *KMT2A* rearrangement has long been associated with a higher risk of lineage switch under chemotherapy and subsequent failure to treatment even before the emergence of immunotherapies [8, 9]. As a monoclonal antibody with bispecificity for both CD19 on B cells and CD3 on cytotoxic T cells, blinatumomab has shown promising therapeutic results in treating refractory or relapsed B-ALL; however, the risk of inducing lineage switch especially in *KMT2A/AFF1* rearranged B-ALL should not be underestimated.

While the exact mechanism of linage switch remains unclear, several possible mechanisms have been proposed [9–14]. Studies have suggested that inherent lineage plasticity of early progenitor cells and immunotherapeutic

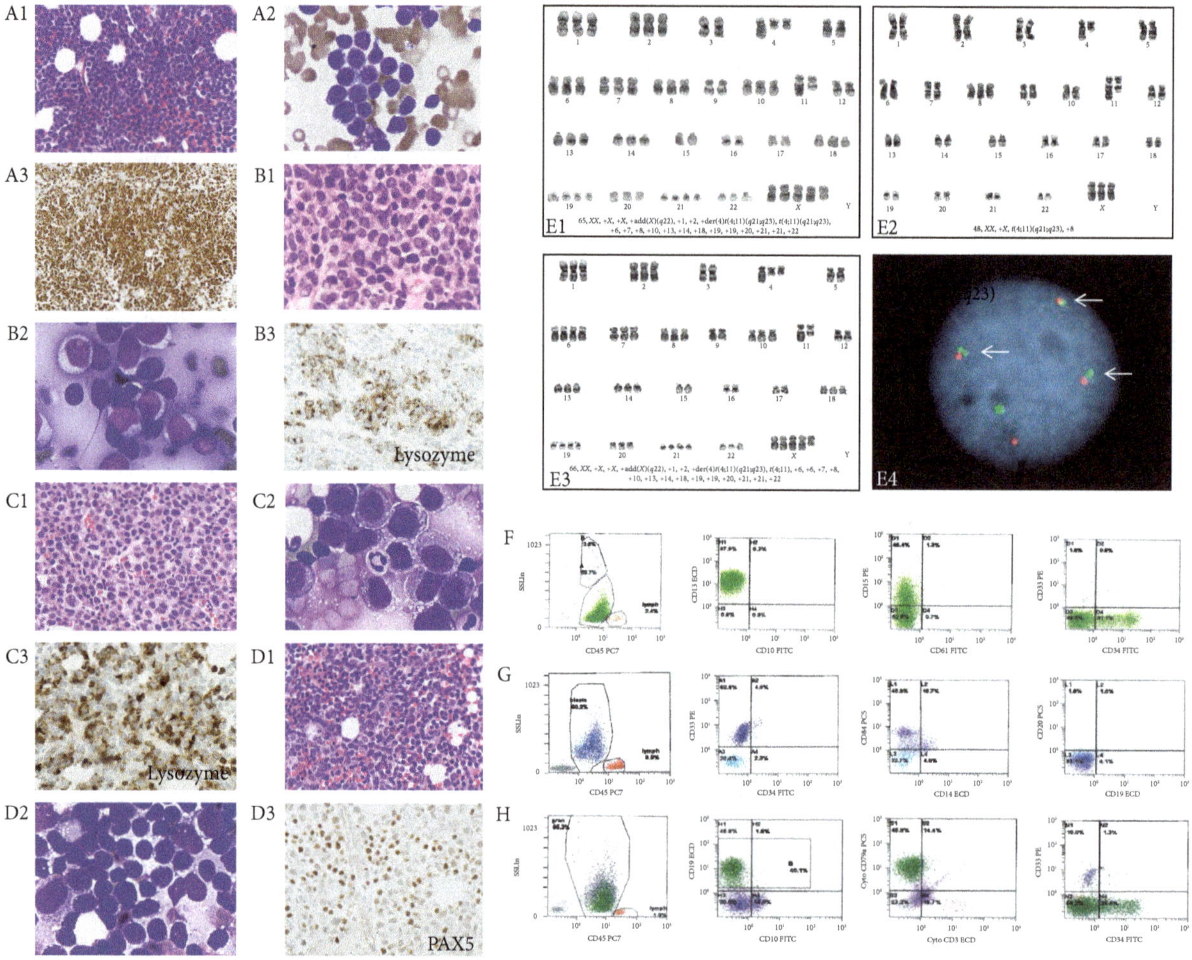

Figure 1: Morphologic, immunohistochemical, flow cytometric, and cytogenetic characteristics of the patient's leukemia. A1–A3 represent bone marrow evaluation at initial diagnosis. Bone marrow biopsy (A1, H&E, 400x) and aspirate (A2, Wright stain 100x, oil) showing numerous small-sized B-lymphoblasts which are strongly positive for PAX5 (A3). B1–B3 represent biopsy of the breast mass (B1, H&E, 400x) and touch imprint (B2, Wright stain, 100x, oil) showing numerous large-sized blasts with monocytic differentiation, which are patchy positive for lysozyme (B3). C1–C3 represent bone marrow biopsy (C1, H&E, 400x) and aspirate (C2, Wright stain, 100x, oil) showing sheets of myeloblasts which are patchy positive for lysozyme (C3). D1–D3 represent bone marrow evaluation six weeks after cessation of blinatumomab. Core biopsy (D1, H&E, 400x) and aspirate (D2, Wright stain, 100x, Oil) show a dimorphic population of blasts: small-sized B-lymphoblasts which are positive for PAX5 (D3) and large-sized myeloblasts which are positive for lysozyme (data not shown here). E1 represents the karyogram of bone marrow specimen at myeloblastic transformation. E2–E4 represent karyograms and *AFF1/KMT2A* fusion of bone marrow specimen with B/myeloid mixed phenotype acute leukemia. F–H represent flow cytometric features of the leukemic blasts. F represents flow cytometry performed on the bone marrow aspirate at the initial diagnosis showing a large population of B-lymphoblasts (green) in dim CD45 region expressing CD19, CD34 (partial), and CD15 (dim), G represents flow cytometry of the bone marrow aspirate while administration of blinatumomab showing a population of myeloblasts (blue) expressing CD33 and CD64 (dim) and was negative for CD19 and CD34. H represents flow cytometry of the bone marrow aspirate six weeks after cessation of blinatumomab showing two populations: B-lymphoblasts (green) expressing CD19, CD34 (dim), and cytoCD79a, and myeloblasts (blue) expressing CD33, CD64 (dim), and MPO (data not shown here).

Table 1: Genetic results obtained at the time of B-ALL diagnosis, transformation to AML following initiation of blinatumomab therapy, and subsequent posttransformation to MPAL upon discontinuation of blinatumomab.

Genetic testing	Diagnosis: B-ALL (10/26/2018)	Transformation: AML (02/25/2019)	Transformation: MPAL (04/18/2019)
Conventional chromosome analysis	48, XX, +X, *t*(4; 11)(*q*21; *q*23), +8 [20]/49, idem, +X, *i*(X) (*p*10)*x*2, −8 [2]/46, XX[1]	63~67, XX, +X, +X, +add(X)(*q*22) *x*1~2, +1, +2, *t*(4; 11)(*q*21; *q*23), +der(4)*t*(4; 11), +6, +7, +8, +10, +13, +14, +18, +19, +19, +20, +21, +21, +22[*cp*10]/46, XX[10]	48, XX, +X, *t*(4; 11)(*q*21; *q*23), +8 [18]/64~66, idem, +X, +add(X)(*q*22), +1, +2, +der(4) *t*(4; 11), +6, +6, +7, +10, +13, +14, +18, +19, +19, +20, +21, +21, +22[*cp*2]
FISH	*KMT2A* rearrangement (93% of 100 interphase nuclei)	Not performed	*AFF1/KMT2A* fusion (92% of 500 interphase nuclei)

B-ALL, B-acute lymphoblastic leukemia; AML, acute myeloid leukemia; MPAL, mixed phenotype acute leukemia; FISH, fluorescence *in situ* hybridization.

pressure-induced lineage reprogramming play important roles [3, 9, 10]. An experimental study demonstrated that cellular microenvironment affects cell fate decisions and lineage interconversions [12]. Other studies hypothesized that immunotherapy-induced cytokine release (notably interleukin 6) may promote myeloid differentiation of a lymphoid clone [1, 3, 13]. Additional studies have postulated that genetic evolutions of leukemic blasts under targeted therapy may contribute to lineage switch [10, 14]. The findings in this case suggest that high biphenotypic potential of *KMT2A/AFF1* rearranged B-ALL blasts, blinatumomab-induced blastic cell reprogramming, clonal evolution, and cytokine release might have played important roles in this lineage switching event.

In conclusion, the lineage switch events indicate that cautious application of immunotherapy in *KMT2A/AFF1*¯ rearranged B-ALL should be advocated in clinical settings. Targeting multiple antigens on leukemia-initiating cells may be a better strategy to reduce the likelihood of lineage switching.

References

[1] R. Gardner, D. Wu, S. Cherian et al., "Acquisition of a CD19-negative myeloid phenotype allows immune escape of MLL-rearranged B-ALL from CD19 CAR-T-cell therapy," *Blood*' vol. 127, no. 20, pp. 2406–2410, 2016.

[2] V. Brower, "Phase 1/2 study of blinatumomab in relapsed paediatric ALL," *The Lancet Oncology*, vol. 17, no. 12, p. e525, 2016.

[3] M. Wölfl, M. Rasche, M. Eyrich, R. Schmid, D. Reinhardt, and P. G. Schlegel, "Spontaneous reversion of a lineage switch following an initial blinatumomab-induced ALL-to-AML switch in *MLL*-rearranged infant ALL," *Blood Advances*' vol. 2, no. 12, pp. 1382–1385, 2018.

[4] E. Fournier, L. Inchiappa, C. Delattre et al., "Increased risk of adverse acute myeloid leukemia after anti-CD19-targeted immunotherapies in KMT2A-rearranged acute lymphoblastic leukemia: a case report and review of the literature," *Leukemia and Lymphoma*, vol. 60, no. 7, pp. 1827–1830, 2019.

[5] C. L. Haddox, A. A. Mangaonkar, D. Chen et al., "Blinatumomab-induced lineage switch of B-ALL with *t*(4:11)(*q*21; *q*23) KMT2A/AFF1 into an aggressive AML: pre- and post-switch phenotypic, cytogenetic and molecular analysis," *Blood Cancer Journal*, vol. 7, no. 9, p. e607, 2017.

[6] A. Rayes, R. L. McMasters, and M. M. O'Brien, "Lineage switch in MLL-rearranged infant leukemia following CD19-directed therapy," *Pediatric Blood and Cancer*, vol. 63, no. 6, pp. 1113–1115, 2016.

[7] C. Mayer, T. Burmeister, D. Gröger et al., "The MLL recombinome of acute leukemias in 2017," *Leukemia*, vol. 32, pp. 273–284, 2018.

[8] J. G. Rossi, A. R. Bernasconi, C. N. Alonso et al., "Lineage switch in childhood acute leukemia: an unusual event with poor outcome," *American Journal of Hematology*, vol. 87, no. 9, pp. 890–897, 2012.

[9] E. Jacoby, S. Nguyen, T. Fountaine et al., "CD19 CAR immune pressure induces B-precursor acute lymphoblastic leukemia lineage switch exposing inherent leukemic plasticity," *Nature Communications*, vol. 7, p. 12320, 2016.

[10] U. Duffner, A. Abdel-Mageed, J. Younge et al., "The possible perils of targeted therapy," *Leukemia*, vol. 30, no. 7, pp. 1619–1621, 2016.

[11] A. C. Winters and K. M. Bernt, "MLL-rearranged leukemias-an update on science and clinical approaches," *Frontiers in Pediatrics*, vol. 5, p. 454, 2017.

[12] J. Wei, M. Wunderlich, C. Fox et al., "Microenvironment determines lineage fate in a human model of MLL-AF9 leukemia," *Cancer Cell*, vol. 13, no. 6, pp. 483–495, 2008.

[13] A. Cohen, D. Petsche, T. Grunberger, and M. H. Freedman, "Interleukin 6 induces myeloid differentiation of a human biphenotypic leukemic cell line," *Leukemia Research*, vol. 16, no. 8, pp. 751–760, 1992.

[14] E. Balducci, V. Nivaggioni, J. Boudjarane et al., "Lineage switch from B acute lymphoblastic leukemia to acute monocytic leukemia with persistent *t*(4;11)(*q*21;*q*23) and cytogenetic evolution under CD19-targeted therapy," *Annals of Hematology*, vol. 96, no. 9, pp. 1579–1581, 2017.

34

Histoplasma capsulatum Infection in an Allogeneic Hematopoietic Stem Cell Transplant Patient Receiving Voriconazole Prophylaxis

Vaibhav Agrawal[1,2] **Bryan J. Brinda,**[3] **and Sherif S. Farag**[1,2]

[1]*Department of Medicine, Division of Hematology and Oncology, Indiana University School of Medicine, Indianapolis, IN, USA*
[2]*Bone Marrow and Blood Stem Cell Transplantation Program, Indiana University, Indianapolis, IN, USA*
[3]*Department of Pharmacy, Division of Hematology-Oncology, University of Kentucky, Lexington, KY, USA*

Correspondence should be addressed to Vaibhav Agrawal; agrawal1@iu.edu

Academic Editor: Tomás J. González-López

Histoplasma capsulatum infection is a rare complication in the allogeneic stem cell transplant patients. Minimal guidance exists on how to appropriately manage histoplasmosis in these patients. We report a patient who developed *Histoplasma* pneumonia while receiving voriconazole prophylaxis at a therapeutic trough level. The patient experienced significant clinical improvement after initiation of itraconazole pharmacotherapy. We recommend a lower threshold for evaluation for histoplasmosis in allogeneic hematopoietic stem cell transplant recipients who live in endemic regions, regardless of their antifungal prophylactic regimen.

1. Introduction

Within the United States, most cases of *Histoplasma capsulatum* infection have been reported in the Ohio and Mississippi River valleys. While an otherwise asymptomatic *H. capsulatum* infection can occur in patients with competent immune systems, it is far more clinically concerning in those who are immunosuppressed [1]. Typical signs and symptoms of *H. capsulatum* infection include fever, chills, myalgias, dry cough, and chest discomfort. In immunocompromised patients, the disease may become disseminated and if untreated, is usually fatal with a reported mortality rate of 67% in allogeneic hematopoietic stem cell transplant recipients [2]. Itraconazole and amphotericin are the first-line therapies for treatment of histoplasmosis; however, other antifungal agents such as voriconazole and posaconazole are thought to be active and have been utilized as salvage therapy [3]. Here, we present a unique case of *H. capsulatum* infection in a matched-unrelated donor stem cell transplant patient who was receiving voriconazole prophylaxis.

2. Case Presentation

A 55-year-old male who was a long-term resident of Indiana with a history of allogenic peripheral stem cell transplantation presented to the bone marrow transplant clinic for routine follow-up. He initially was diagnosed with stage IVB diffuse large B-cell lymphoma in August 2009 and was treated with rituximab, cyclophosphamide, doxorubicin, vincristine, and prednisone (R-CHOP) and achieved complete remission. He relapsed in April 2010 and was treated with rituximab, etoposide, methylprednisolone, high-dose cytarabine, and cisplatin (R-ESHAP) and underwent an autologous peripheral stem cell transplant in July 2010 with the myeloablative preparative regimen of carmustine, etoposide, cytarabine, and melphalan (BEAM). In July 2015, he developed therapy-related myelodysplastic syndrome after his autologous transplant and underwent initial cytoreduction with 5-azacytidine followed by a matched-unrelated donor allogeneic peripheral blood stem cell transplantation in June 2016 at another institution. The patient developed acute graft-versus-host disease (GVHD) involving the skin and gut approximately one month after transplantation, which responded to corticosteroids as well as continuation of calcineurin inhibitor. He continued to be treated intermittently with courses of corticosteroids for presumed chronic GVHD of the liver until day 282 after transplant when he switched his care to our institution. At this point, he was found to have no evidence of active GVHD except for a mild elevation of alkaline phosphatase; corticosteroids were therefore tapered and discontinued on day 329 after transplant. He was also found to have anemia and thrombocytopenia, which was shown to be due to thrombotic microangiopathy, and calcineurin inhibitor therapy was also discontinued and the patient was placed on mycophenolate mofetil to prevent any exacerbations of chronic GVHD.

On day +365 after transplant, he presented to the clinic with a cough productive of whitish sputum, fatigue, weakness, and intermittent fevers with chills. A chest X-ray showed no radiographic abnormalities, and a respiratory viral panel was positive for parainfluenza virus type 3. Blood cultures were negative. No abnormalities were noted in his blood counts or complete metabolic panel. His anti-infectious regimen at the time included prophylaxis with atovaquone 1500 mg daily for prevention of pneumocystis pneumonia, valacyclovir 500 mg daily for prevention of zoster infections, and voriconazole 200 mg twice daily for prevention of fungal infections in the setting of his increased risk secondary to long-term steroid exposure. Initial recommendations were to proceed with supportive care therapeutic strategies for his parainfluenza virus type 3. He returned to the clinic two weeks later and while reporting general improvement in his respiratory symptoms, he continued to experience chills and sweating at night without any documented fever. No antibacterial therapy was prescribed at this time, and continued therapeutic intervention with supportive care was recommended. Five days later, he returned to the clinic with complaints of wheezing, green-yellow sputum production, low-grade fevers, continued fatigue, and nausea. Blood cultures, sputum cultures, and serum cytomegalovirus were all negative. He received nebulized albuterol and a prescription for clarithromycin. A computed tomography (CT) scan of the chest was performed that revealed diffuse peribronchial wall thickening with tree in bud nodularity in the lower lobes, two pulmonary nodules within the left apex each measuring 3 mm, and a 5 mm nodule within the right lower lobe. A repeat respiratory viral panel showed the persistence of both parainfluenza virus 3 and now newly detected respiratory syncytial virus A.

As the patient was not clinically improving and continued to report low-grade fever a week later, bronchoscopy was performed. Bronchoalveolar lavage (BAL) fluid showed pink and cloudy secretions with 6% monocytes, 93% granulocytes, and 1% eosinophils. Calcofluor-white and Gram stains were negative for *Aspergillus* and blastomycosis, as well as for *Histoplasma*. A positive antigen for *Histoplasma* was detected in the bronchoalveolar lavage sample using MiraVista diagnostic testing, but below the limit of quantification (reported as above the limit of detection but <0.4 ng/mL). A urine *Histoplasma* test was negative. At this time, a voriconazole serum trough level was 2.4 mcg/mL (goal 1–5.5 mcg/mL). He was also evaluated in a consultative visit by Infectious Disease to affirm this diagnosis of histoplasmosis. With concern for the patient's worsening clinical condition in his immunocompromised state and the lack of access to molecular testing at the time to support the result of antigen testing, recommendations were made to discontinue voriconazole and commence treatment with itraconazole 200 mg twice daily by mouth and mycophenolate mofetil was discontinued.

The patient returned to the clinic two weeks later and reported resolution of fever, improved well-being, and significant reduction in the frequency and productive nature of his cough. An itraconazole trough level was therapeutic at 0.5 mcg/mL (goal > 0.5 mcg/mL). Over the next two months, the patient reported resolution of all symptoms. He continues on therapeutic itraconazole with the plan of continuing lifelong suppressive therapy after one year of treatment.

3. Discussion

Histoplasma infection is a rare complication in stem cell transplant recipients with very few cases reported to date, and minimal guidance exists on how to appropriately manage this infection in this patient population [3–7].

Infection by *Histoplasma capsulatum* has been reported to occur frequently in the endemic areas of the United States in the Midwest and Central states along the Ohio and Mississippi River valleys. It is the most prevalent endemic mycosis in the United States. In the immunocompetent individual, histoplasmosis generally manifests as an asymptomatic and self-limited presentation with symptoms that are often typical of cough or nonspecific flu-like symptoms. It is reported that fewer than five percent of exposed individuals develop the symptomatic disease of progressive disseminated histoplasmosis, with common risk factors including an immunocompromised state, immunosuppressive medications, or prior solid organ transplantation [8]. In the absence of treatment, and in cases of presentation in immunocompromised individuals, severe complications can arise, including potentially fatal fibrosing mediastinitis, respiratory failure, and progressive fibrosis of lymph nodes [9]. Disseminated histoplasmosis is characterized by the progressive spread of infection to extrapulmonary sites of multiple organs and is fatal unless adequate and timely treatment is administered.

In most patients, histoplasmosis presents as a subacute pulmonary infection and is commonly mistaken as a community-acquired pneumonia or viral infection and is often only considered after there is no initial response to antibacterial therapy [10]. Symptoms typically resolve within a few weeks, but there may be persistent fatigue and asthenia that lasts for several months [11]. While most infections are self-limited, it is estimated that progressive disseminated infection occurs more commonly in immunocompromised patients.

The relationship between an individual's underlying immune function and histoplasmosis severity was elucidated in the early years of the acquired immunodeficiency syndrome (AIDS) epidemic, whereby an increased incidence in symptomatic histoplasmosis was noted [12]. Symptomatic *H. capsulatum* infection is usually accompanied by hematogenous dissemination, which in the normal host is controlled by T-cell-mediated immunity. Immunocompro mised patients are unable to mount adequate immune responses and consequently become symptomatic during the period of acute dissemination [1, 9, 13].

Endemically exposed hematopoietic stem cell transplant (HSCT) recipients may be at increased risk for disseminated histoplasmosis, especially when graft-versus-host disease is managed with long-term corticosteroid therapy [1]. Reactivation of latent *Histoplasma*, rather than a newly acquired infection, is the apparent cause of disseminated histoplasmosis in immunosuppressed patients, particularly in patients from endemic areas [14]. Nevertheless, post-transplantation histoplasmosis is rare even in endemic areas. In solid organ transplant recipients, the largest single-center series reported an incidence of 1 case per 1000 person-years [15]. In a prospectively collected series of solid organ and HSCT patients diagnosed with endemic mycoses, only three of 16,200 HSCT recipients of histoplasmosis were identified (0.02%) of which only one patient underwent an allogeneic transplant [16]. Overall, there have been an estimated seven cases of histoplasmosis reported in the allogenic HSCT population, of which four patients with reported outcomes died [2, 4, 5, 7, 17, 18]. Furthermore, there have been no previously reported cases of histoplasmosis in patients where antifungal prophylaxis with agents that have clinical activity against *Histoplasma* were used as was in our reported case.

Culture of blood, respiratory samples, or bone marrow remains the accepted gold standard for diagnosis, but cultures take weeks to produce result and are often influenced by the extent of disease burden [19]. The presence of organisms in the bone marrow aspirate and biopsy is often the earliest diagnostic approach for early detection in the immunocompromised patient, especially given that the fungus may not be evident in culture for two to three weeks from the initial infection [20]. Serologic studies have not reported to be helpful in diagnosis of histoplasmosis in a prior study of immunocompromised patients, but the sensitivity of detection specifically in the bone marrow transplant population has yet to be studied [21]. Though a definitive diagnosis of histoplasmosis necessitates culture or histopathologic confirmation, a probable diagnosis can still be made in a patient with increased risk secondary to immunocompromised status, compatible clinical picture, and mycological evidence [22].

The diagnostic yield of BAL in confirming the diagnosis of a bacterial or fungal pulmonary infection is often difficult, particularly with the exposure to antibiotic or antifungal prophylaxis. Cytopathologic evaluation of the BAL fluid is relatively noninvasive and has a sensitivity of around 50% for acute pulmonary histoplasmosis; when combined with BAL *Histoplasma* antigen testing, the sensitivity increases to about 97% [23]. Antigen testing is generally accepted as the leading modality to diagnose histoplasmosis. The *Histoplasma* antigen was reformulated into an enzyme immunoassay (EIA) in 1989, and the third generation MiraVista *H. capsulatum* Galactomannan EIA became available in 2007. The MiraVista EIA *Histoplasma* antigen test was found to be the highest in patients with disseminated histoplasmosis (91.8%) and the lowest in patients with subacute histoplasmosis (30%) [24]. Detecting the urine antigen has additionally proven to be slightly more sensitive than the serum across all manifestations of histoplasmosis. In a large retrospective multicenter reviewing the incidence of histoplasmosis in a solid organ transplant population, urine *Histoplasma* antigen detection was the most sensitive diagnostic method with 93% positivity and detection of antibody the least sensitive, positive in 36% of cases [24]. The sensitivity of BAL antigen testing is generally accepted as being superior to both urine and serum (93% vs. 79% and 56%, respectively) [22]. In nondisseminated histoplasmosis, the antigen burden is lower and thus the sensitivity of antigen testing is lower, but combing the results of urine and antigen serum has demonstrated improvement in the sensitivity of detecting pulmonary histoplasmosis [25].

Molecular diagnostic methods have the advantage of higher analytic specificity and shorter turnaround times as compared to other diagnostic methodologies, especially when considering the time needed for colony growth in culture-based diagnosis [26]. There are currently no FDA-approved molecular assays for *Histoplasma* directly applicable to clinical specimens, though laboratory-based PCR assays using a variety of molecular targets have been developed. In prior studies focused in hematology-oncology patients that often have prolonged cytopenias, addition of molecular analysis testing has increased the efficacy of bronchoalveolar lavage in the diagnosis of respiratory infections [27]. In a study of 107 consecutive hospitalized patients with hematologic malignancies and bone marrow transplant recipients who underwent BAL for evaluation of pulmonary infiltrates, the addition of PCR-based *Aspergillus* DNA detection to improve the diagnostic capacity of invasive *Aspergillus* infection decreased mortality from 80 to 35.6% ($P = 0.003$) [28].

Although systemic candidiasis and aspergillosis are more commonly reported as major causes of fungal infections in HSCT recipients, disseminated histoplasmosis presents a threat to the HSCT recipient from an endemic area. Furthermore, the diagnosis of histoplasmosis is especially challenging because empiric or prophylactic antifungal treatment is often administered after HSCT, and this may possibly lead to an underestimation of histoplasmosis. The significant mortality associated with post-transplant histoplasmosis and nonspecific clinical presentation further emphasizes the importance of maintaining a low threshold for considering the diagnosis of histoplasmosis. This accounts for the distinct diagnosis used between definitions of invasive fungal disease in clinical practice compared to clinical research definitions [29].

The Infectious Disease Society of America (IDSA) last published guidelines for the management of histoplasmosis in 2007 [3, 23]. In general, for patients with mild-to-moderate pulmonary histoplasmosis, treatment is not recommended. However, if patients have symptoms for greater than one month, as in the case of our patient, therapeutic itraconazole should be employed for at least one year. While there is no specific recommendation for treatment of histoplasmosis in immunocompromised patients, including recipients of allogeneic HSCT who are receiving immunosuppressive medications, the guidelines recommend that patients who are not immunocompetent should receive suppressive therapy with itraconazole if immunosuppression cannot be reversed. Furthermore, they specifically recommend prophylaxis with itraconazole in HIV patients with CD4 counts <150 cells/mm^3 in endemic areas where the incidence is above 10 cases per 100 patient-years. Indiana, where the patient lived prior to his allogeneic stem cell transplant, is among the states that are endemic for histoplasmosis [30]. Past infection, determined by the skin test reactivity assay, occurs in 50–80% of Indiana residents [31].

Voriconazole has been reported to be successful in the treatment of a small number of patients with varying forms of *Histoplasma* infection [31–33]. The drug has demonstrated *in vitro* activity against *H. capsulatum*, but isolates that became resistant to fluconazole were noted to have elevated minimum inhibitory concentration (MIC) values to voriconazole in patients with AIDS, suggesting that resistance may develop during treatment with voriconazole [34]. IDSA recommends that voriconazole only be utilized as a second-line alternative to itraconazole for treatment of histoplasmosis. In addition, no specific prophylaxis is recommended.

Monitoring of voriconazole blood levels has been advocated as a means to ensure adequate drug exposure in treating patients with invasive mycoses. Freifeld et al. examined nine patients with disseminated histoplasmosis who failed treatment with amphotericin or itraconazole and received voriconazole as secondary therapy where serum trough levels were determined [32]. All patients were deemed to have clinically improved while receiving voriconazole 200 mg twice daily. Of the 20 samples obtained from these patients, serum voriconazole levels ranged from undetectable to 8 mcg/mL. In addition, archived *H. capsulatum* isolates from AIDS patients who had either primary or relapsed histoplasmosis were employed for MIC testing via a modified Clinical and Laboratory Standards Institute (CLIA) assay. The median MIC for primary and relapsed isolates was 0.015 mCg/mL and 0.03 mCg/mL, respectively. Despite two patients having voriconazole levels below the MIC values, no patient relapsed. The authors proposed a threshold voriconazole trough value of 0.125 mCg/mL for the treatment of histoplasmosis [32]. Notably our patient's trough level was higher at 2.4 mCg/mL.

To our knowledge, this is the first case of histoplasmosis reported in an allogeneic stem cell transplant recipient who was receiving voriconazole as antifungal prophylaxis at the appropriate serum drug levels for *Aspergillus* prophylaxis. The detection of *Histoplasma*, despite therapeutic voriconazole levels, is unique to our case. The reason for infection despite seemingly adequate coverage with voriconazole is unclear but may be related to relative resistance, though voriconazole may have contributed to his borderline positive antigen result seen on broncheoalveolar fluid antigen testing. We cannot exclude the possibility that the organism present either was intrinsically resistant or developed resistance to voriconazole due to prolonged drug exposure.

While voriconazole is not a well-validated treatment or prophylactic modality for *Histoplasma* infections, we would recommend caution in using this agent for either approach. Though molecular-based diagnostic methods have the potential to improve the diagnostic sensitivity of *Histoplasma* infections on this unique population, we recommend timely evaluation and high clinical suspicion with the current culture and serologic-based diagnostic methodology. We also recommend a lower threshold for evaluation for histoplasmosis in allogeneic transplant recipients who live in endemic regions, regardless of their antifungal prophylactic regimen.

Disclosure

Vaibhav Agrawal and Bryan J. Brinda are co-first authors.

Authors' Contributions

VA, SF, and BJB contributed to the research and collection of information and participated in the drafting of the report. All authors critically revised the document for intellectual content and approved the final version.

References

[1] C. A. Kauffman, "Diagnosis of histoplasmosis in immunosuppressed patients," *Current Opinion in Infectious Diseases*, vol. 21, no. 4, pp. 421–425, 2008.

[2] M. Natarajan, M. J. Swierzbinski, S. Maxwell et al., "Pulmonary Histoplasma infection after allogeneic hematopoietic stem cell transplantation: case report and review of the literature," *Open Forum Infectious Diseases*, vol. 4, no. 2, p. ofx041, 2017.

[3] L. J. Wheat, A. G. Freifeld, M. B. et al., "Clinical practice guidelines for the management of patients with histoplasmosis: 2007 update by the Infectious Diseases Society of America," *Clinical Infectious Diseases*, vol. 45, no. 7, pp. 807–825, 2007.

[4] S. Haydoura, J. Wallentine, B. Lopansri, C. D. Ford, D. Saad, and J. P. Burke, "Disseminated histoplasmosis in allogeneic bone marrow transplant: a diagnosis not to be missed," *Transplant Infectious Disease*, vol. 16, no. 5, pp. 822–826, 2014.

[5] M. W. Peterson, A. D. Pratt, and K. M. Nugent, "Pneumonia due to Histoplasma capsulatum in a bone marrow transplant recipient," *Thorax*, vol. 42, no. 9, pp. 698-699, 1987.

[6] M. Tomblyn, T. Chiller, H. Einsele et al., "Guidelines for preventing infectious complications among hematopoietic cell transplantation recipients: a global perspective," *Biology of Blood and Marrow Transplantation*, vol. 15, no. 10, pp. 1143–1238, 2009.

[7] T. J. Walsh, R. Catchatourian, and H. Cohen, "Disseminated histoplasmosis complicating bone marrow transplantation,"

American Journal of Clinical Pathology, vol. 79, no. 4, pp. 509–511, 1983.
[8] L. J. Wheat, P. Connolly-Stringfield, R. B. Kohler, P. T. Frame, and M. R. Gupta, "Histoplasma capsulation polysaccharide antigen detection in diagnosis and management of disseminated histoplasmosis in patients with acquired immunodeficiency syndrome," *The American Journal of Medicine*, vol. 87, no. 4, pp. 396–400, 1989.
[9] C. A. Kauffman, "Histoplasmosis: a clinical and laboratory update," *Clinical Microbiology Reviews*, vol. 20, no. 1, pp. 115–132, 2007.
[10] C. A. Hage, K. S. Knox, and L. J. Wheat, "Endemic mycoses: overlooked causes of community acquired pneumonia," *Respiratory Medicine*, vol. 106, no. 6, pp. 769–776, 2012.
[11] R. A. Goodwin, J. E. Loyd, and R. M. Des Prez, "Histoplasmosis in normal hosts," *Medicine*, vol. 60, no. 4, pp. 231–266, 1981.
[12] L. J. Wheat, P. A. Connolly-Stringfield, R. L. Baker et al., "Disseminated histoplasmosis in the acquired immune deficiency syndrome," *Medicine*, vol. 69, no. 6, pp. 361–374, 1990.
[13] A. Porta and B. Maresca, "Host response and *Histoplasma capsulatum*/macrophage molecular interactions," *Medical Mycology*, vol. 38, no. 6, pp. 399–406, 2000.
[14] S. F. Davies, M. Khan, and G. A. Sarosi, "Disseminated histoplasmosis in immunologically suppressed patients. Occurrence in a nonendemic area," *The American Journal of Medicine*, vol. 64, no. 1, pp. 94–100, 1978.
[15] J. Cuellar-Rodriguez, M. Avery Rk Fau - Lard, M. Lard M Fau - Budev et al., "Histoplasmosis in solid organ transplant recipients: 10 years of experience at a large transplant center in an endemic area," *Clinical Infectious Diseases*, vol. 49, no. 5, pp. 710–716, 2009.
[16] C. A. Kauffman, A. G. Freifeld, D. R. Andes et al., "Endemic fungal infections in solid organ and hematopoietic cell transplant recipients enrolled in the Transplant-Associated Infection Surveillance Network (TRANSNET)," *Transplant Infectious Disease*, vol. 16, no. 2, pp. 213–224, 2014.
[17] H. H. Honarpisheh, J. L. Curry, K. Richards et al., "Cutaneous histoplasmosis with prominent parasitization of epidermal keratinocytes: report of a case," *Journal of Cutaneous Pathology*, vol. 43, no. 12, pp. 1155–1160, 2016.
[18] A. Hot, C. Maunoury, S. Poiree et al., "Diagnostic contribution of positron emission tomography with [18F] fluorodeoxyglucose for invasive fungal infections," *Clinical Microbiology and Infection*, vol. 17, no. 3, pp. 409–417, 2011.
[19] P. Couppié, C. Aznar, B. Carme, and M. Nacher, "American histoplasmosis in developing countries with a special focus on patients with HIV: diagnosis, treatment, and prognosis," *Current Opinion in Infectious Diseases*, vol. 19, no. 5, pp. 443–449, 2006.
[20] A. A. Cooperberg and J. Schwartz, "The diagnosis of disseminated histoplasmosis from marrow aspiration," *Annals of Internal Medicine*, vol. 61, no. 2, pp. 289–295, 1964.
[21] C. A. Kauffman, K. S. Israel, J. W. Smith, A. C. White, J. Schwarz, and G. F. Brooks, "Histoplasmosis in immunosuppressed patients," *The American Journal of Medicine*, vol. 64, no. 6, pp. 923–932, 1978.
[22] M. M. Azar and C. A. Hage, "Clinical perspectives in the diagnosis and management of histoplasmosis," *Clinics in Chest Medicine*, vol. 38, no. 3, pp. 403–415, 2017.
[23] C. A. Hage, T. E. Davis, D. Fuller et al., "Diagnosis of histoplasmosis by antigen detection in BAL fluid," *Chest*, vol. 137, no. 3, pp. 623–628, 2010.
[24] C. A. Hage, J. A. Ribes, N. L. Wengenack et al., "A multicenter evaluation of tests for diagnosis of histoplasmosis," *Clinical Infectious Diseases*, vol. 53, no. 5, pp. 448–454, 2011.
[25] J. Guarner and M. E. Brandt, "Histopathologic diagnosis of fungal infections in the 21st century," *Clinical Microbiology Reviews*, vol. 24, no. 2, pp. 247–280, 2011.
[26] S. Simon, V. Veron, R. Boukhari, D. Blanchet, and C. Aznar, "Detection of Histoplasma capsulatum DNA in human samples by real-time polymerase chain reaction," *Diagnostic Microbiology and Infectious Disease*, vol. 66, no. 3, pp. 268–273, 2010.
[27] I. Oren, E. Hardak, T. Zuckerman et al., "Does molecular analysis increase the efficacy of bronchoalveolar lavage in the diagnosis and management of respiratory infections in hemato-oncological patients?," *International Journal of Infectious Diseases*, vol. 50, pp. 48–53, 2016.
[28] E. Hardak, M. Yigla, I. Avivi, O. Fruchter, H. Sprecher, and I. Oren, "Impact of PCR-based diagnosis of invasive pulmonary aspergillosis on clinical outcome," *Bone Marrow Transplantation*, vol. 44, no. 9, pp. 595–599, 2009.
[29] J. P. Donnelly, S. C. Chen, C. A. Kauffman et al., "Revision and update of the consensus definitions of invasive fungal disease from the European organization for research and treatment of cancer and the mycoses study group education and research consortium," *Clinical Infectious Diseases*, 2019.
[30] G. M. Vail, R. S. Young, L. J. Wheat, R. S. Filo, K. Cornetta, and M. Goldman, "Incidence of histoplasmosis following allogeneic bone marrow transplant or solid organ transplant in a hyperendemic area," *Transplant Infectious Disease*, vol. 4, no. 3, pp. 148–151, 2002.
[31] A. Freifeld, L. Proia, D. Andes et al., "Voriconazole use for endemic fungal infections," *Antimicrobial Agents and Chemotherapy*, vol. 53, no. 4, pp. 1648–1651, 2009.
[32] A. Freifeld, S. Arnold, W. Ooi et al., "Relationship of blood level and susceptibility in voriconazole treatment of histoplasmosis," *Antimicrobial Agents and Chemotherapy*, vol. 51, no. 7, pp. 2656-2657, 2007.
[33] R.-K. Li, M. A. Ciblak, N. Nordoff et al., "In vitro activities of voriconazole, itraconazole, and amphotericin B against Blastomyces dermatitidis, Coccidioides immitis, and Histoplasma capsulatum," *Antimicrobial Agents and Chemotherapy*, vol. 44, no. 6, pp. 1734–1736, 2000.
[34] L. J. Wheat, P. Connolly, M. Smedema et al., "Activity of newer triazoles against Histoplasma capsulatum from patients with AIDS who failed fluconazole," *Journal of Antimicrobial Chemotherapy*, vol. 57, no. 6, pp. 1235–1239, 2006.

35

Unusual Presentation with Orbital Mass in a Child with Precursor B-Cell Acute Lymphoblastic Leukemia

Lalita Sathitsamitphong, Rungrote Natesirinilkul, Worawut Choeyprasert, and Pimlak Charoenkwan

Department of Pediatrics, Faculty of Medicine, Chiang Mai University, Chiang Mai, Thailand

Correspondence should be addressed to Lalita Sathitsamitphong; lalita.sat@cmu.ac.th

Academic Editor: Pier Paolo Piccaluga

Orbital involvement is one of the extramedullary manifestations in acute leukemia. It is common in acute myeloid leukemia, but rare in acute lymphoblastic leukemia (ALL). We described a 3-year-old girl who presented with progressive proptosis of the right eye and was later diagnosed with precursor B-cell ALL. Initial blood count showed Hb 6.9 g/dL, WBC 42,000/mm^3, lymphoblast 50%, and platelet count 185,000/mm^3. Bone marrow aspiration revealed 90% lymphoblasts with positivity for CD10, CD19, CD20, CD22, and HLA-DR markers. Computed tomography (CT) scan of the brain and orbit revealed a homogeneous enhancing mass involving the right orbit with intracranial extension. The cytogenetic study showed 46,XX chromosomes. After 4 weeks of induction chemotherapy for very high-risk ALL, although the bone marrow was in remission, the proptosis was partially resolved. CT scan confirmed a decrease in size of the right orbital mass and degree of intracranial extension. Unfortunately, the patient abandoned the treatment after the induction chemotherapy. The actual incidence of orbital involvement in ALL is unknown. Previous case reports describe diverse manifestations of orbital involvement in ALL. The involvement may be unilateral or bilateral, may occur at first diagnosis or at relapse, and may be seen in isolation or with other systemic symptoms. There is no standard treatment protocol. Chemotherapy with or without radiotherapy is generally suggested. The role of upfront hematopoietic stem cell transplantation remains inconclusive. The previously reported prognosis of ALL with orbital involvement is poor.

1. Introduction

Acute lymphoblastic leukemia (ALL), the most common malignancy in childhood, is a clonal proliferation of immature lymphoid progenitor cells. Patients with ALL typically present with fever, pallor, bleeding, bone pain, lymphadenopathy, and hepatosplenomegaly which result from the infiltration of the bone marrow and organs by the lymphoblasts. Orbital involvement, which is a common presentation in acute myeloid leukemia (AML), is rare in ALL.

2. Case Presentation

A 3-year-old girl presented with painless proptosis of the right eye which progressively developed in ten days prior to admission. She did not have eye discharge, fever, or other systemic symptoms. Physical examination revealed marked proptosis with chemosis of the right eye and limited extraocular movement in all directions. A retrobulbar mass of the right eye was suspected. The left eye was normal. The red reflex of both eyes was present. Ophthalmologic examination showed that the retina and optic discs of both eyes were normal. In addition, the patient was pale and enlarged liver and spleen were noted.

3. Materials and Methods

Complete blood count showed hemoglobin 6.9 g/dL, hematocrit 20.7%, white blood cell count 42,000/mm^3 (lymphoblasts 50%), and platelet count 185,000/mm^3. Bone

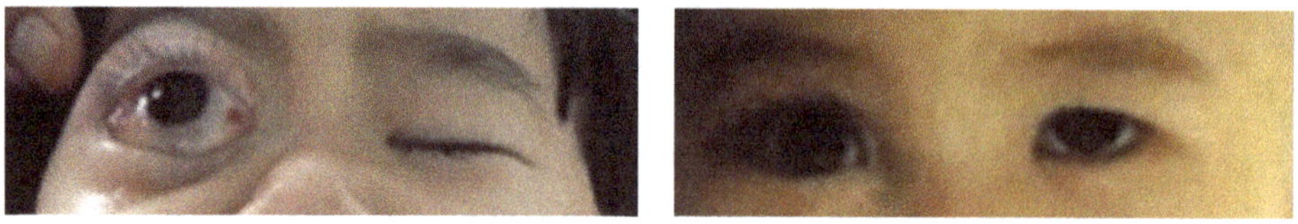

(a) (b)

Figure 1: (a) Photograph demonstrating proptosis of the right eye. (b) After 4 weeks of induction chemotherapy, decrease in the size of proptosis.

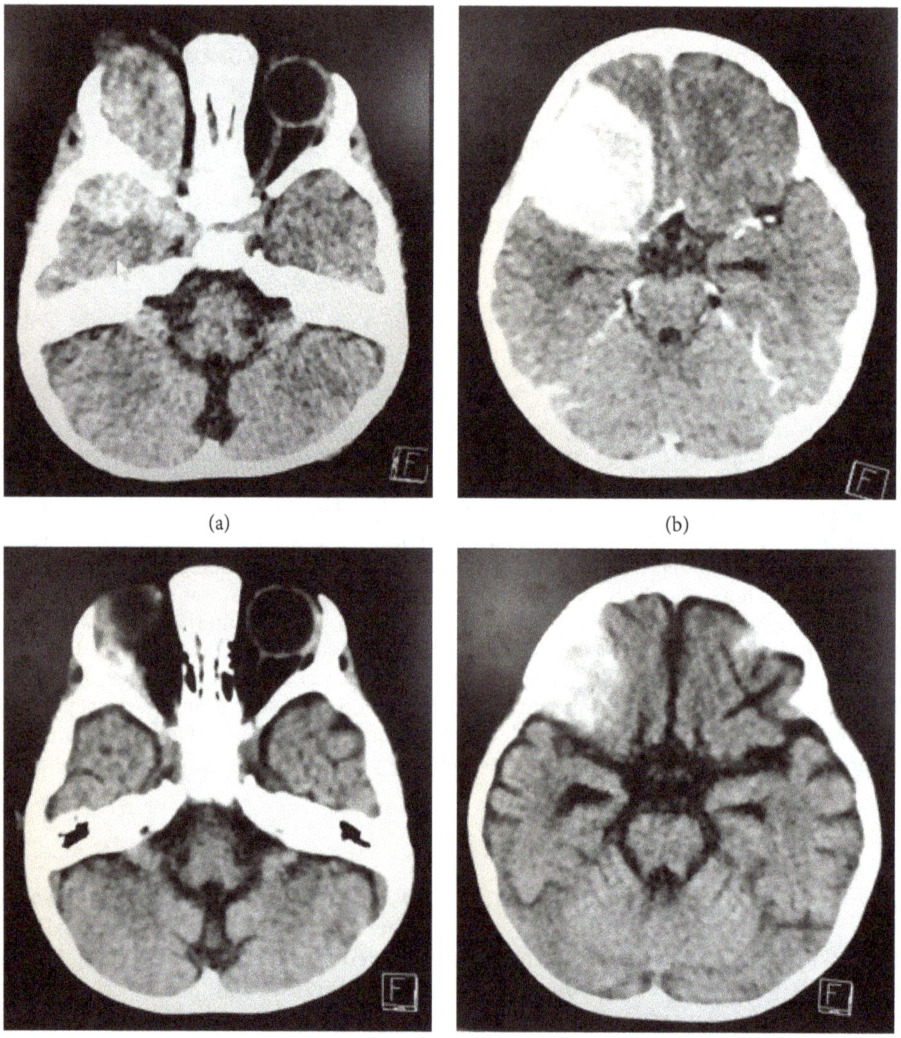

(a) (b) (c) (d)

Figure 2: (a, b) Computed tomography scan revealed a homogeneous enhancing mass involving the right orbit with intracranial extension. (c, d) After 4 weeks of induction chemotherapy, decrease in the size of homogeneous enhancing mass involving the right orbit with intracranial extension.

marrow aspiration showed 90% lymphoblasts. The immunophenotype analysis by flow cytometry showed positivity for CD10, CD19, CD20, CD22, and HLA-DR markers. Precursor B-cell ALL was diagnosed. Computed tomography (CT) scan of the brain and orbits revealed a $5.0 \times 4.2 \times 4.9\,\mathrm{cm}^3$ homogeneously enhancing mass involving superolateral intra- and extraconal components of the right orbit with intracranial extension along the right frontal and temporal convexities. The bone marrow cytogenetic study showed 46, XX chromosomes.

Granulocytic sarcoma or chloroma associated with AML was the provisional diagnosis based on the findings of the orbital mass, hepatosplenomegaly, and blast cells in peripheral blood smear. Other differential diagnoses of benign tumors, such as lymphangioma or dermoid cyst and orbital cellulitis, were less likely with the presence of the blast cells.

However, the diagnosis of precursor B-cell ALL was made according to the blast cell morphology and immunophenotype. The patient was categorized as having very high-risk ALL due to the central nervous system involvement.

4. Results and Discussion

The patient was given a 4-week induction chemotherapy as per the very high-risk ALL protocol composed of vincristine, prednisolone, doxorubicin, and L-asparaginase. Due to the risk of brain herniation, the intrathecal methotrexate was initially deferred and given on the extended 5th and 6th week of induction chemotherapy. Cranial irradiation was planned upon the completion of induction chemotherapy.

After 4 weeks of induction chemotherapy, physical examination showed a decrease in size of proptosis up to 75% and no enlarged liver and spleen (Figure 1). Bone marrow aspiration revealed bone marrow in remission with normal trilineage hematopoiesis. CT scan of the brain and orbits showed a decrease in the orbital mass size measuring $2.9 \times 2.9 \times 2.7\ cm^3$ (Figure 2). Cerebrospinal fluid analysis after 4-week induction chemotherapy revealed no malignant cells. Unfortunately, because of socioeconomic restraints, the patient abandoned the treatment after the induction chemotherapy was completed.

Ophthalmic involvement which consists of orbital and ocular infiltrations is one of the extramedullary manifestations of acute leukemia. While orbital mass is commonly seen in AML and is known as granulocytic sarcoma, it is uncommon in ALL [1]. In a study of 1,264 patients with orbital tumors, 130 were classified as having lymphoid or leukemic lesions. Only two patients were diagnosed with ALL [2].

There are sporadic case reports of patients with ALL who present with an orbital mass, either as an isolated manifestation or seen concomitantly with other systemic manifestations [1, 3–6]. The treatment mostly consists of systemic chemotherapy with or without orbital and craniospinal irradiation [1, 3–9]. The outcomes vary from complete remission after systemic chemotherapy without radiotherapy to relapse and death after chemotherapy and radiotherapy [1, 3–9]. Bidar et al. reported a successful treatment in three patients with hematopoietic stem cell transplantation (HSCT) without radiotherapy [7]. To date, there is no standard treatment protocol for ALL with orbital mass.

Ophthalmic involvement could also be the manifestation of relapsed ALL. Tabata et al. reported a 9-year-old boy who was diagnosed with relapsed ALL and developed an orbital mass post matched unrelated HSCT. The patient achieved engraftment but developed a right orbital mass on day 21 after HSCT and later progressed to systemic relapse [8]. Tayler et al. reported three relapsed ALL cases with ophthalmic involvement, consisted of proptosis, visual acuity impairment, hypopyon, and papilledema. The ophthalmic involvement was bilateral in one patient. All three received chemotherapy and radiotherapy. Two patients achieved complete remission but one had cataract and one had permanent visual acuity impairment [9].

The prognosis in ALL patients with ophthalmic involvement is generally poor. From four previous reports, five of 14 ALL patients with ophthalmic involvement (35.7%) died of disease [6–9]. Three of five patients had ALL at the first diagnosis and two had relapsed ALL [6, 7]. The role of upfront HSCT remains inconclusive. Five of 10 ALL cases at the first diagnosis with orbital involvement attained complete remission without HSCT [1, 3–5, 7]. Among three patients with first-diagnosed ALL who underwent HSCT, one patient died [7]. Another two reports showed that two out of four relapsed ALL cases with orbital involvement who were treated with chemotherapy and did not undergo HSCT were able to achieve remission [8, 9]. Further studies are required to establish the treatment strategies in ALL patients with orbital involvement to improve the outcome and long-term survival.

5. Conclusion

Orbital involvement is an uncommon extramedullary manifestation of ALL, and the actual incidence is unknown. The manifestations of orbital involvement in ALL are diverse. The involvement may be unilateral or bilateral, may occur at first diagnosis or at relapse, and may be seen in isolation or with other systemic symptoms. The prognosis of ALL with orbital involvement is poor. Systemic chemotherapy with or without radiotherapy should be the principal treatment in the first-diagnosed ALL patients with orbital involvement. Radiotherapy may be omitted in patients who achieve complete response to chemotherapy with no residual orbital mass. The role of HSCT may be considered in both relapse ALL patients with orbital involvement and first-diagnosed patients who could not achieve complete response to systemic chemotherapy and radiotherapy. HSCT may improve the treatment outcomes in these patients.

Authors' Contributions

LS was responsible for collection of clinical and laboratory data and wrote the manuscript. RN and WC reviewed clinical and laboratory data. PC reviewed clinical and laboratory data and wrote the manuscript. All authors gave critical comments and revised and approved the final manuscript.

Acknowledgments

The authors would like to thank the Pediatrics laboratory staff for their laboratory supports.

References

[1] J. Ramamoorthy, R. Jain, A. Trehan, A. K. Saxena, and J. Ahluwalia, "Orbital mass in a child with acute lymphoblastic leukemia," *Journal of Pediatric Hematology/Oncology*, vol. 38, no. 8, pp. 646–648, 2016.

[2] J. A. Shields, C. L. Shields, and R. Scartozzi, "Survey of 1264 patients with orbital tumors and simulating lesions," *Ophthalmology*, vol. 111, no. 5, pp. 997–1008, 2004.
[3] I. T. Hossain, M. Moosajee, Y. Abou-Rayyah, and V. Pavasovic, "Orbital mass secondary to infantile acute lymphoblastic leukaemia," *BMJ Case Reports*, vol. 2016, Article ID bcr2016214872, 2016.
[4] M. Thakker, P. Rubin, and E. Chang, "Pre-B-cell acute lymphoblastic leukemia presenting as an orbital mass in an 8-month-old," *Ophthalmology*, vol. 113, no. 2, pp. 343–346, 2006.
[5] S. R. Chaudhry, A. J. Kreis, H. C. Underhill, and S. N. Madge, "Orbital mass secondary to acute lymphoblastic leukaemia in a child: a rare presentation," *Orbit*, vol. 33, no. 6, pp. 421–423, 2014.
[6] H. Kiratli, S. Bilgiç, and S. Emeç, "Simultaneous conjunctival, uveal, and orbital involvement as the initial sign of acute lymphoblastic leukemia," *Japanese Journal of Ophthalmology*, vol. 51, no. 2, pp. 139–141, 2007.
[7] M. Bidar, M. W. Wilson, S. J. Laquis et al., "Clinical and imaging characteristics of orbital leukemic tumors," *Ophthalmic Plastic & Reconstructive Surgery*, vol. 23, no. 2, pp. 87–93, 2007.
[8] Y. Tabata, T. Yoshihara, S. Shirakami, Y. Kohda, S. Hibi, and S. Imashuku, "Letter to the editor: eyelid leukemia as a relapse sign of B-cell type acute lymphoblastic leukemia," *Medical and Pediatric Oncology*, vol. 36, no. 4, pp. 505-506, 2001.
[9] C. W. Taylor, R. E. Taylor, and S. E. Kinsey, "Leukemic infiltration of the orbit: report of three cases and literature review," *Pediatric Hematology and Oncology*, vol. 22, no. 5, pp. 415–422, 2005.

A Case of Acquired Haemophilia A in a Patient with Chronic Myelomonocytic Leukaemia

Takeshi Araki,[1] Shinya Ohata,[1] Kohei Okamoto,[2] Kazuhide Morimoto,[3] Mana Hiraishi,[4] Shinichiro Yamada,[4] Ishikazu Mizuno,[5] and Takeshi Sugimoto[1]

[1]*Department of Hematology and Oncology, Kita-Harima Medical Center, Hyogo, Japan*
[2]*Department of Nephrology, Kobe University Hospital, Hyogo, Japan*
[3]*Division of Laboratory Medicine, Kita-Harima Medical Center, Hyogo, Japan*
[4]*Department of Cardiology, Kita-Harima Medical Centre, Hyogo, Japan*
[5]*Department of Hematology, Hyogo Cancer Center, Akashi, Japan*

Correspondence should be addressed to Takeshi Sugimoto; takeshi_sugimoto@kitahari-mc.jp

Academic Editor: Sudhir Tauro

A 67-year-old male, with a known diagnosis of myelodysplastic syndromes with multilineage dysplasia (MDS-MLD) was admitted to our hospital with a primary complaint of subcutaneous bleeding in his left thigh. Laboratory data showed anaemia and prolongation of activated partial thromboplastin time (85.8 s, normal range 24–39 s) without thrombocytopenia. Coagulation factor VIII (FVIII) activity was less than 1% (normal range 60–150%), and a FVIII inhibitor was identified and quantified at 166 BU/mL to indicate a diagnosis of acquired haemophilia A (AHA). A recent, but sustained circulating monocytosis ($>1 \times 10^9$/L) was observed, which combined with elevated numbers of neutrophil and monocytic cells in the marrow, suggested evolution of MDS-MLD to chronic myelomonocytic leukaemia (CMML), coinciding with AHA. Further analysis revealed a karyotype of 46, XY, *i*(14) (q10), which was the same abnormality previously identified in the patient. To treat bleeding caused by AHA, steroid and activated prothrombin complex concentrate were administered. Azacitidine (AZA) was used to treat CMML. During the clinical course, bleeding partially improved; however, subsequent acute myocardial infarction occurred on day 87. Worsening bone marrow failure was observed 4 months after the original admission, despite administration of AZA therapy, and the patient died due to bleeding from AHA. This case suggests that the evolution of MDS to CMML status can be associated with AHA conferring a bleeding tendency.

1. Introduction

Acquired haemophilia A (AHA) is a bleeding disorder caused by antibodies against coagulation factor VIII (FVIII). The reported incidence of AHA is between 1.0 and 1.5 cases per million population per year [1, 2]. The resulting coagulopathy can be life threatening, and if left untreated, has an overall mortality rate of 7.9%–22% [3]. Almost half of the AHA cases presented are idiopathic; the other half are associated with autoimmune disease, malignancy, dermatological disease, or pregnancy [4, 5]. The case presented herein had AHA with chronic myelomonocytic leukaemia (CMML).

2. Case Presentation

A 67-year-old man presented to our hospital with a primary complaint of subcutaneous bleeding in his left thigh and development of purpura, over the last 3 months. It had been pointed out to him that there was a mild anaemia with haemoglobin level of 10.4 g/dL. He had been diagnosed two years previously with myelodysplastic syndromes with multilineage dysplasia (MDS-MLD) considered in the context of the 2016 World Health Organization (WHO) classification criteria. The 46, XY, *i*(14) (q10) abnormality was detected in 100% of marrow metaphases (Figure 1(a)). The bone marrow blast was 3.3%. He was categorized as low

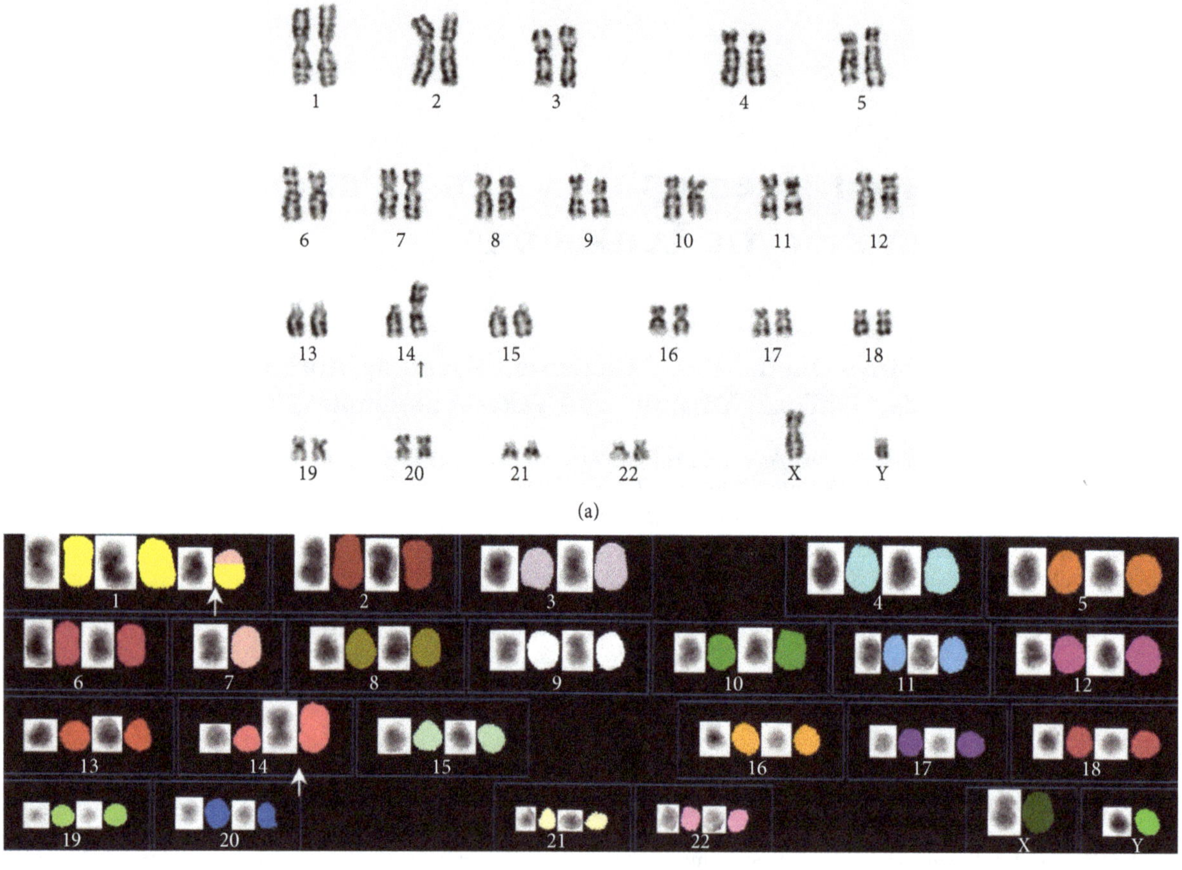

Figure 1: (a) G-banding karyotype showing the *i*(14q) (q10) with a bone marrow aspiration test at two years before admission. (b) Karyotype analysis using spectral karyotyping (SKY) method with a bone marrow aspiration test on day 138. SKY analysis identified an anomaly [idic (14), +1, and der (1; 7) (q10; p10)], which was the same abnormality as the result by G-banding analysis (data not shown).

risk in Revised International Prognostic Scoring System (IPSS-R), and he had not received cytokine therapy or blood transfusion. He had a medical history of hypertension, type 2 diabetes mellitus, spinal canal stenosis, and idiopathic osteonecrosis of the femoral head and underwent right total hip arthroplasty (r-THA).

Physical examination showed conjunctival pallor and a swelling on the left thigh with overlying bruising (Figure 2(a)). Computed tomography revealed a large bleed in the left quadriceps femoris muscle (Figure 2(b)). Laboratory data showed the following: white blood cell count, 13.6×10^9/L (normal range 3.5–9.7×10^9/L); monocyte count, 4.6×10^9/L (monocyte percentage, 33.6%); haemoglobin level, 8.8 g/dL (13.2–17.2 g/dL); haematocrit, 28.1% (40–52%); and platelet count, 258×10^9/L (140–370×10^9/L) (Table 1). On review, the monocyte count on three months previously too had been elevated (3.0×10^9/L). Activated partial thromboplastin time (APTT) was significantly prolonged (85.8 s, normal range 24–39 s). Prothrombin time was within the normal range (10.5–14 s). Mixing studies demonstrated that the prolongation of APTT was not corrected by the addition of an equal volume of pooled normal plasma either instantaneously or over two hours of incubation, indicating the presence of an inhibitor. When coagulation factors of the intrinsic pathway were measured, FVIII activity was less than 1% (normal range 60–150%), and coagulation factors IX, XI, and XII were also found to be reduced. Further tests did not detect lupus anticoagulant antibody. The inhibitor for FVIII was quantified using the Bethesda method and showed a high level of 166 BU/mL, but there was no inhibitory activity against factor IX inhibitor (Table 1). Since the patient's coagulation profile had previously been normal, the current results indicated that he had developed acquired haemophilia A (AHA).

3. Clinical Course

In order to treat bleeding caused by AHA, we administered activated prothrombin complex concentrate (aPCC; FEIBA, Baxalta©) at a loading dose of 50 U/kg. Immunosuppression with oral prednisolone (PSL) at a dose of 1 mg/kg/day was started on day 3 of hospitalization. Once the patient was less hemorrhagic, further investigations were performed: to assess a possible change in the underlying haematological malignancy, bone marrow examination was undertaken 3 weeks after starting PSL therapy. The bone marrow aspirate revealed normocellular marrow (nucleated cell counts (NCC), $29.7 \times 10^4/\mu$L) and normal myeloid/erythroid (M/E)

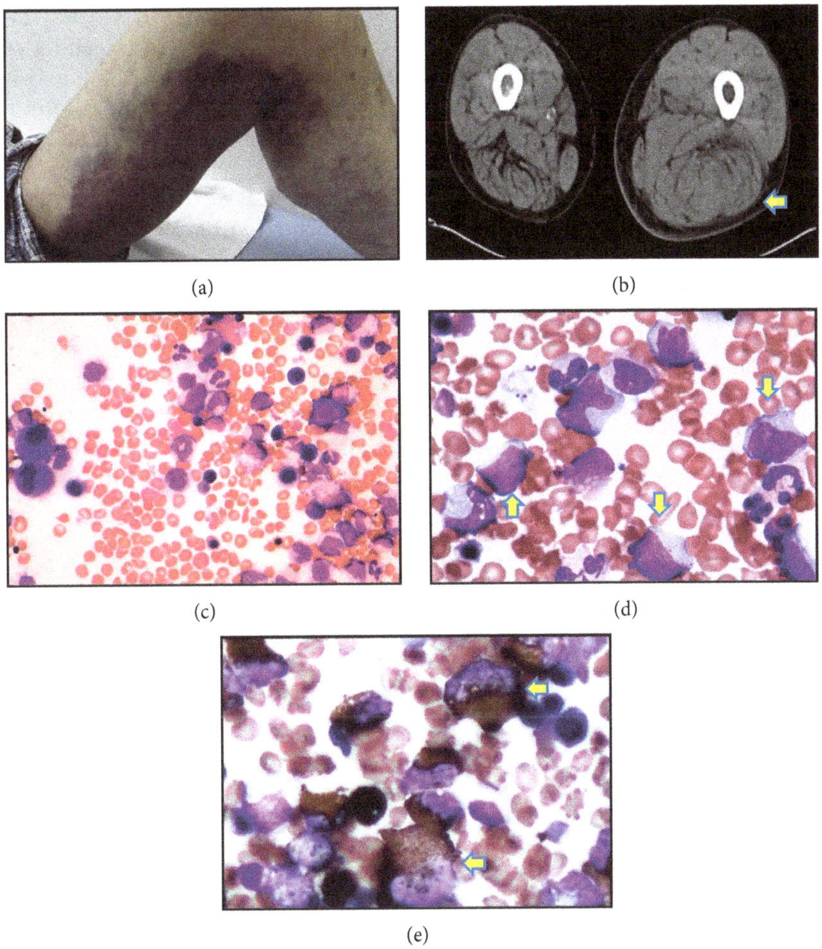

FIGURE 2: (a) Swelling of the left thigh with subcutaneous hemorrhage. (b) Computed tomography showing a large muscle bleed in the left quadriceps femoris muscle (arrow). (c–e) Bone marrow aspiration test on hospital day 24 (HE staining). (c) Normocellular marrow with an adequate proportion of erythrocytes (×400). (d) Granular cells possess a vacuole; 12% of nucleated cell count (NCC) were classified as monocytic cells (×1000, arrow). (e) Abnormal cells stained positive for peroxidase staining (×1000, arrow).

ratio (1.7). Blast cells accounted for two percentage of NCC. Bone marrow aspirate also shown an elevated number of neutrophils and monocytes with cytoplasmic vacuoles (Table 2) with micromegakaryocyte and erythroblast dysplasia, and the karyotype was determined to be 46, XY, *i*(14) (q10), which was the same abnormality as previously identified (Figures 2(c)–2(e)). Polymerase chain reaction was negative for both *bcr/abl1* fusion gene and *JAK2* mutation. Based on the blood monocytosis and marrow appearances, a diagnosis of chronic myelomonocytic leukaemia (CMML-0) was made. He was not eligible for allogeneic stem cell transplantation because of his age and general status. At the time of bone marrow examination, AHA had not remitted on PSL therapy. FVIII activity was still less than 1%, and inhibitor titer was 109 BU/mL (Figure 3). Platelet count was 142×10^9/L, APTT was 90.9 s, and fibrinogen titer was 131 mg/dL. Assuming a causal relationship between CMML and AHA, we decided to initiate treatment of CMML with the hypomethylating agent, azacitidine (AZA; 75 mg/m$^2 \times 7$ days, repeated an intervals of 4 weeks), starting 4 weeks after commencing the patient on PSL therapy. After two months of therapy with PSL, the titer of FVIII inhibitor had reduced to 22 BU/mL, but subcutaneous bleeding in his thigh and hemorrhage at the site where blood was drawn had not settled. The laboratory parameter for coagulation did not improve (platelet count, 36×10^9/L; APTT, 94 s; fibrinogen titer, 185 mg/dL; and FVIII activity level, below 3%). We speculated that hypofibrinogenemia was caused by the consumption of fibrinogen on the bleeding with AHA. Cyclosporine A (100 mg/day) was added in to PSL therapy, which improved bleeding events in the extremities and trunk, and FVIII activity level increased to 6% by day 75. However, the patient now began to complain of chest pain and was diagnosed as angina pectoris and was listed for elective percutaneous coronary artery intervention (PCI). On day 87, prior to PCI, the patient received prophylactic platelet transfusion for his low platelet count (25×10^9/L) and aPCC administration as preoperative treatment to prevent bleeding by PCI, but he suffered an acute myocardial infarction. PCI was urgently performed with successful revascularization and resolution of chest pain. He did not receive antiplatelet agent because of his thrombocytopenia. Bleeding symptoms were not evident until

Table 1: Clinical data on admission.

		Normal range
White blood cell	13.6×10^9/L	(3.5–9.7)
Neutrophil	7.6 (56.1%) $\times 10^9$/L	(38–74%)
Eosinophil	0.16 (1.2%) $\times 10^9$/L	(0–8.5%)
Basophil	0.03 (0.2%) $\times 10^9$/L	(0–2.5%)
Monocyte	4.6 (33.6%) $\times 10^9$/L	(2–10%)
Lymphocyte	1.2 (8.9%) $\times 10^9$/L	(16–50%)
Red blood cell 312	$\times 10^4/\mu$L	(400–550)
Haemoglobin	8.8 g/dL	(13.2–17.2)
Haematocrit	28.1%	(40–52)
MCV	90.1%	(85–103)
Platelet	258×10^9/L	(140–370)
AST	18 IU/L	(13–33)
ALT	12 IU/L	(8–42)
CK	38 IU/L	(62–287)
LD	270 IU/L	(119–229)
Total bilirubin	0.93 mg/dL	(0.2–1.3)
BUN	15.0 mg/dL	(8–20)
Creatinine	0.77 mg/dL	(0.6–1.1)
Total protein	6.4 g/dL	(6.7–8.3)
Albumin	3.7 g/dL	(3.9–4.9)
CRP	2.37 mg/dL	(<0.3)
PT	13.7 s	(10.5–14)
APTT	85.8 s	(24–39)
Fibrinogen	458 mg/dL	(200–400)
FDP	5.6 μg/mL	(<5)
Anticardiolipin β_2GPI	<1.2 U/mL	(<3.5)
Anticardiolipin antibody	<8 U/mL	(<10)
Lupus anticoagulant	1.06 ratio	(<1.3)
Factor VIII activity	<1%	(60–150)
Factor IX activity	34%	(70–130)
Factor XI activity	20%	(75–145)
Factor XII activity	19%	(50–150)
Factor VIII inhibitor	166 BU/mL	(<1)
Factor IX inhibitor	1 BU/mL	(<1)
vWF activity	>200%	(60–170)

Table 2: The results of bone marrow aspiration.

	Two years before admission	Hospital day 24	Hospital day 138
NCC ($\times 10^4/\mu$L)	6.1	29.7	1.2
Megakaryocyte (/μL)	60	156	18
M/E ratio	1.3	1.7	0.1
Erythroid cell (%)	36.8	31.0	71.4
Myeloblast (%)	3.3	2.0	0.8
Promyelocyte (%)	2.9	4.2	0.4
Myelocyte (%)	5.6	8.0	1.0
Metamyelocyte (%)	5.3	4.6	0.2
Stabform cell (%)	8.1	4.8	0.2
Segmented cell (%)	19.8	28.8	6.8
Eosinophilic cell (%)	1.4	0.4	0.8
Basophilic cell (%)	0.2	0.0	0.0
Lymphocyte (%)	9.4	3.0	17.6
Monocyte (%)	6.4	12.0	0.4
Plasma cell (%)	0.2	0.8	0.2

1 month after PCI in which FVIII inhibitor could reach to undetectable level on day 84 and 98 but worsened thereafter coinciding with the appearance of FVIII inhibitor. CyA was switched to 100 mg/day of cyclophosphamide (CPA) with continuous use of PSL on day 117. Prior to the fourth course of AZA therapy, bleeding symptoms emerged and the titer of APTT increased to 100.8 s on day 122, suggesting activation of AHA. Bone marrow reexamination performed on day 138 showed hypocellular marrow, with reduced M/E ratio (1.7 to 0.1). There was no increase in blasts to suggest transformation to acute leukaemic transformation (Table 2). Karyotype analysis, using both G-banding and spectral karyotyping (SKY) methods, revealed an abnormal karyotype, i.e., [idic (14), +1, and der (1; 7)(q10; p10)] (G-banding method [18/20] clone, SKY method [5/5] clone), suggesting clonal evolution (Figure 1(b)) and therefore failure of AZA treatment [6]. AZA was stopped and CPA was replaced with azathioprine 50 mg/day on day 143. He continued on 7.5 mg/day of PSL. He developed recurrent episodes of bruising with APTT index of 100–110 s. Seven months after presenting with AHA, the patient developed gastrointestinal bleeding and died (Figure 3). The response of AHA to treatment was non-CR based on the UK Haemophilia Centre Doctors' Organization criteria [7], despite normalization of FVIII activity and transient disappearance of FVIII inhibitor from hospital day 84 to 98.

4. Discussion

The case presented herein had AHA with evolution of MDS-MLD to CMML, which is classified as a rare cause among haematological malignancies. The relationship between MDS or CMML and autoimmune disease has been previously discussed. Approximately 10%–30% MDS or CMML cases are associated with autoimmune diseases [8–10], of which CMML is the most predominant condition [8]. In terms of haematological autoimmune diseases, idiopathic thrombocytopenic purpura, autoimmune hemolytic anaemia, and pure red cell aplasia are commonly seen. Acquired haemophilia complication as a haematological autoimmune disease is rare in MDS or CMML cases. The reason for this may be due to the rare incidental rate of acquired haemophilia. Several cases of AHA complicated with CMML or MDS have been reported [11–16]. Including our case, four out of eight AHA cases went into remission after treatment; three of these cases were administered a hypomethylating agent (AZA or decitabine) for CMML (Table 3). The No. 1 case [11] treated with AZA and panobinostat (histone deacetylase inhibitor) achieved CR. In the three CMML cases (No. 1, 3, and 4) reached to CR of AHA, bone marrow status was examined in only one case (No. 1), which showed CR of CMML status. Bone marrow assessment for the evaluation of CMML status after treatment will be required. In our case, coagulation bypass therapy involving aPCC was performed to stop the bleeding caused by AHA; immunosuppressive therapy by PSL, involving CyA and CPA, was also initiated to prevent the production of AHA antibody. In addition, AZA was administered to treat CMML, which appeared to be the primary disease underlying AHA. During the clinical course of our case, the bleeding symptoms transiently improved after combination therapy with AZA, PSL, and immunosuppressive drugs (CyA, CPA, and

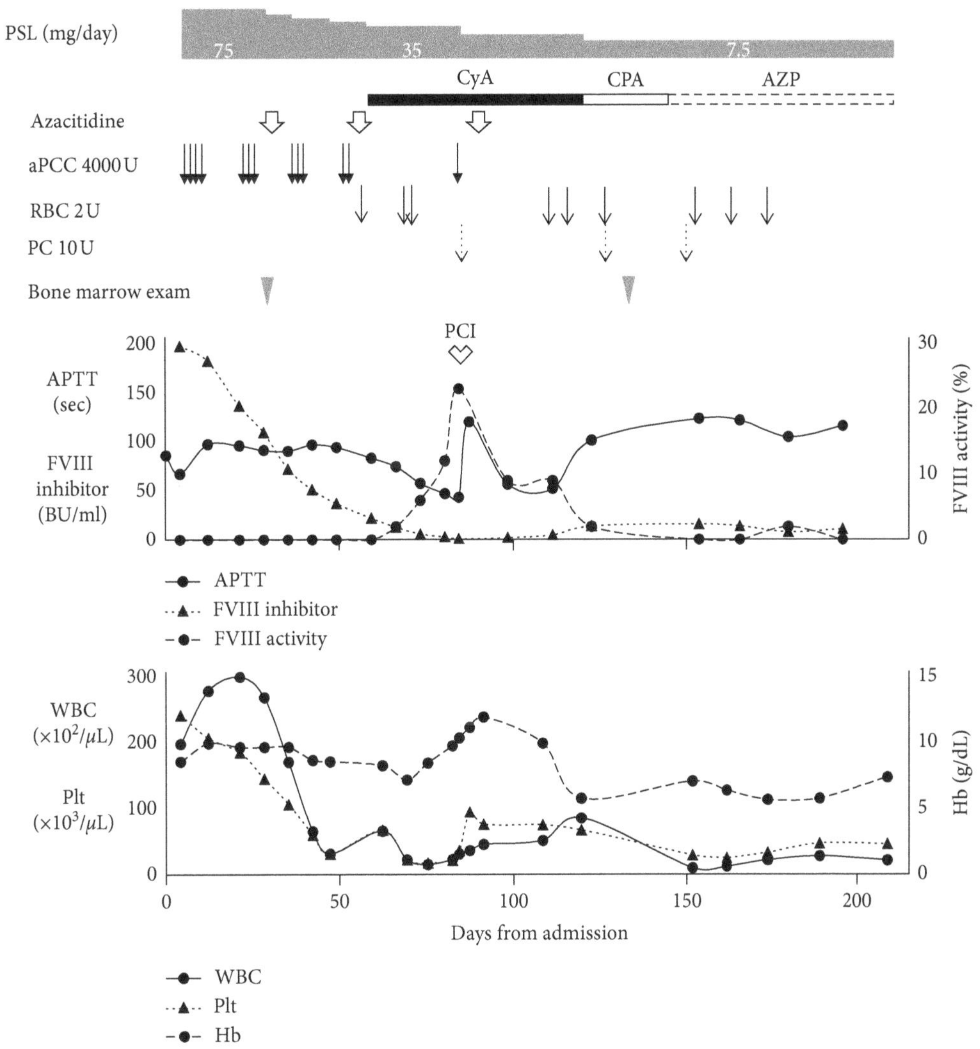

FIGURE 3: The clinical course of our patient. PSL: prednisolone; CyA: cyclosporine A; CPA: cyclophosphamide; AZP: azathioprine; AZA: azacitidine; aPCC: activated prothrombin complex concentrate; RBC: red blood cells; PC: platelet concentrates; PCI: percutaneous coronary artery intervention.

azathioprine); however, bleeding tendency recurred in accordance with a reduction of bone marrow cells. We speculated that this bleeding was caused by both AHA-related coagulopathy and thrombocytopenia. Bone marrow examination on day 138 showed the prevalence of abnormal karyotype, i.e., [idic (14), +1, and der (1; 7)(q10; p10)], even if the effect of cell reduction by AZA might remain. The result of additional cytogenetic abnormality implied that the progression of CMML is related to the AHA condition. In non-CR cases, progressive bleeding such as severe subcutaneous and muscle bleeding in case No. 6 [15], intracranial hemorrhage in case No. 2 [11], or gastrointestinal bleeding in case No. 8 (our case) caused the patient's death. These cases had the ineffective condition for haemostatic treatment in the last part of the clinical course.

The mechanism of secondary AHA due to the presence of CMML or MDS remains unclear. In haematological malignancy complicated by AHA, lymphoid malignancy, including lymphoma, chronic lymphoid leukaemia, or macroglobulinaemia, is more common than myeloid malignancy [17]. However, myeloid malignancy is possible to complicate with AIHA infrequently. CMML is predominant in the eight cases shown in Table 3, indicating that CMML may possess a factor responsible for the development of AHA in myeloid malignancy. It is possible that the reason for this is increased inflammatory cytokines levels such as interleukin-6 (IL-6) or tumor necrosis factor alpha that activates the autoimmune function. However, the precise mechanism responsible is unclear. One possibility is that monocytic cells affect autoimmune diseases via the activation of B-cell activating factor (BAFF). In this scenario, BAFF would suppress the production of monocytic cells via a negative feedback mechanism; under normal conditions, BAFF activation would be strictly controlled [18]. Under the CMML conditions, it is possible that increased proportions of monocytic cells, caused by tumorigenesis, do not decrease if BAFF exerts an influence upon the monocytic cell regulation system; the continuation of BAFF activation facilitates the development of autoimmune diseases, such as AHA.

Table 3: Cases of acquired haemophilia A with chronic myelomonocytic leukaemia or myelodysplastic syndromes.

No	Age/ gender	Disease	Clinical manifestation	APTT (second)	FVIII activity (%)	FVIII inhibitor titer (BU/ ml)	Treatment for bleeding and antibody eradication	Anti-tumor agent	Outcome of AHA	Reference
1	54/M	CMML-1	Large ecchymosis at trunk and extremities	73.4	No data	21	PSL	Azacitidine, panobinostat	CR	[11]
2	41/M	CMML-2	Excessive bleeding	91	No data	107.5	CPA, PSL		Non-CR	[11]
3	58/M	CMML-1	Diffuse ecchymosis and spontaneous iliopsoas hematoma	96.3	<1	>200	APCC, PSL, CPA, rituximab, IVIG	Decitabine	CR	[12]
4	71/M	CMML-1	Gross hematuria	118.6	6.7	7.4	HU, rFVIII	Decitabine, CAG regimen	CR	[13]
5	75/F	MDS	Extensive bruising on body and limbs	71	2	420	PSL, pyridoxine		CR	[14]
6	84/M	MDS (RAEB-1)	Subcutaneous and muscle bleeding	71.8	3	3	rFVIIa, PSL		Non-CR	[15]
7	71/M	MDS/ MPN	Spontaneous hematoma and muscle hemorrhage	64	24	9	rFVIII, rFVIIa, APCC, PSL, CPA, IVIG		Non-CR	[16]
8	67/M	CMML-0*	Subcutaneous and muscle bleeding	85.8	<1	166	APCC, PSL, CyA, CPA, AZP	Azacitidine	Non-CR	Our case

M: male; F: female; CMML: chronic myelomonocytic leukaemia; MDS: myelodysplastic syndromes; PSL: prednisolone; CyA: cyclosporine A; CPA: cyclophosphamide; AZP: azathioprine; HU: hydroxyurea; IVIG: intravenous immunoglobulin; rFVIIa: recombinant factor VIIa; rFVIII: recombinant factor VIII; APCC: activated prothrombin complex concentrate; CR: complete remission; Ref: reference. *Diagnosed by WHO 2016 classification.

Recombinant factor VIIa or aPCC is generally used for the management of bleeding during surgical treatment of AHA. We chose the use of aPCC because these two agents were used as the similar position for haemostasis, and either choice of these agents would be enough for the management of bleeding. In the present case, elective PCI was scheduled for angina pectoris; the use of aPCC as a pretreatment for the prevention of PCI may have triggered the onset of acute myocardial infarction. With regards to the side effects of aPCC, thrombotic diseases such as disseminated intravascular coagulation, acute myocardial infarction, and pulmonary embolism have been reported [19]. The European Acquired Haemophilia Registry reported that the rate of thrombotic adverse events is 4.8% during aPCC treatment for AHA [20]. Our case had additional risk factors for arteriosclerotic coronary artery disease, such as a smoking habit, hypertension, diabetes mellitus, and obesity. We speculate that the existence of AHA prevented the occurrence of coronary artery disease naturally by inhibiting the intrinsic coagulation pathway and that both normalization of FVIII activity and bypass therapy with aPCC may have stimulated thrombosis of the coronary artery in this patient. A similar case complicated by acute myocardial infarction in partial remission of AHA has been already reported [21]. Consequently, the relationship between the use of haemostatic agents and thrombotic event should be studied further.

Concerning abnormal karyotype, isochromosome 14 (q10) is not common but is recognized in myelocytic malignancy, especially in MDS subtypes RA and CMML [22]. This abnormality can exist as a sole abnormality. Another abnormality, der (1; 7) (q10; p10), is observed in about 1–3% of MDS and less commonly in acute myeloid leukaemia (AML) and myeloproliferative disorders [23]. As chromosome 14 abnormality was observed on three sequential bone marrow tests, chromosome 14 abnormality seems to be the potential cause in this case.

In conclusion, we have presented a case of AHA with CMML. The bleeding symptoms improved transiently on a combination therapy with AZA, PSL, and immunosuppressive drugs. The relative contribution of each therapy cannot accurately be established. Because bleeding tendency becomes steadily worse as CMML status advances, it follows that the control of CMML appears to be essential for the management of AHA.

Acknowledgments

The authors would like to thank Enago (http://www.enago.jp) for their English language review.

References

[1] P. Collins, N. Macartney, R. Davies, S. Lees, J. Giddings, and R. Majer, "A population based, unselected, consecutive cohort of patients with acquired haemophilia A," *British Journal of Haematology*, vol. 124, no. 1, pp. 86–90, 2004.

[2] M. Franchini and P. Mannucci, "Acquired haemophilia A: a 2013 update," *Thrombosis and Haemostasis*, vol. 110, no. 12, pp. 1114–1120, 2013.

[3] M. Franchini, G. Targher, M. Montagnana, and G. Lippi, "Laboratory, clinical and therapeutic aspects of acquired hemophilia A," *Clinica Chimica Acta*, vol. 395, no. 1-2, pp. 14–18, 2008.
[4] C. M. Kessler and P. Knöbl, "Acquired haemophilia: an overview for clinical practice," *European Journal of Haematology*, vol. 95, pp. 36–44, 2015.
[5] P. Knoebl, P. Marco, F. Baudo et al., "Demographic and clinical data in acquired hemophilia A: results from the European acquired haemophilia registry (EACH2)," *Journal of Thrombosis and Haemostasis*, vol. 10, no. 4, pp. 622–631, 2012.
[6] F. Onida, G. Barosi, G. Leone et al., "Management recommendations for chronic myelomonocytic leukemia: consensus statements from the SIE, SIES, GITMO groups," *Haematologica*, vol. 98, no. 9, pp. 1344–1352, 2013.
[7] P. W. Collins, S. Hirsch, T. P. Baglin et al., "Acquired hemophilia A in the United Kingdom: a 2-year national surveillance study by the United Kingdom haemophilia centre doctors' organisation," *Blood*, vol. 109, no. 5, pp. 1870–1877, 2007.
[8] T. Braun and P. Fenaux, "Myelodysplastic syndromes (MDS) and autoimmune disorders (AD): cause or consequence?," *Best Practice & Research Clinical Haematology*, vol. 26, no. 4, pp. 327–336, 2013.
[9] D. Peker, E. Padron, J. M. Bennett et al., "A close association of autoimmune-mediated processes and autoimmune disorders with chronic myelomonocytic leukemia: observation from a single institution," *Acta Haematologica*, vol. 133, no. 2, pp. 249–256, 2015.
[10] M. F. Zahid, D. Barraco, T. L. Lasho et al., "Spectrum of autoimmune diseases and systemic inflammatory syndromes in patients with chronic myelomonocytic leukemia," *Leukemia & Lymphoma*, vol. 58, no. 6, pp. 1488–1493, 2017.
[11] N. Uaprasert, S. Wongrakpanich, and P. Rojnuckarin, "Two cases of acquired haemophilia A associated with chronic myelomonocytic leukaemia," *Blood Coagulation & Fibrinolysis*, vol. 24, no. 6, pp. 655–657, 2013.
[12] D. Shah, R. Kumar, and S. Gaikazian, "A rare case of acquired haemophilia in a patient with chronic myelomonocytic leukaemia successfully treated with decitabine," *Haemophilia*, vol. 20, no. 1, pp. e92–e94, 2014.
[13] Y. Liang, R.-N. Lu, R. Wang et al., "Chronic myelomonocytic leukaemia associated with acquired haemophilia A: case report and literature review," *Haemophilia*, vol. 21, no. 4, pp. e341–e343, 2015.
[14] C. K. Lin, R. Liang, H. W. Liu, P. W. T. Tse, and G. T. C. Chan, "Myelodysplastic syndrome and acquired factor VIII inhibitor with severe subcutaneous haemorrhage," *Acta Haematologica*, vol. 85, no. 4, pp. 206–208, 1991.
[15] M. Raval, R. Kallamadi, and D. Bande, "A rare case of acquired hemophilia A associated with myelodysplastic syndrome," *International Journal of Clinical and Experimental Medicine*, vol. 5, no. 3, pp. 262–266, 2012.
[16] T. Biss, L. Crossman, I. Neilly, and J. Hanley, "An acquired factor VIII inhibitor in association with a myeloproliferative/myelodysplastic disorder presenting with severe subcutaneous haemorrhage," *Haemophilia*, vol. 9, no. 5, pp. 638–641, 2003.
[17] M. Franchini, G. Targher, F. Manzato, and G. Lippi, "Acquired factor VIII inhibitors in oncohematology: a systematic review," *Critical Reviews in Oncology/Hematology*, vol. 66, no. 3, pp. 194–199, 2008.
[18] M. Steri, V. Orrù, M. L. Idda et al., "Overexpression of the cytokine BAFF and autoimmunity risk," *New England Journal of Medicine*, vol. 376, no. 17, pp. 1615–1626, 2017.
[19] H. J. Ehrlich, M. J. Henzl, and E. D. Gomperts, "Safety of factor VIII inhibitor bypass activity (FEIBAR): 10-year compilation of thrombotic adverse events," *Haemophilia*, vol. 8, no. 2, pp. 83–90, 2002.
[20] F. Baudo, P. Collins, A. Huth-Kuhne et al., "Management of bleeding in acquired hemophilia A: results from the European acquired haemophilia (EACH2) registry," *Blood*, vol. 120, no. 1, pp. 39–46, 2012.
[21] D. J. M. Routledge, D. Fraser, J. Thachil, and M. J. Nash, "Management of a myocardial infarction in a patient with classical acquired haemophilia patient in partial remission," *Haemophilia*, vol. 21, no. 6, pp. e494–e496, 2015.
[22] J. Welborn, "Acquired robertsonian translocations are not rare events in acute leukemia and lymphoma," *Cancer Genetics and Cytogenetics*, vol. 151, no. 1, pp. 14–35, 2004.
[23] U. Bacher, J. Schanz, F. Braulke, and D. Haase, "Rare cytogenetic abnormalities in myelodysplastic syndromes," *Mediterranean Journal of Hematology and Infectious Diseases*, vol. 7, no. 1, article e2015034, 2015.

37

Portal Vein Thrombosis following Total Colectomy due to Colonic Inertia: A Case Report and Evaluation of Risk Factors

Mohammad Bagher Jahantab, Saadat Mehrabi, Vahid Salehi, Lotfolah Abedini, and Mohammad Javad Yavari Barhaghtalab

Department of General Surgery, Shahid Beheshti Hospital, Yasuj University of Medical Sciences, Yasuj, Iran

Correspondence should be addressed to Mohammad Javad Yavari Barhaghtalab; mj.yavari.barhaghtalab@yums.ac.ir

Academic Editor: Gergely Feher

The portal vein could be occluded by blood clots partially or completely causing portal vein thrombosis (PVT). The acute episode may be asymptomatic or manifested by abdominal pain, increasing body temperature, and unspecific dyspeptic symptoms. The main causes of PVT are categorized into local, acquired, and genetic thrombophilic factors. To our knowledge, this is the 2nd recognized case of PVT following colectomy for colonic inertia successfully treated with an effective anticoagulation therapy. The patient received unfractionated heparin as soon the diagnosis was implemented. The patient was a 34-year-old lady with chief complaint of severe abdominal pain, nausea, vomiting, and anorexia 10 days after the first hospital admission for subtotal colectomy due to colonic inertia. Spiral abdominal CT scan with intravenous (IV) contrast showed thrombosis in main portal vein with its extension to right and left intrahepatic branches. Our case showed that we should keep in mind PVT in patients who present with upper gastrointestinal symptoms several days after a major surgery (open colectomy) as a risk factor and oral contraceptive pills (OCP) usage, postpregnancy, and immobility as other risk factors, that the protein C, S, and FVL deficiencies were secondary, and that the PVT can be managed by low molecular weight heparin plus oral warfarin therapy in the continue.

1. Background

Portal vein could be occluded by blood clot partially or completely causing portal vein thrombosis (PVT). Thrombosis could extend to intrahepatic branches and splenic or superior mesenteric veins (SMV). PVT is the result of a combination of local and systemic risk factors. Local risk factors accounts for about 20–25% of the cases and are categorized to cirrhotic and noncirrhotic patients. Noncirrhotic patients have malignant (solid tumors) or nonmalignant factors. Nonmalignant factors are intra-abdominal infections such as cholecystitis, cholangitis, appendicitis, diverticulitis, pancreatitis, and inflammatory bowel diseases (IBD) and iatrogenic trauma to the portal system (splenectomy, Whipple, gastric bypass, hepatectomy, and liver transplantation), as well as liver and biliary system-related procedures such as cholecystectomy and hepatoportobiliary surgery. Systemic risk factors which account for about 50–60% of cases are acquired thrombophilia (antiphospholipid syndrome and paroxysmal nocturnal hemoglobinuria), inherited thrombophilia (mutations in factor V Leiden (FVL), factor II (prothrombin gene or G20210A), deficiency of protein C, S, plasminogen, and antithrombin III, myeloproliferative neoplasms (MPNs) (polycythemia vera, essential thrombocytemia, and primary myelofibrosis), autoimmune and rheumatologic disorders (autoimmune hepatitis, primary biliary cirrhosis, systemic lupus erythematosus, rheumatoid arthritis, Wegener's granulomatosis, mixed connective tissue disease, and Behcet syndrome), hyperhomocysteinemia, sickle cell disease, nephrotic syndrome, and thrombasthenia thrombocytosis. There are some other risk factors such as recent pregnancy, recent oral contraceptive use, male sex, and low platelet count [1–4]. It is important to know that in PVT pathogenesis, various underlying thrombophilic conditions may be existing [5].

Activated protein C (APC), protein S, and antithrombin are the most important natural anticoagulants [6]. Protein C or protein S deficiency frequency is estimated to be low in general population, but it is estimated to be 1.4–8.6% in venous thromboembolism (VTE) patients. An increased risk of thrombosis in a natural anticoagulant pathway is shown in protein C or S deficiencies. Half of the heterozygote individuals below the age of 50 years would confront a thrombotic event in their lives [7]. Prevalence of protein C and S deficiencies are shown to be 1–9% and 0–7% retrospectively in nonmalignant, noncirrhotic PVT adult patients [8]. FVL has been shown to be in 3–9% of nonmalignant, noncirrhotic PVT adult patients and is the most frequent cause of inherited thrombophilia. Its pattern of inheritance is autosomal dominant [8, 9].

PVT may occur rarely after colorectal procedures such as restorative proctocolectomy (RP) and ileal pouch-anal anastomosis (IPAA) and is associated to inflammatory conditions such as ulcerative colitis (UC) [10–13], and to a lower extent familial adenomatous polyposis and sigmoid cancer [14], and also colonic inertia [15].

Heterogeneity of the PVT clinical manifestations is due to the extent of the obstruction and the speed of its progress. The acute episode may be asymptomatic or manifested by abdominal pain, increasing body temperature, and nonspecific dyspeptic symptoms such as nausea and anorexia. Symptoms may be fewer or absent in partial PVT. Severe and colicky abdominal pain and diarrhea occur when the superior mesenteric vein is involved. With the progression of thrombosis, abdominal pain increases and radiation to the back may occur. In the next steps, ileus, intestinal ischemia, and infarction including hematochezia, ascites, metabolic acidosis, and renal or respiratory failure could be seen [4, 16]. The diagnosis is the absence of flow or the presence of a thrombus in the portal vein demonstrating in Doppler ultrasound, computerized tomography (CT), or magnetic resonance imaging (MRI) [4]. Improvement and increasing trend in the use of noninvasive radiological techniques in the diagnosis of abdominal pain has resulted in progressively more documented cases these days [16].

Colic inertia or slow transit constipation (STC) is a functional bowel pathology which may result in colonic incompetence to change stool consistency to move from the cecum to rectosigmoid for at least once every three days in existence of normal colon intraluminal diameter. If medical treatment fails in severe form of the disease, then several surgical treatment are indicated. These consist of subtotal colectomy with ileosigmoid or cecorectal anastomosis, segmental colectomy, and total abdominal colectomy with ileorectal anastomosis [17–19].

To our knowledge, this is the 2nd recognized case of PVT following colectomy for colonic inertia who successfully treated with an effective anticoagulation therapy. In this study, we evaluated the risk factors for the formation of portal vein thrombosis following total colectomy due to colonic inertia.

2. Case Presentation

The patient was a 34-year-old lady who presented to emergency department with chief complaint of severe generalized colicky abdominal pain not radiating to any quadrant, nausea, not tolerating food ingestion, anorexia, and several episodes of nonprojectile, nonbilious, nonbloody vomiting per day, weakness, and letharginess about 10 days after the first hospital admission for subtotal colectomy due to colonic inertia. The patient had no loose stools and no mucus or blood in feces (melena or hematochezia), hematemesis, jaundice, and fever in days after discharge from the first hospitalization. There was no personal and familial history of venous thromboembolism; but she noted using oral contraceptive pills up to the day before first hospitalization for colectomy, but she denied using them after she was discharged from the 1st hospitalization; she used oral cephalexin, pantoprazole, and acetaminophen after discharge from the 1st admission. The patient had pregnancy about less than one year before the 1st admission but had no previous abortions (G2P2L2A0).

On examination, the patient was oriented to time, place, and person with stable vital sign with a blood pressure of 100/70 mmHg and a pulse rate of 88/min, no icterus, edema, cyanosis or jaundice, and lymphadenopathy, but pale conjunctivae. There were clear breathing sounds and regular heart sounds without murmur. Patient had abdominal tenderness and rebound tenderness in periumbilical and right upper quadrant (RUQ) area, and there was no sign of hepatomegaly, splenomegaly, and wound infection in midline laparotomy site suture. Rectum was empty in rectal examination. Neurologic examination was normal. The patient's weight and height was 55 kg and 154 cm, respectively (body mass index (BMI) = 23.19).

During the 1st hospitalization period, the patient received thromboembolic prophylaxis with heparin 5000 units subcutaneously twice a day, and also, the patient's both lower extremities were compressed by elastic bandages.

Color Doppler ultrasonography showed no blood flow in right portal vein which suggested portal vein and portal confluence thrombosis about 25 mm and 13 mm in length retrospectively. Spiral abdominal CT scan with IV contrast showed thrombosis in main portal vein with its extension to right and left intrahepatic branches and dilatation of small bowel loops with the air-fluid level which suggested partial small bowel obstruction and free fluid in abdomen and pelvic spaces (Figures 1–3).

All laboratory studies were performed in hospital course, and results were as follows: serum blood sugar (BS) = 106 mg/dl, white blood cell (WBC) = 13600, hemoglobin (Hb) = 13.9 g/dl, platelet = 398000 U/L, erythrocyte sedimentation rate (ESR) = 27 mm/hr, C-reactive protein (CRP) = 49.1 mg/l, BUN = 7 mg/dl, creatinine = 0.7 mg/dl, Na^+ = 139 mEq/L, K^+ = 4.5 mEq/L, Mg = 1.74 mg/dl, serum amylase = 84 U/L, aspartate aminotransferase (AST) = 27 U/L, alanine aminotransferase (ALT) = 27 U/L, total protein = 5.2 gr/dl, albumin = 3.1 g/dl, total bilirubin = 0.34 mg/dl, direct bilirubin = 0.13 mg/dl, alkaline phosphatase = 128 U/L, homocysteine = 7.92 micmol/L, lactate dehydrogenase (LDH) = 329 U/L, anticardiolipin immunoglobulin M (IgM) = 1.56 GPLU/ml, anticardiolipin immunoglobulin G (IgG) = 2.55 IgG phospholipid units (GPLU)/ml, anti-B2-glycoprotein (IgM) = 9.48 U/ml, anti-B2-glycoprotein (IgG) = 9.88 U/ml, lupus anticoagulant (PTT-LA) = 38

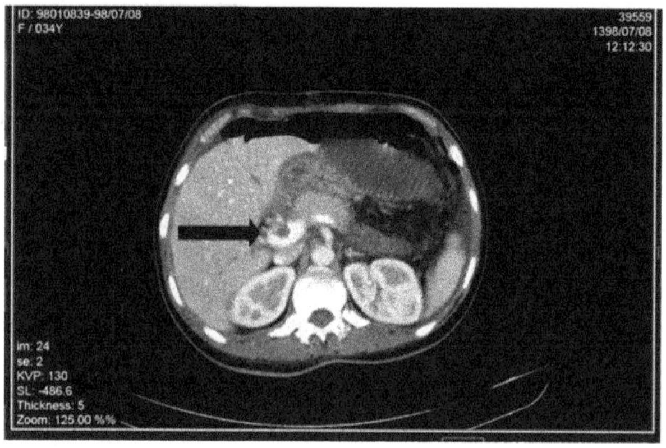

Figure 1: Thrombosis in main portal vein in spiral abdominal CT scan with IV contrast (black arrow).

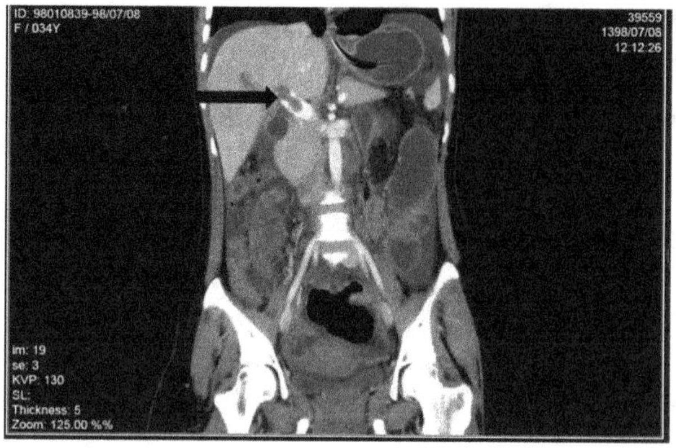

Figure 3: Thrombosis in main portal vein with its extension to right and left intrahepatic branches in spiral abdominal CT scan with IV contrast (black arrow).

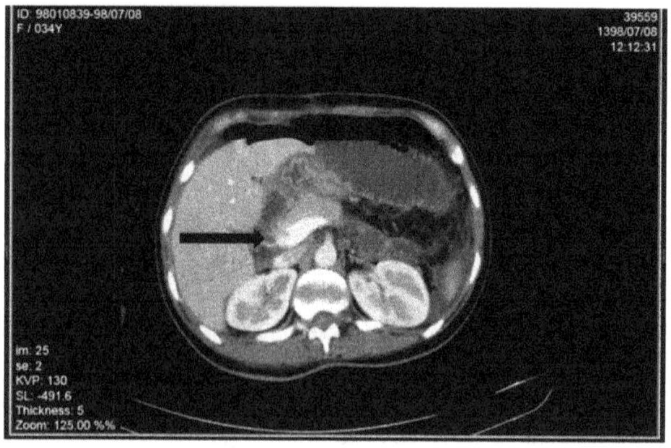

Figure 2: Thrombosis in main portal vein in spiral abdominal CT scan with IV contrast (black arrow).

second, $Ca^{++} = 7.3$ mg/dl (albumin = 3.1 g/dl), phos = 2.7 mg/dl, reticulocyte count = 2.3 corrected 0.95%, antithrombin III = 86%, FVL = 150 second, protein C = 61.57%, and protein S = 47.95%. Analysis of arterial blood gases (ABG) showed pH = 7.471, partial pressure of carbon dioxide (PCO_2) = 31 mmHg, bicarbonate (HCO_3) = 21 mmol/L, and base excess in the extracellular fluid compartment (BEecf) = −1.2 (interpretation = partly compensated respiratory alkalosis).

Heparin was started when results of cell blood count (CBC), activated partial thromboplastin time (aPTT), and prothrombin time (PT) were ready. The patient was administered therapeutic dosing of unfractionated heparin, 80 units/kg (5000 units) IV for loading dose and 1000 units IV continuous infusion for maintenance dose as soon as the diagnosis of PVT was made on the 1st day of hospitalization. In order to monitor unfractionated heparin therapy, aPTT was checked every 6 hours to reach a therapeutic range of 1.5–2.5 times the control value (55–75 seconds). To exclude heparin-induced thrombocytopenia and also finding out if Hb drop occurs, CBC was performed every other day. When aPTT reached the therapeutic level in the 2nd day after heparin administration, warfarin 5 mg daily was started, and afterward, the patient was monitored by aPTT and international normalized ratio (INR). On the 6th day and 4th day after heparin and warfarin administration respectively, INR became more than 2 (therapeutic level), so heparin continued for two other days afterward; then, it was discontinued, and the patient was discharged home in stable vital sign and good condition on the 9th day of hospital admission with warfarin 5 mg daily. In hospital course, there was no adverse or anticipated event.

The patient had follow-up visits on the 7^{th}day and 30th day after discharge from hospital, and there were no complications, and the patient came back to her daily routine activities successfully.

3. Discussion and Conclusions

Portal vein thrombosis is a rare disease with severe complications and would cause variceal bleeding and intestinal ischemia if left untreated. The main causes of PVT are categorized in local, acquired, and genetic thrombophilic factors [20]. In our patient, there were some possible risk factors for developing PVT, a major surgery as a local risk factor (colectomy in this patient), and acquired risk factors as OCP usage, postpregnancy, and immobility, but there were no genetic thrombophilic factors found in this patient.

The risk of PVT after colectomy may be due to ligation of the ileocolic vessels, mobilization of the small intestinal mesentery from the posterior abdominal wall, tension on the mesenteric vessels in the time of bowel loop anastomosis, and direct trauma to the port (it is doubtful because portal vein is located behind the pancreas) [12, 21]. Inflammatory processes such as IBD and diverticulitis are shown to induce PVT after laparoscopic colectomy [22, 23]; however, our patient had no IBD associated with postoperative PVT.

Other risk factors in developing thrombosis include pregnancy or oral contraceptive usage. OCP is a combination of an estrogen (ethinylestradiol) and a progestogen (progestin). Estrogen may cause an increase in procoagulant factors such as prothrombin, VII, X, XII, and XIII, resistance to activated protein C, and fibrinolysis. Progestin may increase the estrogen effect on procoagulant, anticoagulant, and fibrinolytic pathways [24].

In a study performed by Fisher et al. on 29 adult PVT patients, it was found that 18 patients (62%) had deficiencies in one or more of the natural anticoagulant proteins (proteins C, S, or antithrombin), 8 cases (28%) had combined C and S protein deficiency, and 6 cases (21%) had combined deficiency of all three proteins. As far as our knowledge, this report is the first of its own which presents combination of these two protein deficiencies plus FVL deficiency. They proposed that these deficiencies are acquired dominantly, and that is a result of PVT, but a minority of cases have a genetic background for anticoagulant protein deficiency, so a careful evaluation and also consultation of family members (preferably both parents and alternatively siblings) should be conducted [25]. In our case, there was limitation in investigating the patient's family members (her parents and sibling).

Two probable mechanisms were proposed for reduction of these natural anticoagulant proteins in patients who developed PVT: (1) reduction in liver blood flow would cause hepatic atrophy and reduce hepatic protein synthesis (coagulation factors more than albumin). (2) Reduction in coagulation proteins concentration due to increased clearance after shunting of blood from the liver [26].

Nevertheless, there is a related predisposing factor; patients presenting with PVT should be investigated for thrombophilia through checking of CBC, ESR, PT, aPTT, thrombin time (TT), peripheral blood smear (PBS), antithrombin III (AT III), fibrinogen level, proteins C and S, and FLV [20]. In our patient, as we checked proteins C, S, and FVL during the disease process at the hospital course, we could say that the deficiencies in these factors are acquired and could be secondary to the manipulation of the abdomen after the operation.

In conclusion, our case showed that we should keep in mind PVT in patients who present with upper gastrointestinal symptoms several days after a major surgery (open colectomy) as a risk factor; OCP usage, postpregnancy, and immobility as other risk factors, that the proteins C, S, and FVL deficiencies were acquired and secondary to the abdominal operation, and that the PVT can be managed by low molecular weight heparin plus oral warfarin therapy in the continue.

Abbreviations

FVL: Factor V Leiden
IV: Intravenous
OCP: Oral contraceptive pill
PVT: Portal vein thrombosis
SMV: Superior mesenteric veins
IBD: Inflammatory bowel diseases
MPNs: Myeloproliferative neoplasms
APC: Activated protein C
VTE: Venous thromboembolism
RP: Restorative proctocolectomy
IPAA: Ileal pouch-anal anastomosis
UC: Ulcerative colitis
CT: Computerized tomography
MRI: Magnetic resonance imaging
STC: Slow transit constipation
RUQ: Right upper quadrant
BS: Blood sugar
Hb: Hemoglobin
LDH: Lactate dehydrogenase
ABG: Arterial blood gases
ESR: Erythrocyte sedimentation rate
CRP: C-reactive protein
CBC: Cell blood count
PT: Prothrombin time
aPTT: Activated partial thromboplastin time
PBS: Peripheral blood smear
TT: Thrombin time
AT III: Antithrombin III.

Consent

A copy of the written consent is available for review by the editor-in-chief of this journal. Written informed consent was obtained from the patient for publication of this case report and any accompanying images.

Authors' Contributions

MBJ evaluated the patient clinically, operated the patient (main surgeon), and revised the manuscript. SM, VS, and LA revised the manuscript. MJYB evaluated the patient clinically, helped to operate the patient, reviewed the literature, and prepared the manuscript . All authors read and approved the final manuscript.

Acknowledgments

The authors express their gratitude to the patient who kindly gave consent for this case to be presented in this study. The authors also wish to thank Dr. Aida Iraji at the Central Research Laboratory of Shiraz University of Medical Sciences for her assistance in editing this manuscript.

References

[1] H. Samant and K. Garfield, *Portal Vein Thrombosis*, StatPearls Publishing, Treasure Island, FL, USA, 2019.

[2] S. A. Basit, C. D. Stone, and R. Gish, "Portal vein thrombosis," *Clinics in Liver Disease*, vol. 19, no. 1, pp. 199–221, 2015.

[3] N. M. Intagliata, S. H. Caldwell, and A. Tripodi, "Diagnosis, development, and treatment of portal vein thrombosis in patients with and without cirrhosis," *Gastroenterology*, vol. 156, no. 6, pp. 1582–1599, 2019.

[4] J. Hoekstra and H. L. Janssen, "Vascular liver disorders (II): portal vein thrombosis," *The Netherlands Journal of Medicine*, vol. 67, no. 2, pp. 46–53, 2009.

[5] S. R. Shah, A. DasGupta, A. Sharma et al., "Thrombophilic conditions in non-cirrhotic portal vein thrombosis," *Indian Journal of Gastroenterology*, vol. 24, no. 5, pp. 205–210, 2005.

[6] B. Dahlbäck and B. O. Villoutreix, "Regulation of blood coagulation by the protein C anticoagulant pathway: novel insights into structure-function relationships and molecular recognition," *Arteriosclerosis, Thrombosis, and Vascular Biology*, vol. 25, no. 7, pp. 1311–1320, 2005.

[7] F. A. Anderson Jr. and F. A. Spencer, "Risk factors for venous thromboembolism," *Circulation*, vol. 107, no. 23, pp. I9–I16, 2003.

[8] M. Primignani, "Portal vein thrombosis, revisited," *Digestive and Liver Disease*, vol. 42, no. 3, pp. 163–170, 2010.

[9] A. E. Mahmoud, E. Elias, N. Beauchamp, and J. T. Wilde, "Prevalence of the factor V Leiden mutation in hepatic and portal vein thrombosis," *Gut*, vol. 40, no. 6, pp. 798–800, 1997.

[10] M. Millan, T. L. Hull, J. Hammel, and F. Remzi, "Portal vein thrombi after restorative proctocolectomy: serious complication without long-term sequelae," *Diseases of the Colon & Rectum*, vol. 50, no. 10, pp. 1540–1544, 2007.

[11] C. G. Ball, A. R. MacLean, W. D. Buie, D. F. Smith, and E. L. Raber, "Portal vein thrombi after ileal pouch-anal anastomosis: its incidence and association with pouchitis," *Surgery Today*, vol. 37, no. 7, pp. 552–557, 2007.

[12] A. R. Ibele, G. D. Kennedy, D. P. Lund, and P. F. Nichol, "Portal vein thrombus after pediatric proctocolectomy with ileoanal anastomosis," *Journal of Pediatric Surgery*, vol. 45, no. 5, pp. 1026–1029, 2010.

[13] F. H. Remzi, V. W. Fazio, M. Oncel et al., "Portal vein thrombi after restorative proctocolectomy," *Surgery*, vol. 132, no. 4, pp. 655–662, 2002.

[14] A.-W. N. Meshikhes and T. Al-Ghazal, "Portal vein thrombosis after restorative proctocolectomy for familial adenomatous polyposis and sigmoid cancer," *Case Reports in Gastroenterology*, vol. 6, no. 1, pp. 124–130, 2012.

[15] J. Dilday, M. Sirkin, C. McKinnon, and S. Brown, "Portal vein thrombosis after laparoscopic total colectomy for colonic inertia," *Journal of Surgical Case Reports*, vol. 2017, no. 8, p. rjx075, 2017.

[16] G. A. Rodríguez-Leal, S. Morán, R. Corona-Cedillo, and R. Brom-Valladares, "Portal vein thrombosis with protein C-S deficiency in a non-cirrhotic patient," *World Journal of Hepatology*, vol. 6, no. 7, pp. 532–537, 2014.

[17] A. S. G. F. Soares and L. E. R. Barbosa, "Colonic Inertia: approach and treatment," *Journal of Coloproctology*, vol. 37, no. 1, 2017.

[18] P. De Marco, G. Militello, R. Tutino et al., "The management of the slow transit constipation in the laparoscopic era," *Giornale di Chirurgia*, vol. 34, no. 5, pp. 297–302, 2018.

[19] J. McCoy and D. Beck, "Surgical management of colonic inertia," *Clinics in Colon and Rectal Surgery*, vol. 25, no. 1, pp. 20–23, 2012.

[20] H. Nafeh, H. Galal, S. El-Gamal, and E. El-Gezawy, "Factor V Leiden in patients with portal vein thrombosis," *AAMJ*, vol. 6, no. 1, 2008.

[21] N. Ikoma, C. L. Anderson, M. Ohanian et al., "Portal vein thrombosis after laparoscopic cholecystectomy," *JSLS: Journal of the Society of Laparoendoscopic Surgeons*, vol. 18, no. 1, pp. 125–127, 2014.

[22] A. W. James, C. Rabl, A. C. Westphalen, P. F. Fogarty, A. M. Posselt, and G. M. Campos, "Portomesenteric venous thrombosis after laparoscopic surgery," *Archives of Surgery*, vol. 144, no. 6, pp. 520–526, 2009.

[23] R. M. Antiel, Y. Hashim, C. R. Moir, V. Rodriguez, T. Elraiyah, and A. E. Zarroug, "Intra-abdominal venous thrombosis after colectomy in pediatric patients with chronic ulcerative colitis: incidence, treatment, and outcomes," *Journal of Pediatric Surgery*, vol. 49, no. 4, pp. 614–617, 2014.

[24] E. I. Efremidou, G. Kouklakis, O. Tsirogianni, N. Courcoutsakis, K. J. Manolas, and N. Liratzopoulos, "Massive intestinal ischemia, a rare complication of oral contraceptive-induced mesenteric venous thrombosis: a case report and review of literature," *Cases Journal*, vol. 2, no. 1, p. 7416, 2009.

[25] B. K. Choi, S. H. Yang, K. H. Suh et al., "A case of portal vein thrombosis by protein C and s deficiency completely recanalized by anticoagulation therapy," *Chonnam Medical Journal*, vol. 47, no. 3, pp. 185–188, 2011.

[26] N. C. Fisher, J. T. Wilde, J. Roper, and E. Elias, "Deficiency of natural anticoagulant proteins C, S, and antithrombin in portal vein thrombosis: a secondary phenomenon?" *Gut*, vol. 46, no. 4, pp. 534–539, 2000.

38

Spontaneous Epidural Hemorrhage in Sickle Cell Disease, are They All the Same? A Case Report and Comprehensive Review of the Literature

Biplab Saha[1] and **Aditi Saha**[2]

[1]*Division of Pulmonary and Critical Care Medicine, Albany Medical Center, Albany, NY, USA*
[2]*Department of Medicine, Saint Barnabas Medical Center, Livingston, NJ, USA*

Correspondence should be addressed to Biplab Saha; spanophiliac@yahoo.com

Academic Editor: Yusuke Shiozawa

Trauma to the skull causing injury to the middle meningeal artery, middle meningeal vein, or dural venous sinuses is responsible for most cases of epidural hemorrhage (EDH). Spontaneous EDH is a rare entity in clinical practice. Common causes include sinusitis, coagulation abnormalities, dural metastasis, and Langerhans cell histiocytosis. Isolated nontraumatic EDH is an exceedingly rare complication of sickle cell disease (SCD). We report a case of spontaneous EDH in a patient with SCD and review the world literature regarding this rare entity. A 20-year-old African American female with sickle cell disease presented with vaso-occlusive crisis. About 24 hours after hospital admission, the patient had sudden deterioration of her mental status. An emergent CT scan of the head revealed a large right-sided frontoparietal epidural hematoma with midline shift, subfalcine, and uncal herniation. The patient underwent emergent hematoma evacuation but died 24 hours after surgery.

1. Introduction

Sickle cell disease (SCD) is caused by a single amino acid substitution on the beta globin chain resulting in the propensity of the hemoglobin molecule to polymerize in deoxygenated state. The abnormal polymerization is responsible for subsequent RBC injury, hemolysis, microvascular injury, and classical acute and chronic manifestations of the disease. Neurologic manifestations secondary to SCD are common and affect about 35% of patients [1]. Although reports vary [2], existing data suggest that 54% of these patients suffer from ischemic strokes and 34% from intracranial bleeding [1]. Intracerebral, subarachnoid, intraventricular, subdural, and epidural bleeds have been reported, with subarachnoid hemorrhage being the most common, especially in young adults [1–3]. Isolated nontraumatic spontaneous epidural hematoma (EDH) is an exceedingly rare complication of SCD. Other reported etiologies of spontaneous EDH are infectious [4–6], coagulation abnormalities associated with end stage renal disease and hemodialysis [7–9], dural metastasis [10–13], and Langerhans cell histiocytosis [14–16]. We present a case of spontaneous EDH in a sickle cell patient suffering from vaso-occlusive crisis and review the world literature regarding the rare entity.

2. Case Presentation

A 20-year-old African American female with a history of sickle cell disease (HbSS) and multiple previous admissions for vaso-occlusive crisis (VOC) presented to the hospital with severe generalized pain throughout her body. The patient was in severe distress. Her blood pressure was 155/101 mmHg, pulse 117 beats per minute, temperature 37.6 C, respiratory rate 25 breaths per minute, and oxygen saturation 98% on room air. Physical examination revealed poor bilateral air entry on lung auscultation due to splinting and an ejection systolic murmur over the aortic area. Mild-to-

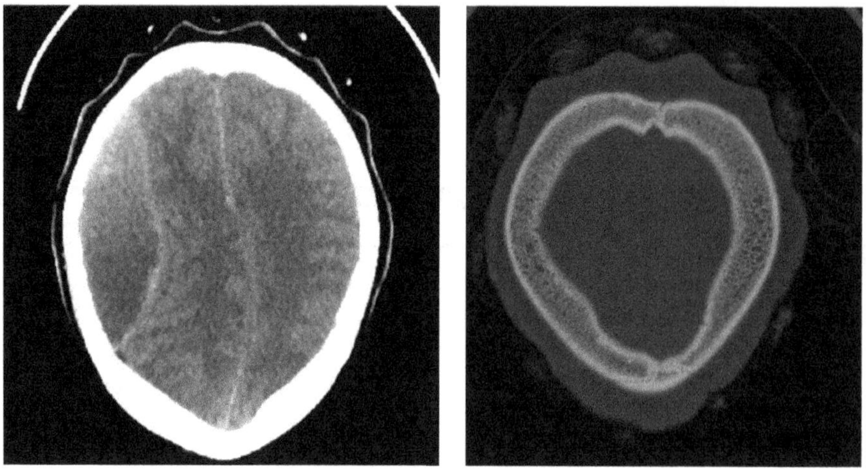

(a) (b)

Figure 1: (a) Mixed density right frontoparietal epidural hematoma with midline shift. (b) Bony window showing massive expansion of the diploic bone from extramedullary hematopoiesis.

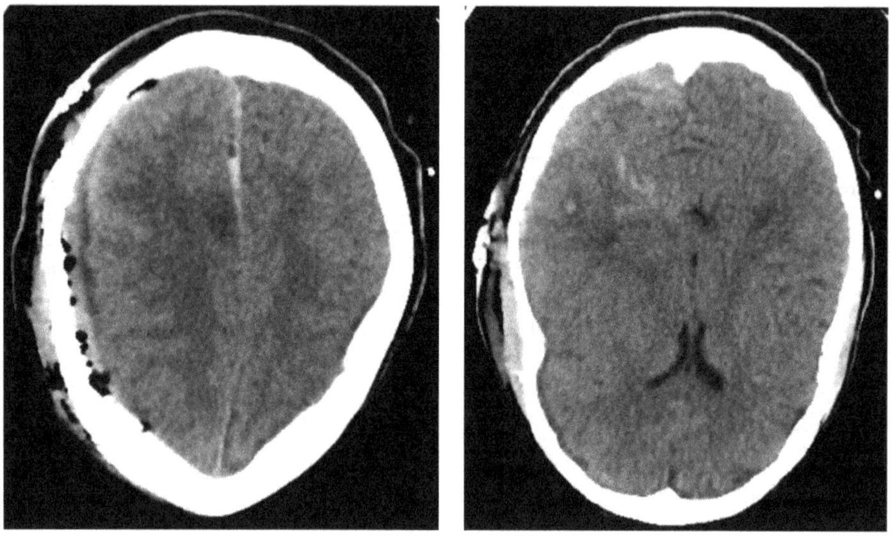

(a) (b)

Figure 2: (a) Postoperative changes following hematoma evacuation with a small collection in the subdural space and significant improvement of midline shift (b) Punctate hemorrhage in the right temporal lobe postop.

moderate tenderness was present over the extremities on palpation. Neurological examination was normal. Blood work showed leukocytosis, 12,800 with 53% neutrophil, 32% lymphocyte, and 1% band, hemoglobin 7.5 gm/dL, hematocrit 22.3%, platelet 181,000/dL, reticulocyte count 13%, lactate dehydrogenase 1144 IU/L, normal blood urea nitrogen, creatinine, and serum electrolyte studies. Liver function tests were normal except a total bilirubin level of 16.2 mg/dL. Chest X-ray was normal. The patient was started on IV hydration; analgesia was achieved by IV narcotics.

About 24 hours after hospital admission, the patient suddenly became unresponsive. Naloxone failed to improve her mental status. An emergent CT scan of the head revealed a large right-sided frontoparietal epidural hematoma with midline shift, subfalcine, and uncal herniation. No subgaleal or subperiosteal collection was noted. There was no noticeable bone infarction overlying the hematoma (Figure 1).

Laboratory data at this time demonstrated a platelet of 45,000/dL, prothrombin time 19.7 Seconds, INR 1.7, activated partial thromboplastin time 43 seconds, and a fibrinogen level of 96 mg/dL, consistent with a diagnosis of disseminated intravascular coagulation (DIC). The patient was emergently taken to the operating room for hematoma evacuation (Figure 2). Intraoperatively, no obvious bony abnormality was noted. Exchange transfusion was performed. The patient, however deteriorated, became hypotensive requiring multiple vasopressors and eventually died about 24 hour after surgical intervention from DIC.

Total 31 cases. R, right; L, left; N/S, not specified; B/L, bilateral; VOC, vaso-occlusive disease; FP, frontoparietal;

Table 1

Case report	Year	Age (years)	Sex	Haplotype	Presentation	Identification of EDH after hospitalization	Location of EDH	Subgaleal hemorrhage	Subperiosteal collection	Skull infarction	DIC present	Outcome
Current case	2019	19	Female	HbSS	VOC	24 hours	R FP	No	No	No (CT/IO)	Yes	Died
Komarla et al. [17]	2018	18	Female	Unspecified	VOC	24 hours	R parietal	No	No	Yes (MRI)	N/S	Survived
		17	Male	Unspecified	Headache	POA	Bifrontal	Yes	Yes	Yes (MRI)	N/S	Survived
Banerjee et al. [18]	2018	Teenage	Male	HbSS	VOC	6 hours	L frontal	No	No	No (MRI)	Yes	Died
Moyen et al. [19]	2018	13	Male	HbSS	Seizure	Imaging not performed till day 8	R FP	No	N/S	No (MRI)	No	Died
Mishra et al. [20]	2017	18	Male	HbSS	VOC	120 hours	R parietal	Yes	No	Yes (IO)	No	Survived
Gajjar and Gupta [21]	2015	20	Male	Unspecified	Headache	POA	L PT	No	No	No (CT)	No	Survived
Hettige et al. [22]	2015	7	Female	HbSS	Coma	POA	B/L parietal	No	No	No (CT/IO)	Yes	Died
Yogarajah at al. [23]	2015	19	Male	HbSC	VOC	24 hours	R PT	No	No	No (CT/IO)	No	Survived
N'dri Oka et al. [24]	2015	19	Male	HbSC	Headache	POA	Occipital	Yes	No	No (CT)	No	Survived
Ilhan et al. [25]	2014	15	Male	HbSS	Headache	POA	Right frontal	Yes	No	Yes (MRI)	No	Survived
Serarslan et al. [26]	2014	19	Female	HbSS	Headache	POA	L FP	No	No	No (CT/IO)	No	Survived
Page et al. [27]	2014	20	Male	HbSS	VOC	48 hours	L frontal	Yes	No	Yes (MRI)	No	Survived
		7	Female	HbSS	Coma	POA	R temporal	No		Yes (MRI)	No	Survived
Babatola et al. [28]	2012	18	Male	HbSS	Headache	POA	R Frontal	No	No	No (CT/IO)	No	Survived
Bolke and Scherer [29]	2012	19	Male	Unspecified	VOC	72 hours	L frontal	No	No	No (CT/IO)	No	Died
Patra et al. [30]	2012	13	Male	Unspecified	Headache	POA	B/L parietal	No	No	No (CT)	No	Survived
Arends et al. [31]	2011	19	Male	HbSC	Headache	POA	R parietal	No	No	Yes (MRI)	No	Survived
Sangle et al. [32]	2011	15	Male	Unspecified	Headache	12 hours	Bifrontal	No	No	No (MRI)	No	Died
Azhar [33]	2010	12	Male	HbSD	VOC	24 hours	L frontal	No	No	N/S (CT)	N/S	Survived
Dahdaleh et al. [34]	2009	18	Male	Unspecified	VOC	12 hours	B/L FP	Yes	No	No (CT/IO)	No	Survived
Kotb et al. [35]	2006	10	Male	Unspecified	Headache	N/S	Bifrontal	Yes	No	Yes (MRI)	N/S	Survived

Table 1: Continued.

Case report	Year	Age (years)	Sex	Haplotype	Presentation	Identification of EDH after hospitalization	Location of EDH	Subgaleal hemorrhage	Subperiosteal collection	Skull infarction	DIC present	Outcome
Kalala Okito et al. [36]	2004	2	Male	HbSS	Coma	POA	R FT	No	No	N/S (IO)	N/S	Died
		12	Male	HbSS	VOC	N/S	L parietal	No	No	Yes (X-ray)	No	Survived
Ganesh et al. [37]	2001	11	Male	HbSS	Proptosis	POA	Bifrontal	Yes	No	Yes (BS)	N/S	Survived
Naran and Fontana [38]	2001	16	Male	Unspecified	Headache	? POA	R Frontal	No	No	Yes (MRI/BS)	No	Survived
Cabon et al. [39]	1997	14	Female	HbSS	Unknown	Unknown	Bifrontal	Unknown	Unknown	Yes	Unknown	Unknown
Resar et al. [40]	1996	14	Male	HbSS	VOC	48 hours	Left parietal and B/L frontal	Yes	Yes	Yes (MRI/BS)	No	Survived
Tony et al. [41]	1995	35	Male	Sickle-thalassemia	Proptosis	POA	Left frontal	No	No	Yes (BS)	No	Survived
Karacostas et al. [42]	1991	19	Male	HbSS	VOC	48 hours	Left frontal	No	No	No (CT)	No	Survived
Mallouh et al. [43]	1987	13	Male	HbSS	Eye swelling	POA	Bifrontal	No	No	Yes	N/S	Survived

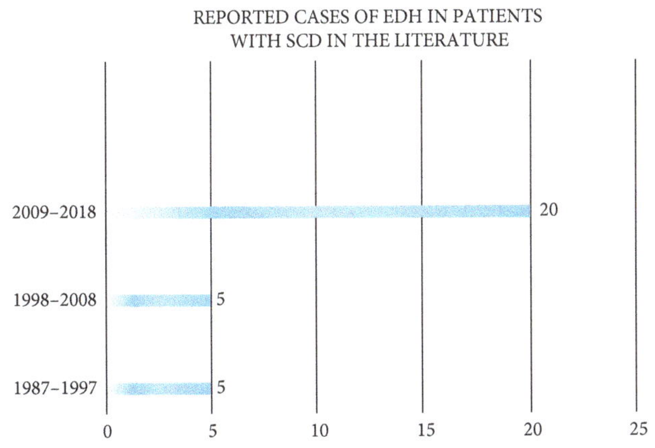

FIGURE 3: Reported cases of EDH in patients with SCD in the literature.

PT, parietotemporal; DIC, disseminated intravascular coagulation; POA, present on admission; BS, bone scan; IO, intraoperatively.

3. Discussion

We have described a patient with SCD suffering from spontaneous EDH is the setting of VOC. Including the present case, we have identified 31 cases described in the literature, which are shown individually in Table 1. Since first reported about 3 decades ago, the reporting incidence has increased precipitously in the last decade possibly due to increased awareness, radiologic advancement, and more opportunities for publication rather than actual increase in incidence (Figure 3).

Most reported cases comprised males 25/31 (80%). The age ranged from 2–35 years (median 16.5) and 7–19 years (median 16), respectively, for males and females. 26/31 (84%) had SCD (17 patients with reported homozygosity and 9 known cases without specified haplotype). Other cases included 3 patients with HbSC disease, 1 with HbSD, and sickle thalassemia each.

Headache was present on admission in 37% (11/30), whereas symptoms consistent with VOC, primarily pain crisis, were the initial complaint in 40% (12/30). Other presenting symptoms were eye swelling, proptosis, seizure, and coma. In patients who presented with a headache, EDH was present on admission in 82% of the time. Patients who presented with VOC, progressed to have EDH within 6–120 hours, with a median of 24 hours after hospital admission.

Unilateral EDH was more common 20/31 (65%). Subgaleal hemorrhage was concurrently present in 9/30 (30%) of patients and associated with bone infarction in (7/9) 78% of cases. 48% of patients (15/31) with EDH showed evidence of overlying bony infarction. The overall mortality among the reported cases was 23% (7/30). Interestingly, patients with evidence of overlying bone infarction had a survival of 100% and patients with DIC had a mortality of 100%.

The most common cause of EDH is trauma causing injury to the middle meningeal artery, middle meningeal vein, the diploic vein, or the dural venous sinuses [44]. Spontaneous nontraumatic EDH is a rare manifestation of SCD and variant sickle cell syndromes. The pathophysiology of this rare occurrence is not completely understood.

Most reported cases in the literature are males. Whether any gender specific etiology is responsible for this discrepancy is not known. Low steady-state hemoglobin and high leukocyte count are known risk factors for hemorrhagic stroke in patients with SCD [1]. Whether this is also true for EDH is not clear. In the landmark study by Ohene-Frempong et al., hemorrhagic strokes were more prevalent in the adult SCD patients in the age range of 20–30 years [1]. However, EDH appears to be more prevalent in the adolescent age group.

Three pathophysiologic explanations have been proposed over the years for the causation of this rare entity: (1) Vaso-occlusion of the haematopoietically active calvarial diploic bone resulting in bone infarction and subsequent leaking of blood and proteinaceous material in the subperiosteal, epidural, or subgaleal space [38–41, 43, 45]. (2) Acute rapid expansion of hematopoiesis with resultant microfracture of already thinned inner cortex and extravasation of blood and hematopoietic tissue [24, 28, 36]. (3) Sludging of sickle cells in the diploic veins hampering venous drainage and oozing of blood due to vascular injury and elevated back pressure. A combination of different mechanisms could also be responsible. Presence of coagulopathy or platelet dysfunction worsens hematoma expansion and portends a dire clinical outcome.

Patients admitted with VOC developed EDH, did so with a median of 24 hours, suggesting early deterioration is expected in this patient population. Patients who suffered from concurrent bony infarction or subgaleal hemorrhage had a survival rate of 100%. This may indicate that vaso-occlusive etiology of the EDH carries better prognosis. This would also explain presence of EDH with contralateral subgaleal hemorrhage as skull bone infarction could be diffused [40]. The identification of bone infarction can be challenging. MRI appears to be the most sensitive tool. CT scan has low yield especially in the acute phase of the disease [18]. Infarcted bone can appear normal intraoperatively although thinning of the inner cortex is frequently seen. In 3 out of 7 patients who succumbed to their disease, an MRI ruled out any bony infarction. In the other 4 cases, no bone damage was noted by CT scan or on intraoperative inspection. We propose that patients without any obvious bony disruption and infarction, most likely suffer from microfracture of the inner table and extrusion of blood and hematopoietic cells in the epidural space due to rapid expansion of hematopoiesis. Presence of coagulopathy as in DIC makes the bleeding significantly worse. Patients who suffered from spontaneous EDH and suffered from DIC had a 100% mortality.

4. Conclusion

The understanding regarding this clinical entity is rapidly evolving in the era of advanced technology and improved awareness among healthcare providers. We believe this review will shed more light on the clinical as well as the pathophysiological aspect of the disease process and help in rapid identification of patients at risk of deterioration and formulate management plan accordingly.

References

[1] K. Ohene-Frempong, S. J. Weiner, L. A. Sleeper et al., "Cerebrovascular accidents in sickle cell disease: rates and risk factors," *Blood*, vol. 91, no. 1, pp. 288–294, 1998.

[2] A. Gueguen, M. Mahevas, R. Nzouakou et al., "Sickle-cell disease stroke throughout life: a retrospective study in an adult referral center," *American Journal of Hematology*, vol. 89, no. 3, pp. 267–272, 2014.

[3] J. J. Strouse, M. L. Hulbert, M. R. DeBaun, L. C. Jordan, and J. F. Casella, "Primary hemorrhagic stroke in children with sickle cell disease is associated with recent transfusion and use of corticosteroids," *Pediatrics*, vol. 118, no. 5, pp. 1916–1924, 2006.

[4] M. C. Papadopoulos, A. Dyer, and C. Hardwidge, "Spontaneous extradural haematoma with sinusitis," *Journal of the Royal Society of Medicine*, vol. 94, no. 11, pp. 588-589, 2001.

[5] G. Moonis, A. Granados, and S. L. Simon, "Epidural hematoma as a complication of sphenoid sinusitis and epidural abscess," *Clinical Imaging*, vol. 26, no. 6, pp. 382–385, 2002.

[6] S. Chaiyasate, S. Halewyck, K. Van Rompaey, and P. Clement, "Spontaneous extradural hematoma as a presentation of sinusitis: case report and literature review," *International Journal of Pediatric Otorhinolaryngology*, vol. 71, no. 5, pp. 827–830, 2007.

[7] K. Shahlaie, A. Fox, L. Butani, and J. E. Boggan, "Spontaneous epidural hemorrhage in chronic renal failure. a case report and review," *Pediatric Nephrology*, vol. 19, no. 10, pp. 1168–1172, 2004.

[8] S. Shimokawa, T. Hayashi, S. Anegawa et al., "Spontaneous epidural hematoma in a patient undergoing hemodialysis: a case report," *No to Shinkei = Brain and Nerve*, vol. 55, no. 2, pp. 163–166, 2003.

[9] F. Zheng and Y. Chao, "Spontaneous intracranial extradural hematoma: case report and literature review," *Neurology India*, vol. 57, no. 3, pp. 324–326, 2009.

[10] S. Anegawa, S. Hirohata, T. Tokutomi, and S. Kuramoto, "Spontaneous epidural hematoma secondary to dural metastasis from an ovarian carcinoma," *Neurologia Medico-Chirurgica*, vol. 29, no. 9, pp. 854–856, 1989.

[11] J. I. McIver, B. W. Scheithauer, C. H. Rydberg, and J. L. D. Atkinson, "Metastatic hepatocellular carcinoma presenting as epidural hematoma: case report," *Neurosurgery*, vol. 49, no. 2, pp. 447–449, 2001.

[12] K. Hayashi, T. Matsuo, M. Kurihara, M. Daikoku, G. Kitange, and S. Shibata, "Skull metastasis of hepatocellular carcinoma associated with acute epidural hematoma: a case report," *Surgical Neurology*, vol. 53, no. 4, pp. 379–382, 2000.

[13] M. S. Shamim, M. E. Bari, and S. A. Enam, "Dural metastases presenting as an extradural hematoma: a rare presentation," *JPMA Journal of Pakistan Medical Association*, vol. 55, no. 11, pp. 509-510, 2005.

[14] D.-Y. Cho, W.-R. Liau, and I.-P. Chiang, "Eosinophilic granuloma with acute epidural hematoma," *Pediatric Neurosurgery*, vol. 35, no. 5, pp. 266–269, 2001.

[15] H. C. Chen, W. C. Shen, D. Y. Chou, and I. P. Chiang, "Langerhans cell histiocytosis of the skull complicated with an epidural hematoma," *AJNR American Journal of Neuroradiology*, vol. 23, no. 3, pp. 493–495, 2002.

[16] J. F. Martinez-Lage, M. Bermudez, E. Martinez-Barba, J. L. Fuster, and M. Poza, "Epidural hematoma from a cranial eosinophilic granuloma," *Child's Nervous System: ChNS: Official Journal of the International Society for Pediatric Neurosurgery*, vol. 18, no. 1-2, pp. 74–76, 2002.

[17] R. Komarla, B. P. Soares, J. J. Chern, and S. S. Milla, "Spontaneous epidural hematoma secondary to bone infarction in sickle cell anemia: case report," *Journal of Neurosurgery: Pediatrics PED*, vol. 22, no. 1, pp. 18–21, 2018.

[18] C. Banerjee, J. Yowtak, D. Fridlyand, and C. Alleyne Jr., "Acute spontaneous intracranial epidural haematoma and disseminated intravascular coagulation in a paediatric sickle cell patient," *BMJ Case Reports*, vol. 2018, 2018.

[19] E. Moyen, J. Kambourou, H. B. Ekouelé-Mbaki et al., "Spontaneous epidural hematoma in a child with sickle cell disease," *Internal Medicine Review*, vol. 4, no. 1, pp. 1–7, 2018.

[20] S. S. Mishra, S. B. Senapati, A. K. Gouda, S. K. Behera, and A. Patnaik, "Spontaneous extradural and subgaleal hematoma: a rare neurosurgical crisis of sickle cell disease," *Asian Journal of Neurosurgery*, vol. 12, no. 1, pp. 47–50, 2017.

[21] R. Gajjar and P. Gupta, "Spontaneous extradural hematoma: a rare neurological crisis in sickle cell disease," *IOSR Journal of Dental and Medical Sciences*, vol. 14, no. 12, pp. 94–96, 2015.

[22] S. Hettige, A. Sofela, S. Bassi, and C. Chandler, "A review of spontaneous intracranial extradural hematoma in sickle-cell disease," *Acta Neurochirurgica*, vol. 157, no. 11, pp. 2025–2029, 2015.

[23] M. Yogarajah, C. C. Agu, B. Sivasambu, and M. A. Mittler, "HbSC disease and spontaneous epidural hematoma with kernohan's notch phenomena," *Case Reports in Hematology*, vol. 2015, Article ID 470873, 3 pages, 2015.

[24] D. N'Dri Oka, A. Tokpa, A. Bah, and L. Derou, "Spontaneous intracranial extradural hematoma in sickle cell disease," *Journal of Neurological Surgery Reports*, vol. 76, no. 1, pp. e97–e99, 2015.

[25] N. Ilhan, C. Acipayam, F. Aydogan et al., "Orbital compression syndrome complicated by epidural hematoma and wide cephalohematoma in a patient with sickle cell disease," *Journal of American Association for Pediatric Ophthalmology and Strabismus*, vol. 18, no. 2, pp. 189–191, 2014.

[26] Y. Serarslan, M. Aras, M. Altaş, H. Kaya, and B. Urfalı, "Nontraumatic spontaneous acute epidural hematoma in a patient with sickle cell disease," *Neurocirugía*, vol. 25, no. 3, pp. 128–131, 2014.

[27] C. Page, K. Gardner, S. Height, D. C. Rees, T. Hampton, and S. L. Thein, "Nontraumatic extradural hematoma in sickle cell anemia: a rare neurological complication not to be missed," *American Journal of Hematology*, vol. 89, no. 2, pp. 225–227, 2014.

[28] B. O. Babatola, Y. A. Salman, A. M. Abiola, K. O. Okezie, and A. S. Oladele, "Spontaneous epidural haematoma in sickle cell anaemia: case report and literature review," *Journal of Surgical Technique and Case Report*, vol. 4, no. 2, pp. 135–137, 2012.

[29] E. Bolke and A. Scherer, "Sickle cell disease," *Canadian Medical Association Journal*, vol. 184, no. 3, p. E201, 2012.

[30] S. Patra, S. Mishra, and S. Das, "A rare case of spontaneous bilateral extradural hematoma in a sickle cell disease child," *Journal of Pediatric Neurosciences*, vol. 7, no. 1, pp. 77-78, 2012.

[31] S. Arends, J. A. Coebergh, J. L. Kerkhoffs, A. van Gils, and H. Koppen, "Severe unilateral headache caused by skull bone infarction with epidural haematoma in a patient with sickle cell disease," *Cephalalgia*, vol. 31, no. 12, pp. 1325–1328, 2011.

[32] S. Sangle, R. Lohiya, S. Karne, and K. Chugh, "Spontaneous epidural hematoma: a rare complication of sickle cell anemia," *Neurology India*, vol. 59, no. 2, pp. 301-302, 2011.

[33] M. J. Azhar, "Extradural hemorrhage: a rare complication and manifestation of stroke in sickle cell disease," *Oman Medical Journal*, vol. 25, no. 4, p. e017, 2010.

[34] N. S. Dahdaleh, T. E. Lindley, P. A. Kirby, H. Oya, and M. A. Howard 3rd, "A "neurosurgical crisis" of sickle cell disease," *Journal of Neurosurgery: Pediatrics*, vol. 4, no. 6, pp. 532–535, 2009.

[35] M. M. Kotb, W. H. Tantawi, A. A. Elsayed, G. A. Damanhouri, and H. M. Malibary, "Brain MRI and CT findings in sickle cell disease patients from Western Saudi Arabia," *Neurosciences (Riyadh, Saudi Arabia)*, vol. 11, no. 1, pp. 28–36, 2006.

[36] J. P. Kalala Okito, O. Van Damme, and L. Calliauw, "Are spontaneous epidural haematoma in sickle cell disease a rare complication? A report of two new cases," *Acta Neurochirurgica*, vol. 146, no. 4, pp. 407–410, 2004.

[37] A. Ganesh, R. R. William, S. Mitra et al., "Orbital involvement in sickle cell disease: a report of five cases and review literature," *Eye*, vol. 15, no. 6, pp. 774–780, 2001.

[38] A. D. Naran and L. Fontana, "Sickle cell disease with orbital infarction and epidural hematoma," *Pediatric Radiology*, vol. 31, no. 4, pp. 257–259, 2001.

[39] I. Cabon, J. P. Hladky, A. Lambilliotte, A. Cotten, and P. Dhellemmes, "Uncommon etiology of extradural hematoma," *Neurochirurgie*, vol. 43, no. 3, pp. 173–176, 1997.

[40] L. M. S. Resar, M. M. Oliva, and J. F. Casella, "Skull infarction and epidural hematomas in a patient with sickle cell anemia," *Journal of Pediatric Hematology/Oncology*, vol. 18, no. 4, pp. 413–415, 1996.

[41] J. Tony, G. Subramanya, K. G. Kallur, A. V. Chalapathy, S. Sheshadri, and B. Lakhkar, "Proptosis, skull infarction and epidural haematoma in sickle thalassemia," *Postgraduate Medical Journal*, vol. 71, no. 837, p. 445, 1995.

[42] D. Karacostas, N. Artemis, M. Papadopoulou, and J. Christakis, "Case report: epidural and bilateral retroorbital hematomas complicating sickle cell anemia," *American Journal of the Medical Sciences*, vol. 302, no. 2, pp. 107–109, 1991.

[43] A. A. Mallouh, M. Young, J. Hamdan, and M. M. Salamah, "Proptosis, skull infarction, and retro-orbital and epidural hematomas in a child with sickle cell disease," *Clinical Pediatrics*, vol. 26, no. 10, pp. 536–538, 1987.

[44] M. R. Bullock, R. Chesnut, J. Ghajar et al., "Surgical management of acute epidural hematomas," *Neurosurgery*, vol. 58, no. 3, pp. S7–15, 2006.

[45] M. Watanabe, N. Saito, R. N. Nadgir et al., "Craniofacial bone infarcts in sickle cell disease," *Journal of Computer Assisted Tomography*, vol. 37, no. 1, pp. 91–97, 2013.

Permissions

All chapters in this book were first published by Hindawi Publishing Corporation; hereby published with permission under the Creative Commons Attribution License or equivalent. Every chapter published in this book has been scrutinized by our experts. Their significance has been extensively debated. The topics covered herein carry significant findings which will fuel the growth of the discipline. They may even be implemented as practical applications or may be referred to as a beginning point for another development.

The contributors of this book come from diverse backgrounds, making this book a truly international effort. This book will bring forth new frontiers with its revolutionizing research information and detailed analysis of the nascent developments around the world.

We would like to thank all the contributing authors for lending their expertise to make the book truly unique. They have played a crucial role in the development of this book. Without their invaluable contributions this book wouldn't have been possible. They have made vital efforts to compile up to date information on the varied aspects of this subject to make this book a valuable addition to the collection of many professionals and students.

This book was conceptualized with the vision of imparting up-to-date information and advanced data in this field. To ensure the same, a matchless editorial board was set up. Every individual on the board went through rigorous rounds of assessment to prove their worth. After which they invested a large part of their time researching and compiling the most relevant data for our readers.

The editorial board has been involved in producing this book since its inception. They have spent rigorous hours researching and exploring the diverse topics which have resulted in the successful publishing of this book. They have passed on their knowledge of decades through this book. To expedite this challenging task, the publisher supported the team at every step. A small team of assistant editors was also appointed to further simplify the editing procedure and attain best results for the readers.

Apart from the editorial board, the designing team has also invested a significant amount of their time in understanding the subject and creating the most relevant covers. They scrutinized every image to scout for the most suitable representation of the subject and create an appropriate cover for the book.

The publishing team has been an ardent support to the editorial, designing and production team. Their endless efforts to recruit the best for this project, has resulted in the accomplishment of this book. They are a veteran in the field of academics and their pool of knowledge is as vast as their experience in printing. Their expertise and guidance has proved useful at every step. Their uncompromising quality standards have made this book an exceptional effort. Their encouragement from time to time has been an inspiration for everyone.

The publisher and the editorial board hope that this book will prove to be a valuable piece of knowledge for researchers, students, practitioners and scholars across the globe.

List of Contributors

Ayrton Bangolo, Trupti Waykole, Bilal Niazi, Chandini Sajja, Mahabuba Akhter and Sameh Elias
Department of Internal Medicine, Hackensack Meridian Health Palisades Medical Center, 7600 River Road, North Bergen, NJ 07047, USA

Bhavna Gupta
Department of Hematology and Oncology, Hackensack Meridian Health Palisades Medical Center, 7600 River Road, North Bergen, NJ 07047, USA

Jui Choudhuri, Yang Shi and Yanhua Wang
Department of Pathology, Montefiore Medical Center/ Albert Einstein College of Medicine, 111 East 210th Street, Bronx 10467, NY, USA

Mohammad Eskandari
Department of Pathology, Altru Health System, 1200 S. Columbia Rd., Grand Forks 58201, ND, USA

Natharina Yolanda, Stefanus Gunawan and Max F. J. Mantik
Department of Child Health, Faculty of Medicine, Sam Ratulangi University, Manado, Indonesia

Anjo J. P. Veerman
Amsterdam University Medical Center, VU University, Amsterdam, Netherlands

Anh Khoi Vo
Section Hematology, Department of Medicine, Haukeland University Hospital, Bergen, Norway

Hilde Kollsete Gjelberg
Department of Pathology, Haukeland University Hospital, Bergen, Norway

Randi Hovland
Department of Medical Genetics, Haukeland University Hospital, Bergen, Norway
Department of Biological Sciences, University of Bergen, Bergen, Norway

Marte Karen Lindstad Brattås
Department of Medicine, Haraldsplass Deaconess Hospital, Bergen, Norway

Øystein Bruserud and Håkon Reikvam
Section Hematology, Department of Medicine, Haukeland University Hospital, Bergen, Norway
Department of Clinical Science, University of Bergen, Bergen, Norway

Daisuke Toyama, Ryosuke Matsuno, Yumiko Sugishita, Ryota Kaneko, Naoko Okamoto, Masaya Koganesawa, Sachio Fujita, Kosuke Akiyama, Keiichi Isoyama and Shohei Yamamoto
Department of Pediatrics, Showa University Fujigaoka Hospital, Yokohama, Japan

Ryan A. Denu
Medical Scientist Training Program, School of Medicine and Public Health, University of Wisconsin-Madison, Madison, WI, USA
Carbone Cancer Center, University of Wisconsin, Madison, WI, USA

Daniel R. Matson
Department of Pathology and Laboratory Medicine, School of Medicine and Public Health, University of Wisconsin-Madison, Madison, WI, USA

Natalie J. Tedford and Christine E. Brichta
Department of Pediatrics, School of Medicine and Public Health, University of Wisconsin-Madison, Madison, WI, USA

Matthew J. Davis, Carol A. Diamond and Margo L. Hoover-Regan
Carbone Cancer Center, University of Wisconsin, Madison, WI, USA
Department of Pediatrics, School of Medicine and Public Health, University of Wisconsin-Madison, Madison, WI, USA

Qurratulain Rizvi, Uzma Zaidi and Tahir Shamsi
Department of Clinical Haematology, National Institute of Blood Diseases & Bone Marrow Transplantation, Karachi, Pakistan

Saba Shahid and Shariq Ahmed
Department of Genomics, National Institute of Blood Diseases & Bone Marrow Transplantation, Karachi, Pakistan

Morgan Bailey, Travis Maestas and Robert Betancourt
Department of Internal Medicine, University of Arizona, Tucson, AZ, USA

Dalia Mikhael
Department of Internal Medicine, Banner University Medical Center-Tucson, Tucson, AZ, USA

Hani M. Babiker
Department of Hematology-Oncology, University of Arizona Cancer Center, Tucson, AZ, USA

Damodaran Narayanan, Patricia Ruegsegger and William Nicholas Rose
Department of Pathology, University of Wisconsin Hospital, 600 Highland Ave Madison, WI 53792, Madison, USA

Noreen B. Hogan and Karen A. Schaser
Department of Nursing, University of Wisconsin Hospital, 600 Highland Ave Madison, WI 53792, Madison, USA

Tarig Omer, Naresh Mullaguri, Pravin George and Christopher R. Newey
Department of Neurointensive Care, Cerebrovascular Center, Cleveland Clinic Foundation, 9500 Euclid Avenue, Cleveland, Ohio 44195, USA

Øystein Sefland
Section of Hematology, Department of Medicine, Haukeland University Hospital, Bergen, Norway

Ulla Randen
Department of Pathology, Akershus University Hospital, Lørenskog, Norway

Sigbjørn Berentsen
Department of Research and Innovation, Haugesund Hospital, Haugesund, Norway

Anna Schuh and Julie Makani
Department of Haematology and Blood Transfusion, Muhimbili University of Health and Allied Sciences, Dar-es-Salaam, Tanzania

Mboka Jacob
Department of Radiology and Imaging, Muhimbili University of Health and Allied Sciences, Dar-es-Salaam, Tanzania

Jamila Makame, Mclean Abisay and Mbonea Yonazi
Department of Haematology, Muhimbili National Hospital, Dar-es-Salaam, Tanzania

Ahmad Al-Sabbagh and Feryal Ibrahim
Department of Laboratory Medicine and Pathology, National Center for Cancer Care and Research, Hamad Medical Corporation, Doha, Qatar

Dina Sameh Soliman
Department of Laboratory Medicine and Pathology, National Center for Cancer Care and Research,Hamad Medical Corporation, Doha, Qatar
Clinical Pathology Department, National Cancer Institute, Cairo University, Cairo, Egypt
Clinical Pathology and Laboratory Medicine, Weill-Cornell Medicine, Doha, Qatar

Amna Gameil, Mohamed Yassin and Halima El-Omri
Department of Hematology and Medical Oncology, National Center for Cancer Care and Research, Hamad Medical Corporation, Doha, Qatar

Clarisse Mpinganzima and Alf Haaland
Department of Haematology, Oslo University Hospital, Oslo, Norway

Anne Guro Vreim Holm
Department of Orthopedic Surgery, Oslo University Hospital, Oslo, Norway

Swee Lay Thein
Sickle Cell Branch, National Heart Lung and Blood Institute, National Institutes of Health, Bethesda, MD, USA

Geir Erland Tjønnfjord
Department of Haematology, Oslo University Hospital, Oslo, Norway
Institute of Clinical Medicine, University of Oslo, Oslo, Norway

Per Ole Iversen
Department of Haematology and Blood Transfusion, Muhimbili University of Health and Allied Sciences, Dar-es-Salaam, Tanzania
Department of Haematology, Oslo University Hospital, Oslo, Norway
Department of Nutrition, Institute of Basic Medical Sciences, University of Oslo, Oslo, Norway
Division of Human Nutrition, Stellenbosch University, Tygerberg, South Africa

Christophe Cisarovsky and Pierre-Alexandre Bart
Division of Internal Medicine, Department of Medicine, Lausanne University Hospital and University of Lausanne, Rue du Bugnon 46, CH-1011 Lausanne, Switzerland

Marie Théaudin
Division of Neurology, Department of Clinical Neurosciences, Lausanne University Hospital and University of Lausanne, Rue du Bugnon 46, CH-1011 Lausanne, Switzerland

Grégoire Stalder and Lorenzo Alberio
Service and Central Laboratory of Hematology, Department of Oncology and Department, Laboratories and Pathology, Lausanne University Hospital and University of Lausanne, Rue du Bugnon 46, CH-1011 Lausanne, Switzerland

Mirko Farina, Federica Cattina, Nicola Polverelli, Michele Malagola and Domenico Russo
Chair of Hematology, Unit of Blood Diseases and Stem Cell Transplantation, Department of Clinical and Experimental Sciences, University of Brescia, ASST Spedali Civili di Brescia, 25123 Brescia, Italy

Simona Bernardi, Camilla Zanaglio, Federica Re and Chiara Foroni
CREA Laboratory (Centro di Ricerca Emato-Oncologica AIL), ASST Spedali Civili di Brescia, 25123 Brescia, Italy

Francesca Schieppati
Unit of Transfusion Medicine, ASST Papa Giovanni XXIII, 24127 Bergamo, Italy

Andrew J. Dunbar
Department of Medicine, Leukemia Service, Memorial Sloan Kettering Cancer Center, New York, NY, USA

Hassan Alshehri, Mohammad Alnomani, Mubarak Alghamdi, Ibrahim Motabi, Imran Tailor, Nawal Alshehry, Abdul Rehman Z. Zaidi, Syed Altaf and Syed Z. A. Zaidi
Department of Adult Hematology and BMT, King Fahad Medical City, Riyadh, Saudi Arabia

Mansour Alfayez
Department of Adult Hematology and BMT, King Fahad Medical City, Riyadh, Saudi Arabia
Department of Leukemia, $e University of Texas MD Anderson Cancer Center, Houston, TX, USA

Azizah AlSwayyed and Ammar AlSughayyer
Department of Pathology and Clinical Laboratory Medicine, King Fahad Medical City, Riyadh, Saudi Arabia

Heidi A. Worth, Zachary Marlette, David Aljadir and Ronald Lands
Department of Medicine, Division of Hematology/ Oncology, University of Tennessee Medical Center, Knoxville, TN, USA

Lydie Ocini Ngolet and Josue Simo Louokdom
Department of Medical Hematology, Brazzaville Teaching Hospital, 13 Avenue Auxence Ikonga, BP 32, Brazzaville, Congo

Nelly Guembo
Department of Pediatry, Brazzaville Blanche Gomes Hospital, Sassou Nguesso Boulevard, Brazzaville, Congo

Ocko Ngokaba Thibault
Department of laboratory, Brazzaville Teaching Hospital, 13 Avenue Auxence Ikonga, BP 32, Brazzaville, Congo

Douglas Tremblay, Ronald Hoffman and John O. Mascarenhas
Tisch Cancer Institute, Icahn School of Medicine at Mount Sinai, New York, NY, USA

Juan Putra and Maria Isabel Fiel
Department of Pathology, Icahn School of Medicine at Mount Sinai, New York, NY, USA

Alexander Vogel and Adam Winters
Department of Medicine, Icahn School of Medicine at Mount Sinai, New York, NY, USA

Thomas D. Schiano
Department of Medicine, Division of Liver Diseases, Recanati/Miller Transplantation Institute, Icahn School of Medicine at Mount Sinai, New York, NY, USA

Jan Braune, Kathrin Rieger and Olga Blau
Department of Hematology, Oncology and Cancer Immunology, Charité-Universitätsmedizin Berlin, Freie Universität Berlin and Humboldt-Universität zu Berlin, Berlin, Germany

Ulrich Keller, Lars Bullinger and Jan Krönke
Department of Hematology, Oncology and Cancer Immunology, Charité-Universitätsmedizin Berlin, Freie Universität Berlin and Humboldt-Universität zu Berlin, Berlin, Germany
German Cancer Consortium (DKTK) Partner Site Berlin and German Cancer Research Center (DKFZ), Heidelberg, Germany
Berlin Institute of Health (BIH), Berlin, Germany

Gaurav Shah
Internal Medicine, University of Alabama at Birmingham, Birmingham, AL, USA

Fady M. Mikhail and Andrew J. Carroll III
Department of Genetics, University of Alabama at Birmingham, Birmingham, AL, USA

Matthew Kutny
Division of Hematology/Oncology, Department of Pediatrics, University of Alabama at Birmingham, Birmingham, AL, USA

Nikolaos Papadantonakis
Division of Hematology/Oncology, Department of Medicine, University of Alabama at Birmingham, Birmingham, AL, USA

Calum Slapnicar and Peter Vadas
Division of Allergy and Clinical Immunology, St. Michael's Hospital, University of Toronto, Toronto, Ontario, Canada

Martina Trinkaus and Lisa Hicks
Division of Hematology, St. Michael's Hospital, University of Toronto, Toronto, Ontario, Canada

Zachary Ciochetto, Maria Georgen, Adam Hadro, Lauren Jurkowski, Adam Wooldridge, Nathan Gundacker and Javeria Haque
Medical College of Wisconsin Affiliated Hospitals, Milwaukee, WI, USA
Zablocki VA Medical Center, Milwaukee, WI, USA

Kimberly Ridolfi
Zablocki VA Medical Center, Milwaukee, WI, USA

Ashley C. Eason and Himalee S. Sabnis
Department of Pediatrics, Aflac Cancer and Blood Disorders Center, Children's Healthcare of Atlanta and Emory University, Atlanta, GA, USA

Silvia T. Bunting
Department of Pathology, Children's Healthcare of Atlanta, Atlanta, GA, USA

Jess F. Peterson
Division of Laboratory Genetics and Genomics, Department of Laboratory Medicine and Pathology, Mayo Clinic, Rochester, MN, USA

Debra Saxe
Department of Pathology and Laboratory Medicine, Emory University, Atlanta, GA, USA

Ali Mala, Yameena Noman Khan, Akbar Ahmed, Naema Khayyam and Kanwal Aftab
Indus Hospital and Health Network, Plot C-76, Sector 31/5, Opposite Darussalam Society Korangi Crossing, Karachi 75190, Pakistan

Jianping Zhang, Minghua Li and Peihua Lu
Bone Marrow Transplantation (BMT) Unit, Hebei Yanda Ludaopei Hospital, Sanhe, China

Guangxu Ren and Suqin Yi
Institute of Food and Nutrition Development, Ministry of Agriculture, Beijing, China

Sherine J. Thomas
Hematology and Oncology, Northside Hospital Cancer Institute, Georgia Cancer Specialists, Atlanta, GA, USA

D. P. Dash
Molecular Oncology & Genetics (MOGL), Versiti Wisconsin (Formerly Known as Blood Center Wisconsin), Milwaukee, WI, USA

Cilomar Martins De Oliveira Filho and Alexander Gavralidis
Mass General Brigham, Salem Hospital, Salem, MA, USA

Motoharu Shibusawa
IMS Group, Shinmatsudo Central General Hospital, Department of Hematology, Chiba, Japan

Xiangyang Pu and Shengyong Deng
Ministry of Education Key Laboratory of Child Development and Disorders, Chongqing, China
Department of Pediatric Respiratory Medicine, Qianjiang Central Hospital of Chongqing, Chongqing, China

Nange Yin
Ministry of Education Key Laboratory of Child Development and Disorders, Chongqing, China
Department of Pharmacy, Children Hospital of Chongqing Medical University, Chongqing, China

Lin Song
Department of Pharmacy, Children Hospital of Chongqing Medical University, Chongqing, China
National Clinical Research Center for Child Health and Disorders, Chongqing, China
China International Science and Technology Cooperation Base of Child Development and Critical Disorders, Chongqing 400014, China

Xiangling He
Department of Pediatric Hematology and Oncology, Children's Medical Center of Hunan Provincial People's Hospital (2e First-Affiliated Hospital of Hunan Normal University), Changsha, China

Jianwen Xiao
Ministry of Education Key Laboratory of Child Development and Disorders, Chongqing, China
Chongqing Key Laboratory of Pediatrics, Chongqing, China
Department of Hematology, Children Hospital of Chongqing Medical University, Chongqing, China

Kanda Fanhchaksai
Research Cluster of Thalassemia and Red Blood Cell Disorders, Faculty of Medicine, Chiang Mai University, Chiang Mai 50200, Thailand

Suphara Manowong, Lalita Sathitsamitphong, Rungrote Natesirinilkul, Worawut Choeyprasert and Pimlak Charoenkwan
Department of Pediatrics, Faculty of Medicine, Chiang Mai University, Chiang Mai 50200, Thailand

Rui R. He and Kimberly Woodward
Department of Pathology, Inova Fairfax Hospital, Falls Church, VA, USA

Zacharia Nayer
School of Medicine, George Washington University, Washington, DC, USA

Matthew Hogan
School of Medicine, Virginia Commonwealth University, Richmond, VA, USA

Raymund S. Cuevo and David Heyer
Inova Schar Cancer Institute, Inova Fairfax Hospital, Falls Church, VA, USA

Christine A. Curtis
Department of Cytogenetics, Quest Diagnostics Nichols Institute, Chantilly, VA, USA

Vaibhav Agrawal and Sherif S. Farag
Department of Medicine, Division of Hematology and Oncology, Indiana University School of Medicine, Indianapolis, IN, USA
Bone Marrow and Blood Stem Cell Transplantation Program, Indiana University, Indianapolis, IN, USA

Bryan J. Brinda
Department of Pharmacy, Division of Hematology-Oncology, University of Kentucky, Lexington, KY, USA

Takeshi Araki, Shinya Ohata and Takeshi Sugimoto
Department of Hematology and Oncology, Kita-Harima Medical Center, Hyogo, Japan

Kohei Okamoto
Department of Nephrology, Kobe University Hospital, Hyogo, Japan

Kazuhide Morimoto
Division of Laboratory Medicine, Kita-Harima Medical Center, Hyogo, Japan

Mana Hiraishi and Shinichiro Yamada
Department of Cardiology, Kita-Harima Medical Centre, Hyogo, Japan

Ishikazu Mizuno
Department of Hematology, Hyogo Cancer Center, Akashi, Japan

Mohammad Bagher Jahantab, Saadat Mehrabi, Vahid Salehi, Lotfolah Abedini and Mohammad Javad Yavari Barhaghtalab
Department of General Surgery, Shahid Beheshti Hospital, Yasuj University of Medical Sciences, Yasuj, Iran

Biplab Saha
Division of Pulmonary and Critical Care Medicine, Albany Medical Center, Albany, NY, USA

Aditi Saha
Department of Medicine, Saint Barnabas Medical Center, Livingston, NJ, USA

Index

www.ingramcontent.com/pod-product-compliance
Lightning Source LLC
LaVergne TN
LVHW082232200926
848484LV00008B/2338